THE BLACK BUTTERFLY

THE
BLACK
BUTTERFLY

*The
Harmful Politics
of Race and Space
in America*

LAWRENCE T. BROWN

JOHNS HOPKINS UNIVERSITY PRESS

BALTIMORE

Johns Hopkins Paperback edition, 2022
4 6 8 9 7 5 3

Johns Hopkins University Press
2715 North Charles Street
Baltimore, Maryland 21218
www.press.jhu.edu

Library of Congress Cataloging-in-Publication Data

The Library of Congress has cataloged the hardcover edition of this book as follows:

Names: Brown, Lawrence T., 1978– author.
Title: The black butterfly : the harmful politics of race and space in America /
Lawrence T. Brown.
Description: Baltimore : Johns Hopkins University Press, [2021] | Includes
bibliographical references and index.
Identifiers: LCCN 2020013107 | ISBN 978-1-4214-3987-7 (hardcover) |
ISBN 978-1-4214-3988-4 (ebook)
Subjects: LCSH: African Americans—Maryland—Baltimore—Social conditions. |
African Americans—Segregation—Maryland—Baltimore—History. | African American
neighborhoods—Maryland—Baltimore. | African Americans—Maryland—Baltimore—
Civil rights. | Historical trauma—United States—African Americans—Case studies. |
Segregation—United States—Case studies. | African Americans—
Social conditions—21st century.
Classification: LCC F189.B19 N395 2021 | DDC 323.1196/07307526—dc23
LC record available at https://lccn.loc.gov/2020013107

A catalog record for this book is available from the British Library.

ISBN 978-1-4214-4544-1 (paperback)

*Special discounts are available for bulk purchases of this book. For more information,
please contact Special Sales at specialsales@jh.edu.*

May the rhythm of my heart stir music that enslaves darkness.

May I stand in the midst of celestial fire until my heart is molten gold.

Awakening Osiris: The Egyptian Book of the Dead

Contents

THE BLACK BUTTERFLY

Introduction to Racial Equity

We had been drugged nearly to death
by proslavery compromises.
A radical change was needed
in our whole system.
Nothing is better calculated
to effect the desired change
than the slow, steady and certain
progress of the war.

Frederick Douglass, *The Mission of the War*, January 13, 1864

The first bloodshed of America's Civil War occurred on April 19, 1861, during a deadly riot on Pratt Street in Baltimore when the city's Confederate sympathizers attacked Union Army troops passing through the city. The blood spilled that day near the intersection of Pratt and Light Streets belonged to 4 Union soldiers and 12 members of a pro-Confederate mob.[1] In the aftermath, President Abraham Lincoln had to consider how to respond since Marylanders willing to kill Union soldiers would certainly be willing to join the Confederate States of America, thus leaving Washington, DC, completely surrounded by Confederates to the south (Virginia) and Confederates to the north (Maryland). When Baltimore's business leaders and residents demanded that Lincoln stop dispatching Union troops through the city—heading south to war with their Confederate friends—Lincoln snapped back: "Go home and tell your people that if they will not attack us, we will not attack them;

but if they do attack us, we will return it and that severely."[2] And with that, Lincoln placed Baltimore City under martial law.

Throughout its long history, Baltimore has been a city defined by striking conflicts that threaten to tear the city apart. Traitorous Confederates vs. loyal Unionists. White Baltimore police vs. Black people grieving after Martin Luther King Jr.'s assassination. The Baltimore Police Department vs. Black high school students grieving on the day Freddie Gray was laid to rest. Ever since blood was spilled during the Pratt Street Riot, Baltimore has been a city warring with itself, just as America has remained in turmoil over the question of whether Black Lives really matter.

Since 2015, the term *racial equity* has increasingly become a popular buzzword in many philanthropic and government circles, coinciding with the rise of the Movement for Black Lives and #BlackLivesMatter. It has become fashionable, even popular, for public officials and philanthropic organizations to place the label "racial equity" on their work while having little understanding of the precise ways Black neighborhoods were redlined or how racial segregation has been enforced and maintained. After declaring themselves to be staunch racial equity advocates, both politicians and philanthropists happily laud themselves for doing "good work" without clarity concerning what racial equity means.

Given the persistence and permanence of American racism, clarity about what racial equity is and why it is needed to make Black neighborhoods matter is vitally important. The reason government and organizations must foster racial equity across the nation is not to "help" Black neighborhoods nor out of a fuzzy sense of moral obligation. Racial equity is required to dismantle American Apartheid, which continues to damage thousands of Black neighborhoods across the nation.

Throughout America's history, Black communities, cities, and economic districts have been repeatedly disrupted, deprived, demolished, and destroyed. Before the Civil War, free Black and maroon communities were threatened by the clutches of enslavers and slave traders along with the deployments of slave catchers and patrols.[3] After the Civil War, the safety of Black communities was pierced by lynchers and white supremacist mobs who destroyed entire Black cities and business districts.[4] In the 1910s, as the Great Migration commenced, cities began using racial zoning, and White residents began using racially restrictive covenants to stop the "Negro invasion." In the 1930s, the federal government partnered with local governments and real estate agents to draft Residential Security Maps, which deliberately redlined and underdeveloped Black neighborhoods in more than two hundred cities.[5] In response to Black political activism and urban uprisings of the 1960s, the US government intensified police repression and authorized a war on Black communities—under color of the War on Drugs—instead of fixing the damage that the federal government caused in those communities.

Today, many Black neighborhoods at the core of hypersegregated metropolitan areas remain deeply redlined and are confronted with everything from urban apartheid to toxic pollution. As evidence of America's antipathy toward Black neighborhoods, both a Democrat and a Republican took turns demonizing and denigrating majority Black jurisdictions in Maryland within a span of several months in 2019. Their acidic language illustrates how Black neighborhoods are often viewed with disgust by elected officials and how America's abusive treatment of Black neighborhoods continues. Maryland Delegate Mary Ann Lisanti, a Democrat representing Harford County, called Prince George's County—the nation's wealthiest concentration of Black affluence—a "nigger district."[6] Just months later, Republican President Donald Trump lobbed an attack on Representative Elijah Cummings by tweeting that Baltimore is "a disgusting, rat and rodent infested mess. If he spent more time in Baltimore, maybe he could help clean up this very dangerous & filthy place."[7]

In their stigmatizing language, neither Lisanti nor Trump acknowledged how local, state, and federal governments inflicted severe damage on Black neighborhoods and spaces through devastating policies, practices, systems, and budgets. This damage sustained from intentional government actions explains the conditions of such neighborhoods today. But Trump and Lisanti are not alone in devaluing Black neighborhoods. Research reveals that many White Americans harbor stereotypes about Black areas and devalue the real estate prices of homes in Black neighborhoods, even when they do not hold negative views about Black people.[8]

This discursive redlining has devastating consequences because it undergirds and underwrites policies, practices, systems, and budgets that impact Black neighborhoods.[9] Lisanti's and Trump's racist rhetoric reveals how "race has been understood in spatial terms . . . that bound individuals and groups in place, classify them according to their geographical locations, and arrange them in a spatio-temporal hierarchy."[10] Because of America's spatial racism, White neighborhoods and spaces are imagined as thriving and superior while Black neighborhoods and spaces are deemed as doomed and inferior.[11] Whether Black populations reside in wealthier places such as Prince George's County or less wealthy places such as Baltimore City, where majority Black populations reside does not matter.

To chart a path forward so that Black neighborhoods can thrive, an honest examination of American history is needed. Racial equity is needed to dismantle spatial racism (a process) and produce spatial equity (the outcome).[12] Racial equity is *required* to restore Black neighborhoods, underdeveloped by deliberate public and private policies, practices, systems, and budgets. An authentic racial equity strategy will foster healing from past harms and support collective self-determination for the future. Implementing racial equity as a process or a strategy means building community wealth and boosting health without displacing existing residents. It means establishing budgets that equitably fund infrastructure, schools, recreation centers, and emergency preparedness. Producing racial equity as an outcome means restructuring policies, practices, systems, and budgets at the neighborhood level to foster spatial equity for redlined Black neighborhoods.[13]

To implement a robust racial equity strategy, government officials, philanthropies, corporations, and nonprofits must follow these five steps:

1. Obtain a deep understanding of historical trauma inflicted on Black neighborhoods.
2. Identify and stop all forms of ongoing historical trauma affecting Black neighborhoods.
3. Make decision making participatory and deeply democratic for existing residents in redlined communities.
4. Ensure a meaningful community ownership and wealth-generating stake in all projects, programs, developments, and interventions using collective economics.
5. Make corrective and equitable budget allocations and funding choices to repair the damage caused by ongoing historical trauma on redlined neighborhoods.

Each step must be implemented to foster healthy and wealthy Black neighborhoods. Racial equity starts with a reckoning. If an official, an entity, or an institution cannot explain the specific ways Black communities have been damaged or if they have not deeply reflected on damage they may have inflicted—personally or institutionally—then they are incapable of effectively undertaking the work needed to foster the development of healthy and wealthy Black neighborhoods.

Book Organization

This work is organized according to the five steps to implement a robust racial equity approach and designed to walk the reader through the types of reflection, analysis, and actions needed to develop thriving Black neighborhoods.

Step 1
> Track 1. The Trump Card
> Track 2. This Is America
> Track 3. The "Negro Invasion"

Step 2
> Track 4. Ongoing Historical Trauma
> Track 5. Black Neighborhood Destruction

Steps 3 and 4
> Track 6. Make Black Neighborhoods Matter

Step 5
> Track 7. Healing the Black Butterfly

The "outro" is written to inform the work of activists and organizers as they push for racial equity. Everybody has a role to play. Governments, systems, institutions, organizations, philanthropies, nonprofits, and public officials must engage in a serious, critical, and iterative process of reflection and truth telling, followed by shifting budgets and implementing corrective action. Residents living in Black neighborhoods must become deeply engaged in urban planning and neighborhood design to chart their future. Residents in redlined Black neighborhoods and throughout the city must *organize* to confront ongoing historical trauma and engage in the work needed to restore Black neighborhoods.

Methods and Outline

Using redlined Black neighborhoods as my unit of analysis, I deploy multiple methods to arrive at the strategies, approaches, and recommendations in this volume. In Track 1, I analyze county-level racial demographic data, discuss recent urban uprisings, and offer an analysis of the current national political moment. In Track 2, I conduct a condensed historical analysis and policy review to lay bare the multiple ways that America has erected its own system of apartheid that damages redlined Black communities. In Track 3, I analyze the spatial policies and practices of Baltimore City and Baltimore County to reveal how the jurisdictions created an urban apartheid system of government-enforced racial segregation and forced displacement.

In Track 4, I briefly discuss the concept of historical trauma and use Michelle Sotero's conceptual model of historical trauma to analyze how its effects are ongoing in redlined Black neighborhoods. In Track 5, I explain how ongoing historical trauma leads to Black neighborhood destruction and contextualize how the harms and damages sustained at the neighborhood level culminate in community health crises and catastrophes.

In Track 6, I conduct a racial equity analysis of various systems in Baltimore to demonstrate how they play a role in perpetuating historical trauma. Following this, I discuss how each system can do its part to help dismantle Baltimore Apartheid and make Black neighborhoods matter. In Track 7, I lay out eight citywide strategies that can foster and promote the healing of redlined Black Butterfly neighborhoods. I present an analysis of the city budget and discuss how various solutions can be financed.

Baltimore looms large in this book because its history is intimately linked to the spread of American Apartheid in large urban areas. More broadly, however, this book illuminates the crises and catastrophes occurring in America's Category 5 hypersegregated metropolitan areas and cities. Baltimore, Chicago, St. Louis, Birmingham, Flint, Detroit, Cleveland, and Milwaukee are all sister cities in the most intense and devastating category of racial hypersegregation. Since the Baltimore metropolitan area created the template for urban apartheid nationwide, perhaps it can construct the template for how other hypersegregated metropolitan areas can dismantle their apartheid systems and make Black neighborhoods truly matter.

Each of these eight metropolitan areas (and other jurisdictions) can replicate this type of racial equity analysis and approach to fostering concrete solutions by asking key questions:

- How did all parties contribute to the development of government-enforced racial segregation in this county, city, or area?
- How has serial forced displacement been carried out in this city or area?
- What are the policies, practices, systems, and budgets that inflict ongoing historical trauma on redlined Black neighborhoods in this city or area?
- What racial equity solutions are being implemented, how well did they work, and what future solutions should be deployed?

These and other questions should be front and center for virtually every jurisdiction in the nation.

Key Terms: Origins and Definitions

Here are key terms or phrases that I use throughout the book, along with their origin and definition:

American Apartheid. As defined by Mindy Fullilove and colleagues, American Apartheid is "both a system of separation and serial forced displacement."[14] Hence, American Apartheid includes the government enforcement of both segregation by race and repeated forced uprootings of colonized and enslaved people.

Baltimore Apartheid. A term I coined to describe the city government's enforcement of both segregation by race and the repeated forced uprootings of Black people and neighborhoods.

The Black Butterfly. A term I coined to describe the geographic clustering of Black Baltimoreans. The phrase denotes not only where Black Baltimoreans are geographically clustered but also where capital is denied and structural disadvantages have accumulated due to the lack of capital access. Hence, the Black Butterfly is more than a demographic description; it is a political, economic, and sociocultural description.

Just as a butterfly's wings often have spots of varying colors, the same is true for the Black Butterfly. There are White enclaves in the Black Butterfly, such as northern Park Heights and the two historically segregating universities that sit in East Baltimore (Johns Hopkins medical campus) and West Baltimore (University of Maryland Baltimore).

Category 5 hypersegregation. I use hurricane categories as an analogy to describe metropolitan areas corresponding to the Massey-Tannen scheme of hypersegregation.[15] Hence, I refer to metropolitan areas highly segregated along all five dimensions as *Category 5 hypersegregated cities.* There are eight Category 5 hypersegregated metropolitan area core cities: Baltimore, Chicago, Detroit, Flint, St. Louis, Cleveland, Birmingham, and Milwaukee.

Equity. A term I define as doing more for those communities that have less wealth and health due to ongoing historical trauma. Equity is a process of repairing damage and making communities whole.

Gentrification. Many urbanists attempt to define gentrification without accounting for its racist and classist dimensions. The California-based group Causa Justa :: Just Cause has written such a definition in their report *Development without Displacement* where they articulate:

> We define gentrification as a profit-driven racial and class recon-
> figuration of urban, working-class and communities of color that

have suffered from a history of disinvestment and abandonment. The process is characterized by declines in the number of low-income, people of color in neighborhoods that begin to cater to higher-income workers willing to pay higher rents. Gentrification is driven by private developers, landlords, businesses, and corporations, and supported by the government through policies that facilitate the process of displacement, often in the form of public subsidies.[16]

The beauty of this definition is that it connects modern displacement with a "history of disinvestment and abandonment." It is that very history that gives potency to the processes of gentrification. The other thing this definition acknowledges is that gentrification is not merely the private markets at work. It is supported by public subsidies and constitutes a government policy or practice similar to urban renewal or highway construction through Black neighborhoods.

The Great Rebellion. I define the contemporary period as the "Great Rebellion"—from 2014 to 2020. I argue that urban uprisings between 2014 and 2017 were the first wave, while the uprisings and mass protests following the killing of George Floyd constitute the second wave. This naming convention follows the tradition of activists and historians who coined labels for other eras of racial upheaval.

Such labels help Americans to contextualize and commemorate the nation's history of racialized violence and turmoil. Historian Douglas Egerton called post–Civil War violence the "Wars of Reconstruction" roughly covering the period between 1866 and 1876. Activist James Weldon Johnson coined the phrase "Red Summer" which took place in 1919. A larger period of racial violence actually stretches roughly from 1917 (riot in East St. Louis) to 1923 (the destruction of Black Wall Street in Tulsa and Rosewood, Florida). Historian Peter Levy called urban uprisings during the Civil Rights and Black Power eras the "Great Uprising" stretching from 1963 to 1971.

Historical trauma. A conceptual framework first articulated by Maria Yellow Horse Brave Heart. Historical trauma was advanced as a public health conceptual framework by Michelle Sotero who described historical trauma as "the premise . . . that populations historically subjected to long-term, mass trauma exhibit a higher prevalence of disease even several generations after the original trauma occurred."[17] Mass traumas include war, imperialism, genocide, apartheid, slavery, and caste. I conceptualize *ongoing historical trauma* as the intergenerational effects of past mass traumas combined with the contemporary structural violence that continue to inflict damage on vulnerable racial and ethnic groups and impose spatial inequity on their land or in their neighborhoods. This damage is transmitted through public and private policies, practices, systems, and budgets.

Hyperpolicing. A term I coined to discuss a system of aggressive racial profiling and militarized policing based on a combination of US Supreme Court decisions, presidential executive orders, and federal laws that authorize the disproportionate policing strategies in Black neighborhoods. Because of its aggressiveness and resulting brutality, hyperpolicing breeds mistrust as police do not "protect and serve" Black neighborhoods with the same courtesy and respect afforded to other communities. Hence, Black neighborhoods are often paradoxically hyperpoliced yet underprotected.

Hypersegregation. A concept developed by Douglas Massey and Nancy Denton. According to Massey and Tannen, hypersegregation "describe[s] metropolitan areas in which African Americans were highly segregated on at least four of the

five dimensions" of spatial racial segregation. Here are the five
dimensions according to Massey and Tannen:

> *Unevenness* is the degree to which blacks and whites are unevenly
> distributed across neighborhoods in a metropolitan area; *isolation* is
> the extent to which African Americans live in predominantly black
> neighborhoods; *clustering* is the degree to which neighborhoods
> inhabited by African Americans are clustered together in space;
> *concentration* is the relative amount of physical space occupied by
> African Americans within a given metropolitan environment; and
> *centralization* is the degree to which blacks reside near the center of a
> metropolitan area."[18]

Racial equity. A term I define as taking restorative actions to
help redlined Black communities organize themselves in order
to heal from ongoing historical trauma. This requires fully
acknowledging and stopping all manifestations of ongoing
historical trauma. Hence, racial equity is not simply a "lens" or
a "perspective." Racial equity is a *process* comprising five steps
outlined earlier and described in more detail throughout this
book. In a racially segregated society, racial equity as an *outcome*
is contingent on achieving spatial equity—where resources and
amenities are intentionally deployed based on demonstrated
neighborhood needs while disamenities are removed or
dismantled based on disproportionate neighborhood harms.
There can be no racial equity without spatial equity.

Redlining. Denying Black neighborhoods equitable access to
private financial capital *and* equitable spending on public goods.
Redlining is an ongoing process of wealth denial practiced in
Black neighborhoods across the country. Private bank redlining
was formalized with the drafting of Residential Security Maps
in nearly 250 cities by the federal government with the aid of
local governments. The maps featured four color codes—red,

blue, yellow, and green—to help the federal government and banking institutions determine which communities received capital access (green, blue, and yellow) and which did not (red).[19] The differential spending on public goods in segregated cities from the early 1900s onward—particularly in Black neighborhoods—is an often unrecognized form of redlining.[20]

Serial forced displacement. A term coined by researchers Mindy Fullilove and Rodrick Wallace that includes public and private policies and practices such as "segregation, redlining, urban renewal, planned shrinkage/catastrophic disinvestment, deindustrialization, mass criminalization, gentrification, HOPE VI, and the foreclosure crisis."[21] I view serial forced displacement as the forced uprooting of people and communities in concert with land seizures. It can sometimes take the form of withdrawing critical resources in communities, such as mass school closures, school takeovers, recreation center closures, and the demolition and privatization of public housing.

Segrenomics. A term coined by Noliwe Rooks as "the business of profiting specifically from high levels of racial and economic segregation."[22] Although she examines segrenomics from an education lens, I find her term useful to explain how Black neighborhoods are denied equitable spending on public goods and private capital (e.g., redlining) and how economic exploitation is practiced in Black neighborhoods (e.g., subpriming or predatory lending and taxation). In some instances, I equate segrenomics with the internal colonization of Black neighborhoods in America (through wealth extraction). In short, segrenomics is the economic weaponization of government-enforced racial segregation.

Whitelash. A term dropped by Van Jones on CNN on election night in November 2016 that combines *white* and *backlash*.[23] As

Jones articulated regarding the results of the election: "This was a whitelash against a changing country. It was whitelash against a Black president in part. And that's the part where the pain comes." I define whitelash as the racist American tradition of backlash against Black progress rooted in a zero-sum framework.

The White L. A description of the geographic clustering where White Baltimoreans live. The White L describes not only where White Baltimoreans live but also where access to capital is most readily available and structural advantages have accrued due to that capital access. Hence, the White L is more than a demographic description but a political, economic, and social-cultural description. There are also historically Black enclaves in the White L, such as Sharp Leadenhall, Hoes Heights, and Cross Keys Village.

White supremacy. An ideological, philosophical, and theological perspective that spawns institutions, policies, practices, systems, and budgets that incur structured advantages for White people and neighborhoods and create structured disadvantages for Black, Brown, and Native people and neighborhoods. Structural advantages include material wealth, access to capital, high-quality public goods, respectful policing, and landownership, while structured disadvantages include wealth extraction, lack of access to capital, poor quality public goods, hyperpolicing, and forced displacement or uprootings.

A new vision for public health must emerge. Public health cannot simply focus on the health of generalized populations. Public health must evolve and uplift community health—with emphasis on the particular spaces and places where people live. This means adopting an explicitly spatiotemporal framework that views community health as deeply informed by history and influenced by previous policies, practices, systems, and budgets. In a nation founded on the colonization of Native nations' lands and the current rise of what Samuel Stein calls the "real estate state," spatial racism is alive and well.[24] In America, Black neighborhoods are treated as places for pilfering and profiteering, as spaces for extraction and exploitation. This work is an interruption and an intervention that posits that it is impossible to make Black Lives matter without making Black neighborhoods matter.

Why tracks instead of chapters? Because the work of bolstering community health is as much about fusing art and storytelling as it is about conveying science. I often listen to music while I am writing and suffuse my writing with spoken word, poetry, rhythm, and song. While I draw heavily from research and social science, I also draw from the wellspring of Black speculative visions, ranging from Parliament-Funkadelic's Mothership to *Black Panther*'s Wakanda. This book is infused with *Afrofuturistic ecological thinking*—a mode of thinking that says healthy Black people and thriving Black neighborhoods exist in the future! It is up to this nation, along with its cities and counties, to make this future a functional reality.

Finally, some readers may ask, "Why should I care about urban Black neighborhoods since I live in a safe and secure suburb or exurb?" To these persons, I would respond that people living in all areas of America should care because the social and economic advantages involved in the creation and maintenance of suburbs and exurbs help exacerbate many of the disadvantages that exist in urban areas and Black neighborhoods.

I also present the thinking of President Lincoln when he offered his analysis of a bitterly divided nation while running for Congress in 1858:

A house divided against itself cannot stand.
I believe this government cannot endure,
permanently half slave and half free.

I do not expect the Union to be dissolved—
I do not expect the house to fall—
but I do expect it will cease to be divided.
It will become all one thing or all the other.

Lincoln was partially wrong. By 1861, the Union was dissolved. The house did fall. America was soon ensnared in a brutal and bloody war. Although formal hostilities ceased, the nation still wrestles with its structural and spatial sins. In 2020, COVID-19 snatched over 200,000 lives and the Great Rebellion engulfed the nation in the flames of uprisings, riots, and looting after police killed George Floyd in Minneapolis. The nation is currently teetering on its axis as American Apartheid threatens to tear the nation apart. America is splintering politically because it is fractured spatially. The nation cannot endure by denying spatial equity and maintaining urban apartheid. Either the nation will make racial equity a reality or succumb to the infernal outcomes of American Apartheid. It will become all one thing or the other.

A radical change is needed in our whole system. America will not move forward until there is a great reckoning where Americans fully acknowledge the legacy of white supremacist violence and terrorism unleashed during the Wars of Reconstruction (1866–1876) and again during the period encompassing the Red Summer (1917–1923). The nation will not know tranquility until it addresses the root causes of the Black pushback during the Great Uprising (1963–1971) and more recently during the Great Rebellion (2014–2020). If we, the people of the United States of America, wish to bequeath to posterity a thriving nation, the nation must undergo a reckoning with its wrongs and make amends for its past. Only this reckoning followed by radical change can make racial equity a concrete reality and make Black neighborhoods matter.

The Trump Card

> Excuse me: could I please ask a favor?
> Could we really integrate like the layers of a flavor?
> Could a Black girl that's urban
> Have suburban girls as neighbors?

Martina Lynch, "Fences"

> They're celebrating our deaths like it's a badge of honor
> And all of those degrees don't mean a damn thing
> Every time I see a video or hear a gunshot . . . I feel that in my chest
> And I can't sleep because my soul can't rest
> 'Cause I can't help but think . . .
> . . . WHAT IF THAT WAS ME!?

Aja Cross, "Officer Don't Shoot"

Whitelash

"Trump triumphs" read the stunning headline on November 9, 2016. After the election of Barack Obama in 2008, pundits and demographers declared that the demographic destiny of the United States was in favor of the Democratic Party. By 2042 or thereabouts, America would be "majority minority," and America would reach its status as a multicultural oasis and postracial promised land.

But America's true demographic destiny was revealed on November 9, 2016, in the early hours after the election. There are 3,142 counties across the nation. Out of these, 413 counties are 98% or more White in population. Another 1,413 counties are between 90% and 97.99% White, while 504 counties are between 80% and 89.99% White. This means that, in nearly three-fourths of all counties in the United States, White people are 80% of the population or more (table 1.1). By contrast, over 80% of all Black people in the United States live in the remaining 791 counties. Perhaps nothing captures the capacity for future political dominance better than the fact that 1,847 counties are 90% or more White, but only 185 counties are 10% White or less.[1] Unsurprisingly, Trump did best in the demographically whitest counties.[2]

Currently, 21 metropolitan areas in the United States are hypersegregated, and another 32 are classified as highly segregated. The 21 hypersegregated metro areas contain 26% of the nation's Black population, and approximately 22.5 million Black people live in the nation's top 50 largest cities—roughly 53% of the entire Black population.[3] The spatial clustering of people by race is both a national phenomenon and a metropolitan phenomenon. While Black America is spatially clustered in highly or hypersegregated urban areas, White Americans are the supermajority in three-fourths of all counties in the United States—many of them rural counties. Asian Americans are also highly concentrated in the 719 counties that are less than 80% White, while Native Americans are concentrated disproportionately on reservations.

This translates into a high degree of White demographic power in the realm of politics. By being the supermajority population in so many counties and in so many rural areas, White America will

Table 1.1. Number of counties by percentage of White America

Percentage White	Number of Counties	Description of Counties
98% or more	413	Demographically dominant
90%–97.99%	1,413	Highly hegemonic
80%–89.99%	504	Supermajority white
Less than 80%	791	Comparatively diverse

be ensured significant advantages in electing the majority of senators to Congress and the president by means of the Electoral College. The ability to win elections with a minority of the popular vote and the election of two Senators per state—regardless of population size—gives significant advantages to rural areas and states with smaller populations.[4] Even as America becomes a true rainbow nation, two of the most powerful political entities can potentially remain in the hands of White Americans. And since the president nominates US Supreme Court justices and the Senate confirms Supreme Court nominees, the three major political branches of government can possibly be run by a White minority population because of American Apartheid.[5]

Donald Trump's election in 2016 reveals the way that American Apartheid will continue to give outsized power and influence to White voters seeking to maintain white privilege and power. Trump was electorally supported by 81% of White evangelical born-again Christians, 63% of White male voters, 53% of White female voters, 49% of White college graduates, and 48% of all voters earning over $100,000.[6] He also won all of these categories over Democratic candidate Hillary Clinton. With overt appeals to bigotry and the slogan Make America Great Again, especially after eight years of the first Black president, Trump's election embodied a whitelash against perceived Black progress.

But whitelash is nothing new. It is a time-honored tradition in American history. America is notorious for backsliding on progress benefiting Black Lives. The slogan Make America Great Again echoes the politics animating White Redemption designed to roll back Black Reconstruction in the 1870s and recalls the Southern Strategy designed to unravel the progress of the Civil Rights and Black Power movements in the 1970s and 1980s. America is now in a moment where White Redemption in national politics is being deployed for the third time. Each deployment has had disturbing aims:

- First American Whitelash—dismantle and diminish Black Reconstruction
- Second American Whitelash—reverse gains obtained by Civil Rights and Black Power movement activists
- Third American Whitelash—repeal and replace President Barack Obama's policies and legacy

The Trump presidency is the culmination of the third iteration of whitelash. Nearly every policy that President Barack Obama passed or pushed has been systematically targeted for elimination, nullification, or repeal by the Trump administration. But the broader national animus directed against Obama's legacy can be explained with political science data. Research revealed that White Americans with more fear of immigrants causing cultural displacement had an increased likelihood of supporting Trump.[7] A Reuters survey revealed that Trump supporters were significantly more likely to view Black people as less intelligent, more lazy, more rude, more violent, and more criminal than Clinton supporters or even other Republican candidates (e.g., Ted Cruz and John Kasich).[8] Still other analyses highlight the centrality of racism in Trump's ascendance and governance.[9] As Francis Cress Welsing remarked shortly before her death: "Donald Trump's trump card is the race card in the system of racism/white supremacy."[10]

The Reduction in Protection under the Law

Although many people expressed alarm over the election of Donald Trump, the Supreme Court was already at work stripping away the legal protection of Black Lives and the enforcement of Black people's civil rights. In 2005, President George W. Bush nominated John Roberts to the Supreme Court to serve as the chief justice. Under the Roberts Court, the great 1960s Civil Rights Acts and previous *Brown v. Board of Education* decisions have been systematically undermined.[11] As just one example, the 2016 *Utah v. Strieff* Supreme Court decision undermined the Fourteenth Amendment's equal protection clause and earned a stinging rebuke from Supreme Court Justice Sonia Sotomayor, who wrote in dissent:

> This Court has allowed an officer to stop you for whatever reason he wants—so long as he can point to a pretextual justification after the fact. That justification must provide specific reasons why the officer suspected you were breaking the law, but it may factor in your ethnicity, where you live, what you were wearing, and how you behaved. The officer does not even need to know which law you might have broken so long as he can later point to any possible infraction—even one that is minor, unrelated, or ambiguous.[12]

This judicial retrenchment is conjoined with the Republican Party's political ascendance. The GOP–Tea Party has been ramping up toward the current moment, especially after the 2008 election of President Obama. On October 23, 2010, Kentucky Senator Mitch McConnell gave voice to the GOP–Tea Party's aim: "The single most important thing we want to achieve is for President Obama to be a one-term president."[13] Although McConnell failed to stop an Obama second term, President Trump would succeed in rolling back Obama's policy legacy.[14] By refusing to confirm Merrick Garland, Obama's pick for the Supreme Court, the GOP–Tea Party flipped the high court and ensured conservative judicial dominance for the foreseeable future.

Urban Uprisings and Historical Trauma

Just as Trump's triumph and the future political dominance of White Americans can be explained by America's enduring apartheid, so can the urban uprisings Americans have witnessed since the killing of Mike Brown in Ferguson, Missouri, during the presidency of Barack Obama. During the first wave of the

Great Rebellion, urban uprisings erupted in six metropolitan areas—Ferguson, Baltimore, Minneapolis, Baton Rouge, Charlotte, and St. Louis. If Americans understand "a riot is the language of the unheard"—as once described by Martin Luther King Jr.—then it behooves the nation to learn to interpret that "language" and listen to what the unheard have been attempting to convey.

Black people in the United States have long endured historical trauma since their arrival as indentured servants on American shores over 400 years ago. But it is equally important to remember that the history of African Americans has not just been one of victimization in the face of unrelenting trauma, violence, and brutality; it is also one of resilience, resistance, and revolution in opposition to race-based exploitation and domination. However, historical trauma does inflict lasting damage in redlined Black neighborhoods. Public health scholar Michelle Sotero outlined four ways that ongoing historical trauma damages community health: (1) segregation/forced displacement, (2) physical/psychological violence, (3) economic destruction, and (4) cultural dispossession.[15] These four components of historical trauma have devastating impacts on the health of African Americans in the United States. Explaining further, researcher Sarah Malotane argues: "Historical trauma is not an event, but a series of lived events over time—a process that requires systemic rather than only individual intervention."[16] Without systemic intervention, the symptoms of historical trauma will remain unchecked and unresolved.

Since a large proportion of Black people in America are demographically clustered in metropolitan areas and core urban areas, understanding the impact of the four main components of historical trauma can only be ascertained by examining core urban areas' policies, practices, systems, and budgets that damage Black neighborhoods and hurt and harm Black Lives. This volume elucidates how hypersegregated cities have functioned as the tip of the American Apartheid spear in the lives of millions of African Americans, leading to militant protests and community-police confrontations in cities such as Ferguson, Baltimore, Minneapolis, Baton Rouge, Charlotte, Milwaukee, and St. Louis during the first wave of the Great Rebellion from 2014 to 2017. Urban uprisings do not erupt out of thin air. They occur after a community has been pushed to the edge.

The Baltimore Uprising

By the afternoon of April 27, 2015, Baltimore was on fire. That fateful morning, a West Baltimore man named Freddie Gray was being funeralized and laid to rest in the afternoon. His death by hyperpolicing occurred after he was chased and then arrested by Baltimore police officers on April 12. Freddie Gray was denied immediate medical attention although he was writhing and screaming in pain as he was placed in the police van. He was in a coma for a week and died on April 19.

A little over a week later, at 11:39 a.m. on the morning of April 27, Baltimore police officials released a memo of a "credible threat" that local gangs were uniting to kill cops and claimed that Black youth were getting together to conduct a lawless purge after they got out of school at 3 p.m. These police claims would later be classified as unsubstantiated or disproven, but the fear-mongering had already been done. As a result of salacious reports, the Baltimore Police Department (BPD) deployed police in riot gear and stopped high school students from going home by shutting down buses adjacent to Mondawmin Mall in West Baltimore. Grieving, frustrated, and unable to go home, Black youth began throwing rocks at the police. Baltimore police responded by launching rocks, rubber bullets, and tear gas at the teenage students. Afterward, the situation devolved. Looting commenced, stores and police cars were set afire, and, by nightfall, the city was under a state of emergency.

Although the events of April 27 unfolded rapidly, the uprising erupted against a bubbling historical backdrop: the street shutdowns and protests against police brutality along with the emerging Movement for Black Lives protests the previous year. On September 15, 2014, a Black police officer was captured on camera pummeling a cowering victim with his fists in Baltimore. On September 28, 2014, *Baltimore Sun* reporter Mark Puente published a hard-hitting investigative story called "Undue Force," highlighting how the BPD had brutalized many victims. The reporting sparked the City of Baltimore to request a "collaborative review" with the US Department of Justice (DOJ) regarding police violence.

Roughly two months later, on November 24 and December 3, 2014, Ferguson and New York prosecutors announced that Officer Darren Wilson and New York Police Department officers would not be indicted for their actions involving the deaths of Mike Brown and Eric Garner, respectively. Mourners around the nation joined together in solidarity to protest and express their outrage that the law enforcers responsible for the killings of Brown and Garner would not be charged or called to account. On December 16, 2014, after days of rolling protests and street shutdowns, a 19-year-old Black male (Donte Jones) shot a West Baltimore police officer, reportedly out of fear that he would be killed like recent victims of police shootings.[17]

While tensions simmered over the winter months, the DOJ convened a meeting on April 16, 2015—four days after Freddie Gray was arrested and ended up in a coma—where roughly 300 Baltimore residents spoke out about their grievances against the BPD. Two days later, residents of Gilmor Homes—a public housing community where Gray lived—began marching down to and assembling at the Western District Police Station to protest the police brutality that led to Freddie Gray's hospitalization. Therefore, when Freddie Gray died on April 19, months of anger and frustration boiled over and were punctuated with moving protests, many of which spread from the Western District, snaked through traffic crossing Martin Luther King Jr. Boulevard, and arrived downtown resulting in business shutdowns.

On April 23, Gene Ryan, head of the Baltimore Fraternal Order of Police, publicly declared that peaceful protesters "looked like a lynch mob," introducing inflammatory rhetoric that reflected and escalated BPD's tactical deployment against protesters.[18] Thousands of Baltimore residents and protesters would hold massive marches during this weekend, demanding justice for Freddie Gray. On Saturday, April 25, after a gathering and speech held by Malik Shabazz in front of City Hall, a mixed crowd of protesters and predominantly White Baltimore Orioles fans clashed as windows of cars and buildings near the baseball stadium were smashed in what the *Baltimore City Paper* dubbed the "Clash at Camden Yards." Later that night, Baltimore police officers swarmed and attacked protesters near the Western District, including reporter Baynard Woods. The *Baltimore City Paper* dubbed it "The Battle of Sandtown-Winchester."

Thus, when fires burned in multiple locations across the city on April 27, it was the culmination of months of street protests, inflammatory rhetoric, and concussive clashes between city protesters and suburban residents or police. In the span of eight days, the city had gone from the death of Freddie Gray (April 19) to the Clash at Camden Yards and the Battle of Sandtown-Winchester (April 25–26) to the Mondawmin Mall bus shutdown by police and subsequent uprising (April 27). The city would be placed under curfew for five days following the April 27 civil disturbance, causing stress and strain particularly for late-night workers and businesses. On Friday, May 1, Baltimore City State's Attorney Marilyn Mosby proclaimed that the six BPD officers involved in the death of Freddie Gray would be indicted. There was an eruption of jubilation and joy as many Black Baltimoreans celebrated that possibility that there might actually be justice for Freddie Gray. That catharsis would soon subside as none of the officers involved in the death of Freddie Gray would be found guilty.

Crises and Catastrophes in Hypersegregated Cities

Why did several Black communities explode into shutdowns and uprisings between 2014 and 2017? Examining data on racial hypersegregation in a metropolitan area provides an explanation. The core urban cities in the 21 hypersegregated metropolitan areas contain redlined Black neighborhoods that have been deeply damaged by apartheid policies and practices that result in devastating resource deprivation. At the same time, predominantly White neighborhoods benefit from an influx of public dollars and private capital. Therefore, hypersegregation results in the hyper-allocation of resources to White neighborhoods and the hyper-deprivation of resources in Black neighborhoods.

Starving neighborhoods of critical resources fosters places where crime and violence are likely to fester. Instead of responding to crime and violence by reversing economic and resource deprivation, most municipalities respond to crime and violence in redlined Black neighborhoods with hyperpolicing. The legal framework for hyperpolicing in redlined Black neighborhoods has been structured by several pivotal but little-known Supreme Court decisions—*Terry v. Ohio* (1968), *Graham v. Connor* (1989), *Illinois v. Wardlow* (2000), and *Utah v. Strieff* (2016). These decisions established case law that authorized discriminatory police practices, including stop-and-frisk, the killings of unarmed people if officers claim fear for their lives, differential policing in neighborhoods deemed "high crime areas," and the legalization of unlawful investigatory stops.

These Supreme Court decisions, along with other pieces of congressional legislation and presidential executive orders, collectively create the legal basis for hyperpolicing Black neighborhoods. Hyperpolicing elevates the likelihood that police-citizen interactions will escalate into scenarios where police, who often are not residents of the cities they patrol, bring their racial biases and stereotypes with them when they encounter Black residents living in redlined neighborhoods damaged by apartheid. Instead of blaming the conditions in redlined Black communities on national, state, and local urban policies, police officers most often ascribe conditions to the residents. The toxic stew of resource apartheid, racial biases, and hyperpolicing contribute to police brutality and the fatal police shootings of Black persons such as Mike Brown, Aiyana Stanley-Jones, Tamir Rice, Philando Castile, Korryn Gaines, and Freddie Gray. The police killings of unarmed Black people—followed by the lack of indictments and convictions—often lights the match that sparks the fire of an urban uprising.

After SARS-CoV-2—commonly called the novel coronavirus—began spreading rapidly across the nation in February 2020, America was once again on the edge. In mid-March, governors across the nation ordered people to shelter in place and businesses closed. The toll of the coronavirus soon became clear. In a period of less than three months, over 100,000 Americans died due to COVID-19 and 40 million people were thrown into unemployment. Black Americans died at a disproportionate rate as SARS-CoV-2 took root in redlined neighborhoods in the nation's cities with legacies of hypersegregation.[19] In doing so, COVID-19 exposed the fault lines embedded within American Apartheid.

While COVID-19 radically altered American life, another pandemic was also stalking Black Lives. The stories of the vigilante killing of Ahmaud Arbery in Brunswick, Georgia, and the police killing of Breonna Taylor in Louisville, Kentucky, began circulating more widely throughout March and April. By late May, Black America was set to explode. When Minneapolis police officers killed George Floyd by kneeling on his neck for over 8 minutes and 46 seconds on Memorial Day, Black America was thunderstruck with intense grief. The video of the slow and deliberate police killing of Floyd elicited fire and fury. After viewing the video, South Minneapolis exploded in riot, protest, fires, and looting. Los Angeles, Denver, Memphis, and Atlanta exploded next by the same means by the end of the week.

By mid-June, over 3,200 cities had erupted in protests.[20] The National Guard was activated in over 25 states. In some cities, protests were often followed by rioting—setting police vehicles on fire, looting, and property destruction. In Minneapolis, where George Floyd was killed by Minneapolis officer Derek Chauvin, protesters and city residents were so insistent in their militance that they overwhelmed the Minneapolis police and forced them to abandon their Third Precinct building.

The nationwide riotous turmoil in 2020 echoed the Holy Week Uprisings in 1968. Historian Peter Levy dubbed the period from 1963 to 1971 the *Great Uprising*, an era which witnessed over 750 uprisings. The Great Uprising is an appropriate phrase that helps convey the totality of the frustration and anger that Black people experienced as well as the conditions to which they were responding. In a similar vein, I call the period from 2014 to 2020 the *Great Rebellion* to explain the era of urban uprisings that took place between 2014 and 2017 (Wave 1) and nationwide protests and uprisings in 2020 (Wave 2).

American Apartheid is the root cause for both the Great Uprising and the Great Rebellion. Hypersegregation breeds hyperpolicing. Civic leaders continually ignore hypersegregation while elected officials repeatedly authorize hyperpolicing that leads directly to fatal police shootings. Spatial racism sparks the fires of crises and catastrophes burning in many urban communities.

During the first wave of the Great Rebellion, urban uprisings took place largely in Category 5 hypersegregated metropolitan areas, signaling the depths of despair and frustration simmering in many American cities. The cascading crises and catastrophes that rock redlined Black neighborhoods in each of the Category 5 hypersegregated core cities are presented in table 1.2.

Table 1.2. Crises and catastrophes in the eight Category 5 hypersegregated cities

Category 5/City	Issues and Crises
Baltimore	Mass protests for Freddie Gray in mid-April 2015; police occupation and April 27, 2015, Mondawmin uprising; second in 2017 murder rate, second in rental evictions
Flint	2016 ongoing lead poisoning crisis; under emergency management by state
Detroit	Third in 2017 murder rate, first in rental evictions; mass school closures, teacher sickouts, under emergency management by state
Chicago	Fifth in 2017 murder rate; protests against violence; mass school closures; school funding crisis; South Shore residents clash with police after shooting of Harith Augustus on July 14, 2018; potential uprising averted after former officer Van Dyke was judged guilty in the killing of Laquan McDonald in August 2018
St. Louis and Ferguson	Mass protests for Mike Brown, police occupation and 2014 Ferguson Rebellion, 2017 St. Louis Uprising, mass protests in the city; first in 2017 murder rate
Birmingham	Three straight years of increasing murder rate; school resegregation, White school district separation; spike in drug overdose deaths
Cleveland	May 23, 2015, uprising in response to not guilty verdict of Officer Michael Brelo; police killing of 12-year-old Tamir Rice on November 22, 2014, and protests after nonindictment of Officer Timothy Loehmann; lead poisoning crisis
Milwaukee	August 14–15, 2016, Sherman Park uprising after killing of Sylville Smith by police; high homicide rates, 2018 lead poisoning crisis

If the first wave of the Great Rebellion was the stunning prelude, then the second wave was the smashing crescendo. The crises of hypersegregation and hyperpolicing that simmered beneath the surface began bubbling and boiling over from large hypersegregated cities and started spilling into protests and demonstrations for racial justice in smaller communities.[21] The profound anguish and rage unleashed during the Great Rebellion revealed that hypersegregated cities are linked with suburbs, small towns, and rural communities. The same is true with COVID-19, which also first spread heavily in hypersegregated cities. In the early 1900s, White Americans attempted to cordon off Black people into redlined urban neighborhoods. But ultimately what starts in redlined neighborhoods spills over into the rest of the nation. By June 2020, the cauldron of racial and spatial inequity boiled over leaving no part of the nation unscathed nor unscarred.

Conclusion

Perhaps it is the constant crises and catastrophes or the sense of being under attack that provoked Baltimore City spoken word artists Aja Cross and Martina Lynch to pointedly question and critique America. In "Officer Don't Shoot," Aja Cross—a trauma nurse and Morgan State University graduate—narrates the ominous shadow of death that impacts the mental health of Black people in America due to police brutality.

> Every time I see a video or hear a gunshot . . .
> I feel that in my chest
> And I can't sleep
> because my soul can't rest

In her piece "Fences," Lynch pointedly asks if a Black girl born in Baltimore City can be neighbors with a White girl in one of Baltimore County's suburbs. Listening to Aja and Martina, one can hear the voices of thousands of Baltimore's Black children—especially those that grow up in deeply redlined Black neighborhoods—wondering whether peace, safety, and suburban spaces are meant for them.

Are safe and healthy neighborhoods meant for a Black child growing up in redlined neighborhoods in hypersegregated cities like Baltimore? Should Black children have to aspire to leave their neighborhoods to find safety and security? Martina and Aja should not have to question America—and the allocation of resources and safety in urban versus suburban spaces—in the "land of the free and home of the brave." If America is to ever move forward as a nation, everyone should question why many Black people feel unsafe. Americans can start by asking, *How did America become a nation so characterized by devastatingly deep spatial and racial divides?*

This Is America

If the Freedom Democratic Party is not seated now,
I question America.
Is this America?
The land of the free
and the home of the brave,
where we have to sleep
with our telephones off the hooks
because our lives be threatened daily,
because we want to live
as decent human beings,
in America?

Fannie Lou Hamer, *Testimony at the Democratic National Convention*,
August 22, 1964

When Thomas Jefferson drafted the Declaration of Independence, the terror of enslavement was already enshrined in the law of the British colonies. White British colonizers—who would become Americans after the Revolutionary War in 1776—participated actively in the Transatlantic Slave Trade until 1820. These settlers became slave traders and enslavers, transporting approximately 388,000 Africans to the new nation as cargo in the form of property in the attempt to make America "great."[1] Enslaved Africans originated in the "Bantu-speaking regions of west-central Africa" (34%), Senegambia (20%), the Gold Coast (15%), and Sierra Leone (15%). The remaining 16% of enslaved Africans mostly came from the Bight of Biafra and the Windward Coast.[2]

American slavery imposed a system of terror on Black Lives by splitting apart Black families without warning. Black people were auctioned, purchased, sold, traded, rented, leased, and mortgaged in city squares and markets for White profit. Black children were ripped out of their parents' arms. Africans' various cultures, languages, and customs were continually demonized and suppressed by White slave traders and slave masters as enslaved Africans and people of African descent in America were forced to assimilate and abandon their ways of life in a strange land. In spite of this attempted cultural dispossession imposed by the violent traumas of the Middle Passage, the auction blocks, slave trading, enslavement, and community surveillance, Black people resisted and proceeded to Africanize the thirteen colonies. Although descendants of Africans enslaved in the United States would be torn from Africa, Africa could not be torn from them.[3]

Sugar, tobacco, rice, and other crops became lucrative commodities for White planters and plantation owners. White American slave traders forcibly relocated Black people time and again to supply plantation owners with an enslaved labor force. A new slave trade arose within America's borders—the Domestic American Slave Trade—after international slave trading became outlawed in 1820 as cotton became a primary cash crop in the Deep South. To meet the rising global demand for cotton, White slave owners in the Chesapeake and mid-Atlantic regions engaged in a process of breeding Black people like horses or dogs to genetically engineer a commodity of enslaved field hands.[4] Nearly 1.2 million enslaved Black people were shipped or transported from the East Coast to the Deep South in the Domestic American Slave Trade.[5] Freedom fighter and abolitionist Frederick Douglass testified about the nature of the trade:

> Behold the practical operation of this internal slave-trade, the
> American slave-trade, sustained by American politics and American

religion. Here you will see men and women reared like swine for the market. You know what is a swine-drover? I will show you a man-drover. They inhabit all our Southern States. They perambulate the country, and crowd the highways of the nation, with droves of human stock. You will see one of these human flesh-jobbers, armed with pistol, whip and bowie-knife, driving a company of a hundred men, women, and children, from the Potomac to the slave market at New Orleans. These wretched people are to be sold singly, or in lots, to suit purchasers. They are food for the cotton-field, and the deadly sugar-mill. Mark the sad procession, as it moves wearily along, and the inhuman wretch who drives them. Hear his savage yells and his blood-chilling oaths, as he hurries on his affrighted captives![6]

Douglass vividly illustrated the geographic scope of the infernal Domestic American Slave Trade, which saw "man-drovers" forcibly and violently transporting enslaved Black workers as cargo from cities such as Baltimore and Washington, DC, to slave markets in New Orleans.[7] He also alluded to its economic underpinnings. Many American banks and insurance companies obtained wealth and profits from the commodification of enslaved people as Black children, women, and men were traded, sold, leased, rented, collateralized, mortgaged, and securitized.[8] Medical examiners certified the fitness of the Black enslaved property for enslavers.[9] The trustees and founders of America's Ivy League and state land-grant universities in Northern states often derived their wealth from chattel slavery practiced in Southern states.[10] Nearly every part of the nation's economy was intertwined with the commoditization of Black people's flesh and the wealth extraction of Black people's labor—particularly Black women's labor via the practice of human breeding.

The Coming of War

Despite the commodification of human beings and the toll of psychological terror, the enslaved descendants of African people would strike back—stealing (themselves) away, plotting insurrections, and engaging in other means of slave system sabotage. Enslaved people constructed a clandestine Underground Railroad and engaged in militant abolitionist resistance. Still American slavery grew in scope and scale. Beginning in the 1850s, enslaved Black workers labored and began producing 3 million bales of cotton most years. By 1861, their labor produced a staggering 5 million bales of cotton.[11] When the US Congress passed the Fugitive Slave Act of 1850, it signaled the coming war, as it forced Northerners to return escaped slaves, or "property," to their former masters.

Many Northern abolitionists resisted this expansive police act that nullified Northern states' rights, and thus the militant abolitionist movement swelled.[12] In 1854, Congress passed the Kansas-Nebraska Act, which prevented future congressional representatives from prohibiting slavery in any new states or territories. This sparked fighting such as the Kansas-Missouri Border War, where abolitionists sparred with enslavers, leading to the killing of 56 people.[13]

Two years later, the US Supreme Court handed down *Dred Scott v. Sandford*, one of the most explicit articulations of white supremacy and racial domination in American history. Chief Justice Roger B. Taney, a Marylander and former slave owner, wrote the decision where he explained with striking clarity:

> The question is simply this: can a negro whose ancestors were imported into this country and sold as slaves become a member of the political community . . . and as such become entitled to all the rights, and privileges, and immunities, guaranteed by [the Constitution of the United States] to the citizen. . . . The question before

us is whether the class of persons described in the plea in abatement compose a portion of this people, and are constituent members of this sovereignty?

We think they are not, and that they are not included, and were not intended to be included, under the word "citizens" in the Constitution, and can therefore claim none of the rights and privileges which that instrument provides for and secures to citizens of the United States . . . and, whether emancipated or not . . . had no rights or privileges but such as those who held the power and the Government might choose to grant them.[14]

And thus just four years before the Civil War, the supreme American court protected the rights of White planters, slave traders, and enslavers while denying the rights and humanity of Black people—slave or free. The chief justice of the Supreme Court had articulated a doctrine of absolute white supremacy, one so clear that it could be used as language to inspire the future Confederacy and terrorist groups, such as the Ku Klux Klan, White Knights, White League, and Red Coats. Chief Justice Taney went as far as to articulate the justification for American slavery and the inferiority of Black people in America:

They had for more than a century before been regarded as beings of an inferior order, and altogether unfit to associate with the white race, either in social or political relations; and so far inferior, that they had no rights which the white man was bound to respect; and that the negro might justly and lawfully be reduced to slavery for his benefit. He was bought and sold, and treated as an ordinary article of merchandise and traffic, whenever a profit could be made by it. This opinion was at that time fixed and universal in the civilized portion of the white race.[15]

By 1859, militant abolitionist John Brown had seen enough. A veteran of the Kansas-Missouri War, Brown devised a plan to incite an insurrection to end America's slave system once and for all. His revolutionary band would lead a doomed yet heroic raid on the US armory in Harpers Ferry, Virginia (now West Virginia), and he was executed after being captured by US Army Colonel Robert E. Lee.

The Fugitive Slave Act (1850), the Kansas-Nebraska Act (1854), and the *Dred Scott v. Sandford* decision (1856) had each increased the power of White enslavers and slave traders. They enjoined Northern police officers and citizens to apprehend runaway Black people and return them to their legal owner. There was no justice to be found, no end to slavery in sight. Each pivotal legislation and Supreme Court decision constituted a call to war. And so the war came.

On April 14, 1861, nearly two years after John Brown's failed raid, the nation would be torn asunder at Fort Sumter in South Carolina. Southern Confederates withdrew from the United States to protect slavery as their means of economic production and "way of life."[16] The first blood spilled during the Civil War occurred during a violent riot on Pratt Street in Baltimore on April 19, 1861. Twelve civilians were killed when Confederate sympathizers attacked a detachment of Massachusetts soldiers heading south to confront the Confederate rebellion.[17]

At first, President Abraham Lincoln, as the commander in chief of the Union Army, simply wanted to bring the Confederate rebels back into the fold. But the Civil War soon became a hellish and bloody affair. As the war wore on, Black soldiers were eventually admitted into the fighting ranks of the Union Army. Some 180,000 Black men answered the call to war and to reunite a broken nation. A Black woman from Maryland also answered the call of the Union Army. She was a master spy, a nurse, and a field general. Her name? Harriet Tubman.[18]

The Civil War was utterly destructive and exacted a terrible toll. Over 750,000 men were killed in the bloody conflict—more than American soldiers killed in both world wars combined. In 1864, Union Army generals Ulysses S. Grant and William T. Sherman devised and prosecuted a strategy that demoralized the Confederate rebels—gathering up Southern planters' infrastructure and burning plantations down to the ground. When General Sherman's battalions burned Atlanta down and marched to the sea, Confederate territory was fully occupied. The Confederate spirit was broken and Confederate General Robert E. Lee arrived at a courthouse in Appomattox, Virginia, on April 9, 1865, to surrender and cease hostilities.

The First American Whitelash

The formal War Between the States was won by the Union Army with the assistance of Black soldiers and Black people militarily classified as contraband. President Lincoln and the Grand Army of the Republic were victorious, but Lincoln was assassinated the very next week on April 15, 1865, by a Confederate lover, native Marylander, and stage actor named John Wilkes Booth. Although the Civil War had ceased, the War of Reconstruction had just begun. The Thirteenth Amendment—which ended chattel slavery—was ratified on December 6, 1865. Less than three weeks later, the white supremacist terrorist group known as the Ku Klux Klan was founded on December 24, 1865, by former Confederate general Nathan Bedford Forrest. Chattel slavery had been abolished, but former Confederate traitors were intent to make the Confederate States of America great again for former enslavers and slave traders.

The ratification of Black freedom provoked the response of white supremacist terrorism. Black people in Memphis and New Orleans suffered violent massacres at the hands of former Confederates in 1866. In the same year, Southern states passed Black Codes to curtail Black freedom. Soon it was clear that federal troops would be needed to help protect the newly free but domestic refugee Black population until the Fourteenth Amendment was ratified on July 28, 1868, conferring citizenship. Months later, during the 1868 presidential election, the Democratic candidate Horatio Seymour ran on an unabashedly white supremacist slogan against the Republican candidate Ulysses S. Grant. Seymour's campaign motto: "This is a White Man's Country; Let White Men Rule."[19]

In spite of the rising whitelash, Black people would make many strides during Reconstruction. Landownership and building schools and churches became top priorities for freedwomen and freedmen. Black farmers began buying land and by 1910 owned nearly 15 million acres. Black urban designers and planners built Black economic districts and Black cities.[20] Black men were elected to Congress under Reconstruction governments in Southern states.[21] It was a time of social and political advancement for a people bursting forth into the muted light of freedom.

But Black Reconstruction would eventually come to an end. A major victory in the War of Reconstruction was won by the former Confederates in the Compromise of 1876 when the Dirty South was able to secure the withdrawal of federal troops from the former Confederacy. Local battles for control of city governments closed the door on Black political governance. One example of this was the Wilmington Massacre in North Carolina as white supremacist Democrats led a brutal coup d'état and slaughtered scores of Black people to restore city government to all-White governance in 1898.

White Redemption was America's violent reprisal to Black Reconstruction.[22] During Reconstruction, between 1865 and 1876, over 2,000 Black people were lynched by white supremacist terrorists.[23] Between 1877 and 1950, over 4,400 Black people were lynched in communities all over the nation.[24] Not one White person was ever convicted or punished by the legal system for any of these racial terror lynchings.[25] In her 1893 speech "Lynch Law in All Its Phases," anti-lynching crusader Ida B. Wells highlighted the reign of racial terror. She contended that lynchings were deployed to destroy Black Reconstruction and often prosecuted under the guise of false rape accusations. Making matters worse, White-owned newspapers hyped alleged Black criminality to justify White vigilante violence.[26]

The rise of White Redemption—the First American Whitelash—foreclosed Black freedom, autonomy, and participation in government. When President Grant dispatched federal troops to crush the Ku Klux Klan in 1871, other white supremacist terrorists groups emerged: the Red Coats, White Liners, and White Man's League served as the paramilitary arms of the Democratic Party. They sought to dismantle the emancipation work of Radical Republicans, such as Charles Sumner and Thaddeus Stevens. White supremacists not only lynched Black people but also unleashed large-scale mob violence to decimate Black independent districts and cities. Between 1877 and 1950, nearly 300 Black communities, business districts, and independent towns would be destroyed by white supremacist mob violence, or what Liam Hogan calls "collective punishment."[27]

This history—America's history—underscores the multiple successive ways by which Black people have been displaced and uprooted by slavery, slave trading, and white supremacist violence. These uprootings can be categorized as the first three great displacements in African American history:

- *The Transatlantic Slave Trade* (1619–1820s), which includes the capture and transportation of roughly 388,000 Africans on European and American slave ships for the purpose of forced labor
- *The Domestic American Slave Trade* (1820–1861), which includes the breeding of Black people and transportation of

enslaved Black people from the Chesapeake region to the Deep South to satisfy the demands for Black labor to pick cotton on Southern plantations

- *Black Exodus during the War of Reconstruction* (1866–1909), which includes the rapid outflow of Black people from cities after white supremacist terrorists engaged in barbaric acts of violence against individuals (lynchings) or communities (mob violence, pogroms, coup d'états)

In the aftermath of lynchings and the destruction of Black places, Black people often fled in droves. The 1870s witnessed the Exoduster Movement when as many as 40,000 Black people fled the Deep South and migrated west to Kansas, Oklahoma, and Colorado.[28] As the push for White Redemption picked up steam between 1877 and 1925, another 25,000 or so Black people fled Black neighborhoods destroyed or disturbed by white supremacist violence.

Ida B. Wells barely escaped the clutches of White lynchers in Memphis in 1892 after a mob of White people captured the three Black owners of Peoples Grocery and lynched them. Wells connected the lynchings of Black people with the dispossession of land, wealth, security, and opportunity. She wrote in her autobiography that lynchings were nothing more than "an excuse to get rid of Negroes who were acquiring wealth and property and thus keep the race terrorized and 'keep the nigger down.'"[29]

Beyond white supremacist violence, the political wing of the White Redemption movement engineered racial segregation. State and local governments enforced racial segregation in one system after another, starting with transportation and education. Black and White people rode in different railcars and trolley lines. They attended different schools and churches. Even places such as parks and amenities such as swimming pools were segregated by law. During this period, sundown towns proliferated in number as the American Apartheid system of Jim Crow was brought online. If a Black person was caught in a sundown town after dusk, they were subject to be killed. Sundown towns were created with actual and implied violence, the force of legal codes, and other contractual arrangements. Thousands of towns went sundown between 1890 and 1930 during the imposition of White Redemption.[30]

Laws excluding where Black people could live were not only found in the South. When the territory of Oregon gained statehood in 1859, the state's constitution explicitly forbid Black people from living, working, and owning property in Oregon, and Black people could not legally move there until 1926 or vote until 1927.[31] It is not surprising then that White families with Confederate sympathies would find Oregon to be a refuge for white supremacy:

> Whites looking to escape the South after the end of the Civil War flocked to Oregon, which billed itself as a sort of pristine utopia, where land was plentiful and diversity was scarce. In the early 1900s, Oregon was a hotbed of Ku Klux Klan activity, boasting over 14,000 members (9,000 of whom lived in Portland). The Klan's influence could be felt everywhere, from business to politics—the Klan was even successful in ousting a sitting governor in favor of a governor more of its choosing. It was commonplace for high-ranking members of local and statewide politics to meet with Klan members, who would advise them in matters of public policy.[32]

The legal codification of White Redemption resulted in the ratification of American Apartheid. American Apartheid was erected with the combination of white supremacist terrorism, racial segregation in nearly all public spaces, land dispossession, exploitative labor arrangements (e.g., convict leasing and sharecropping), and racial cleansing or Black expulsions in sundown towns. Historian James M. Smallwood summarized the situation succinctly: "You can say the North won the Civil War. But the South won the War of Reconstruction."[33]

In 1896, the Supreme Court further solidified and concretized white supremacy, this time in *Plessy v. Ferguson*, which gave sanction to what scholar Kaye Whitehead calls "Jim and Jane Crow." Separate but equal was the supreme law of the land. Racial segregation pervaded all areas of American life, including the realm of religion. In *W. E. B. Du Bois, American Prophet*, Edward Blum describes how White clergy and theologians promulgated white supremacy theology, positing that Black people did not have souls.[34] W. E. B. Du Bois would strike back in 1903 against this theological distortion with his masterpiece *The Souls of Black Folk*.

By 1910, the First American Whitelash was virtually complete. For the next 50 years, state-sanctioned policies, practices, and terrorist violence congealed to inflict severe damage on Black people living in separate, unequal, and redlined Black neighborhoods.[35] White city leaders delayed the building of public sewer and water systems and the paving of streets and alleys in areas where Black people lived.[36] Black neighborhoods also received separate and inferior public goods and services, ranging from public school, library, and recreational facilities, sanitation and street cleaning, and public health programs.[37] In short, the municipalization of racial segregation constrained the amount and quality of public goods and services that flowed into Black neighborhoods, contributing to a greater burden of disease and illnesses among Black residents—particularly infectious diseases such as tuberculosis, typhoid fever, cholera, yellow fever, and pneumonia.[38]

The Rise of American Apartheid

White supremacists were at war with the very presence of Black people, as evidenced in government-enforced racial segregation in education and transportation, propaganda preached in pulpits and disseminated in newspapers, and potent punctuations of mob

violence, lynchings, pogroms, and coup d'états. Many Black Southerners were reduced to sharecroppers or domestic maids during
what Douglas Blackmon called an "age of neoslavery," when
many Black prisoners were subjected to the convict leasing system and leased out as hyper-cheap labor to companies.[39]

In 1910, nearly 90% of African Americans lived in the Deep
South. Given the life-draining environment that Black people faced
below the former Mason-Dixon Line, 6.5 million African Americans were compelled to head for seemingly greener pastures and
headed West, Midwest, and North only to find American Apartheid
was being erected and enforced all across the nation. Just as during
the period between the Thirteenth and Fourteenth Amendments,
the descendants of Africans enslaved in the United States would
become an internally displaced people in their own nation.[40]

After 1910, Black communities faced four major subsequent
waves of forced displacement:

- *Black Land Dispossession* (1910–1980), which included the
  dispossession and loss of millions of acres of farmland and
  waterfront property owned by Black farmers and
  landowners[41]
- *The Great Migration* (1910–1970), which ran concurrent with
  Black land dispossession and involved the movement of
  6.5 million Black people from the Deep South to states in the
  North, West, and Midwest regions of the United States
- *The Great Urban Displacement* (1940–1974), the destruction
  of Black neighborhood villages, which included massive
  policies of displacement and disruption of Black
  neighborhoods—slum clearance, urban renewal and
  university-led displacement (Housing Act of 1954), and
  highway construction through Black neighborhoods
  (Federal Highway Aid Act of 1956); the introduction of the
  War on Drugs[42]

- *Resource Withdrawal and Neighborhood Destabilization*
  (1975–present), which includes the demolition of a quarter of a
  million public housing units (HOPE VI); the rise of mass
  incarceration; mass foreclosures due to subprime lending to
  Black homeowners and mass eviction of Black renters;
  gentrification due to local incentives and public housing
  demolition; New Orleans evacuees displaced by Hurricane
  Katrina and levee destruction; national mass Black school
  closures, mass reduction of Black teachers, and school
  pushout[43]

No matter where Black people tried to go to escape the clutches of Jim and Jane Crow, they could not escape violence visited by white supremacists. East St. Louis erupted in racist violence in 1917 that resulted in the deaths of Black workers. Later that year, an entire battalion of Black soldiers stationed in Houston, Texas, was court-martialed and 13 Black soldiers executed without appeal after a Black soldier was arrested for attempting to stop the arrest of a Black woman by a Houston police officer that resulted in rioting and 20 deaths.[44] In 1919, over 25 cities exploded in white supremacist urban violence, often triggered by racist reactions against Black homebuyers moving into White areas or Black men returning home from World War I and proudly wearing their uniforms.[45] Cities such as Washington, DC, Chicago, Illinois, and Longview, Texas, erupted in large-scale racial violence during the Red Summer of 1919.[46]

In the deadliest massacre of Red Summer, white supremacists brazenly murdered approximately 150 Black women, men, and children while they were meeting in a church attempting to organize a farmers union in Elaine, Arkansas. Black farmers were organizing to take advantage of the rising price of cotton on September 30, 1919, when "five automobile loads of white men stopped in front of the church and immediately fired a volley of shots into the building."[47] The bloodletting would not stop there.

[The] next day white men from all over Phillips County and even from Mississippi set the church on fire, burning up several persons who were killed the night before, and then began a systematic man-hunt, killing colored men indiscriminately, driving others from their homes, and then taking from these abandoned homes the produce saved by the farmers for their winter use. Thousands of dollars worth of property was destroyed and stolen and cotton by the bale which the [Black] farmers had refused to sell was boldly carried away by [White] members of the mob.[48]

Black communities in Tulsa, Oklahoma (1921), and Rosewood, Florida (1923), would suffer a similar destructive fate. In the 1930s, white supremacists attacked the Black Sharecroppers' Union in Tallapoosa County, Alabama, to undermine their labor efforts and visited violence upon Black organizers of the interracial Southern Tenant Farmers' Union in an attempt to break up the union.[49] From 1945 to 1960, white supremacist urban violence characterized many eruptions in cities such as Chicago, Detroit, Philadelphia, Miami, Los Angeles, Orlando, Dallas, Birmingham, Atlanta, and Norfolk.[50] In 1951, approximately 4,000 White segregationists rioted in Cicero—a Chicago suburb—to keep a Black family from moving in. If racial segregation laws were used to keep Black people locked into redlined Black communities, more overt forms of intimidation and violence were deployed to keep Black homebuyers out of White communities.[51]

Public schools and public universities were often the sites of dramatic White desegregation resistance to Black student integration. Education sites such as Central High School in Arkansas and state universities in Mississippi and Alabama became pitched battlegrounds when crowds of White people assembled to block the entrance of Black students into all-White educational institutions during the 1950s and 1960s. White desegregation resistance was so fierce that President Dwight Eisenhower had to federalize the National Guard to quell White dissent and allow Black students to enter these schools.

However, federal intervention to oppose racist policies and practices was a rare occurrence before the 1960s. More commonly, the US government was a powerful enforcer of Jim and Jane Crow—using the Department of Defense (segregated military units), the Federal Housing Administration (segregated housing), the Veterans Affairs (racially disparate GI Bill), and the Department of Agriculture (disparate treatment of farmers by race).[52] According to a 1968 report published by the National Commission on Urban Problems, chaired by Senator Paul H. Douglass of Illinois, the Federal Housing Administration played a powerful role in the creation of suburbs and urban sprawl:

FHA [the Federal Housing Administration] has also been a vital factor in financing and promoting the exodus from the central cities and in helping to build up the suburbs. That is where the vast majority of FHA-insured homes have been built. The suburbs could not have expanded as they have during the postwar years without FHA. Superhighways constructed at Government expense have also opened up the areas outside the cities and supported the exodus of a large proportion of the white middle class.[53]

By mentioning subsidized superhighways, the report invokes another FHA—the Federal Highway Administration. Both FHAs played a powerful role in creating and shaping what came to be known as "the ghetto"—or more accurately, the redlined, subprimed, and demonized urban areas where lower-income Black people in America were concentrated. Both FHAs helped give working-class Whites discriminatory suburban subsidies in the form of mortgage lending for housing and highway construction to facilitate transportation to those newly constructed homes. This would be one of the greatest federal instances of affirmative action in American history for the benefit of White people (along with the Homestead Act of 1862).[54]

When Congress passed the Federal-Aid Highway Act of 1956 at a cost of $25 billion, it provided a direct pathway for White flight out of America's increasingly Black urban areas. Given the value of roughly $160 billion in home loan insurance and home improvement loans by the Federal Housing Administration ($67.8 billion in home loans insured and $18.2 billion in home improvement loans), Fannie Mae ($3.2 billion in home loans insured), and Veterans Affairs ($70.6 billion in home loans insured), White Americans were given discriminatory access to subsidized suburban housing and jobs (as many companies also relocated to the suburbs).[55] By 1968, the US government's expenditures on highway construction, home improvement loans, and insurance on home loans totaled an estimated $184.8 billion. That amount in 1968 dollars is equivalent to roughly $1.4 trillion in 2019 after adjusting for inflation.[56] Hence, the US government handed out an estimated $1.4 trillion White flight and suburban housing affirmative action package, fostering the rise of a stable White middle class after World War II.[57]

Even as the federal government doled out White affirmative action in housing and transportation dollars to subsidize racially exclusionary suburbs (i.e., structural economic advantage), the Federal Housing Administration actively participated in the intensification of redlined neighborhoods (i.e., structural economic disadvantage). The Federal Housing Administration joined local governments in deploying racially restrictive covenants, which barred Black people from buying homes owned by Whites.

> Until 1948, when restrictive covenants or written agreements not to sell to Negroes were declared unconstitutional by the Supreme Court, FHA actually encouraged its borrowers to give such guarantees and was a powerful enforcer of the covenants. The FHA

definition of a sound neighborhood was a "homogeneous" one—one that was racially segregated.[58]

Hence, the Federal Housing Administration was a primary enforcer of redlining and greenlining, shaping the landscape of America's metropolitan areas and solidifying spatial racism.[59] While Black people wrestled with residential racial segregation and the rapid succession of uprootings in urban areas, Black farmers were facing land dispossession in rural areas in large part due to the racist actions (or, in some cases, inactions) of the Department of Agriculture, causing Black farmers to go from owning nearly 16 million acres of land by 1920 to 3 million acres of land by the 1990s.[60] In short, the US government lifted up White exclusive suburbs while putting down Black neighborhoods. Redlined communities were derisively dubbed "the ghetto" in the vernacular of the 1970s, but little blame was assigned to federal agencies that played a powerful role in the ghettoization of Black neighborhoods and the suburbanization of White communities.

The Case of Crittenden County, Arkansas

Events in Crittenden County, Arkansas, reveal how the destiny of a Black community could be severely undermined by white supremacist violence and land dispossession. In 1888, White residents in Crittenden County armed themselves with Winchester rifles and expelled the county's Black political leadership at gunpoint—overthrowing the county's Black leaders. Included in the group of Black exiles was a Black man named York Byers who owned over 200 acres of land. Out of the 15 Black exiles, 12 owned property.[61]

Over 65 years later, another wealthy Black landowner and World War I veteran would suffer a more gruesome fate. Isadore Banks reportedly owned over 1,000 acres of land, was a part of the Grant Co-op Gin, and was instrumental in helping other Black farmers with loans and the local Black school with supplies.[62] Isadore Banks was lynched by a group of White residents in Crittenden County in early June 1954. His body was found mutilated. He had been doused with gasoline and set afire. His family was forced to flee in terror, and his land was dispossessed.[63] Because of the 1888 coup d'état and the 1954 lynching of Isadore Banks and subsequent dispossession of his land, the political and economic development of Black residents in Crittenden County was severely undermined.

In terms of social relations, Black residents of Crittenden County would live in a state of quiet fear that meant not challenging White authority or stepping out of line. Just as Ida B. Wells concluded after the 1892 lynching across the Mississippi River in Memphis, Tennessee, the brutal 1954 lynching of Isadore Banks eliminated a wealthy Negro and undercut Black economic empowerment. His lynching sent a powerful signal to the broader Black community: *stay in your place.*[64]

Black Freedom Movements Strike Back

Black freedom fighters refused to surrender to fear or submit to white supremacist terrorism. In ways big and small, from the 1940s through the 1960s, Black people once again engaged in nationwide but locally rooted struggles to defeat the interlocking systems of Jim and Jane Crow. Black activists, such as Mae Mallory, Walter Percival Carter, Ella Jo Baker, and Bayard Rustin, worked entire lifetimes to boost Black Lives and empower Black communities. Hundreds of thousands of others joined the Black Freedom Movement.

Black women also spoke out against the sexual violence they endured at the hands of White men. Often, White men would rape Black women and never face legal charges, much less a trial or a conviction.[65]

The fight to stop the unpunished rape and attacks on Black women would help animate a movement. A young Rosa Parks would serve as an investigator on behalf of Recy Taylor, who was raped by multiple White men.[66] Parks would later spark a boycott to end transportation segregation in Montgomery, Alabama. The movement to stop sexual violence committed against Black women catalyzed the push for racial and gender justice in Black communities. At the same time, militant Black activists—usually students from historically Black colleges and universities[67]—entered the emerging Civil Rights and Black Power Movements to secure freedoms and access to opportunities denied by American Apartheid.

The Baltimore Freedom Movement provided the spark. Black students at Morgan College—known today as Morgan State University—engaged in mass struggle starting in 1947 to desegregate Northwood community eateries. Over a 16-year period, Morgan College students filled the jails in mass direct actions and protests to defeat segregation in various establishments, including the Ford Theater in 1952. Students successfully desegregated the Northwood Plaza to the west of Morgan College's campus one after the other: Read's Drug Store (mid-1950s), Arundel Ice Cream (1959), the Rooftop Restaurant (1960), and the Northwood Theater (1963).[68] Morgan College students and their allies succeeded in toppling Jim and Jane Crow in Baltimore. Other Baltimore activist groups such as the NAACP, Congress of Racial Equality (CORE), the Goon Squad, and Activists for Fair Housing Inc. would also work to bury Jim and Jane Crow, winning desegregation campaigns for equal access to housing, parks, and government representation. Because of their organizing efforts, Baltimore City would pass Ordinance 103, a municipal civil rights ordinance in 1964 to further help address and remediate instances of racial discrimination in Baltimore City.

Amid the rising Baltimore Freedom Movement, the sit-in movement took off like wildfire across the Deep South as Black college students in Greensboro, North Carolina, kicked off a campaign to desegregate lunch counters and ensure access to public spaces. Under the sage guidance of the supreme organizer Ella Baker, the Student Nonviolent Coordinating Committee (SNCC) was founded in April 1960 at Shaw University. Soon, SNCC organizers began to coordinate spirited Freedom Rides from the North to Southern states to help organize rural Black sharecroppers and mobilize voting drives to break the back of Jim and Jane Crow.

But change for many urban Black neighborhoods was slow in materializing in spite of the civil rights victories that were beginning to be won. This was especially the case outside of the Deep South. While overt Jim and Jane Crow was being defeated in Southern states, the more subtle American Apartheid still ruled the prospects of Black Lives in areas outside the old Confederate South.

Soon, those urban Black communities began to erupt and explode. Black Harlem in 1964. Black Watts in 1965. Black Cleveland in 1966. Black Newark and Detroit in 1967. It was the time of Great Uprising—when working-class Black folks in cities large and small struck back, rebelling against American Apartheid nationwide. According to historian Peter Levy, a staggering number of Black uprisings took place between 1964 and 1971. There were over 750 altogether in cities large and small.[69] Hundreds of cities burned in fury as Black America grieved in response to the assassination of Dr. Martin Luther King Jr. after April 4, 1968. Just seven days later, President Lyndon Johnson signed the landmark 1968 Fair Housing Act, the third of the great civil rights bills to pass into law in the 1960s.

The Second American Whitelash

By the 1970s, America hit a wall in advancing Black political demands for freedom and economic justice. As with the case after Black Reconstruction, the Second American Whitelash emerged to stymie gains won during the Civil Rights and Black Power Movements. The US government's security apparatus, known as the Counter Intelligence Program, or COINTELPRO, spearheaded vicious and violent reprisals against Black radical organizing. COINTELPRO, a program of the FBI, coordinated with local police forces to neutralize, kill, or exile Black leaders deemed as radical or revolutionary.[70] By the end of the 1960s, many Black freedom fighters—women and men—were incarcerated, exiled, or murdered by the agents and activities of COINTELPRO.

In addition, the local American police apparatus would become more militarized and assumed an active war footing against redlined Black neighborhoods due to President Johnson's law enforcement acts to quell the Great Uprising.[71] Law enforcement militarization and mass incarceration escalated with President Nixon's executive order, which commenced what many have called the "War on Drugs." But as Nixon domestic policy chief John Ehrlichman revealed, the US government responded to the Civil Rights and Black Power Movements and the Great Uprising with what can more accurately be called a "war on Black communities." Ehrlichman remarked:

> The Nixon campaign in 1968, and the Nixon White House after
> that, had two enemies: the antiwar left and black people. You
> understand what I'm saying? We knew we couldn't make it illegal
> to be either against the war or black, but by getting the public to
> associate the hippies with marijuana and blacks with heroin. And
> then criminalizing both heavily, we could disrupt those communi-
> ties. We could arrest their leaders, raid their homes, break up their

meetings, and vilify them night after night on the evening news. Did we know we were lying about the drugs? Of course we did.[72]

Although the old version of Jim and Jane Crow had been defeated because of the organizing efforts of Southern Black activists and organizations such as SNCC, CORE, SCLC (Southern Christian Leadership Conference), and the Deacons for Defense and Justice, the New Jim Crow emerged and supplanted the previous version. Progress would still come in the form of the 1974 Equal Credit Opportunity Act (to end credit denials based on race), the 1975 Home Mortgage Disclosure Act (to make mortgage data by race public), and the 1977 Community Reinvestment Act (to combat bank redlining), but America's war on Black communities gave rise to entrenched police repression and mass incarceration as a response to the Great Uprising of 1963–1971.

Desegregation efforts came to a screeching halt with the pitched anti-busing battles in Boston, Massachusetts, during the 1970s and the bombastic White resistance to deconcentrating public housing in Yonkers, New York, in the late 1980s and early 1990s. But Black political organizing and protests would continue. Black women's organizing would emerge in efforts such as the Black Panther Party in the 1970s, the Combahee River Collective from 1974 to 1980, and the struggle for welfare rights among lower-income Black women in public housing.[73] As Rhonda Williams details in her book *The Politics of Public Housing*, lower-income Black women were pivotal in the struggle to improve policies that affected the lives of public housing residents. Black women in public housing fought for tenants' rights, engaged in cooperative economics, staged rent strikes, and advocated for their inclusion in the governance of public housing communities in the 1960s and 1970s.

Arising out of the devastation of American Apartheid in the Bronx in New York City, hip-hop culture was born in the late 1970s, giving voice to lower-income and working-class Black, Puerto

Rican, and Caribbean youth. In the 1980s, hip-hop became a cultural and political movement for redlined Black communities at the same moment that the crack cocaine and HIV/AIDS epidemics exploded.[74] Black activists joined the international movement against apartheid in South Africa in the late 1980s and 1990s, helping lead to the formal fall of apartheid in South Africa. In spite of America's whitelash against the urban uprisings, Black protest and pushback continued well after the 1960s.

Many struggle to understand why there remains a plethora of social ills that disproportionately affect Black people in America over 150 years after chattel enslavement has ended. The answer: Black communities have been subjected to unrelenting and ongoing historical trauma. Black communities have collectively faced seven successive waves of uprootings, disruptions, dispossessions, and displacements (see appendix A). White Redemption disrupted and destroyed Black Reconstruction. White supremacist violence—consisting of unchecked lynchings, rapes, mob violence, programs, coups d'états, and expulsions of Black people in thousands of smaller sundown towns—decimated and destabilized successful Black communities and burgeoning Black economic efforts during the reign of Jim and Jane Crow.

During and after the Great Uprising and the movements for Civil Rights and Black Power (1954–1968), even as Black people secured landmark legislative achievements, America waged a spatial war on Black communities. Black neighborhoods were being torn apart repeatedly. Black rural farmland and waterfront properties were being lost to dispossession in the fourth wave of uprooting. Meanwhile, urban Black neighborhoods were shocked and rocked by the sixth and seventh waves of serial forced displacement, which included destructive policies and practices such as slum clearance, urban renewal, highway construction, post-industrialization, planned shrinkage, mass incarceration, and stripping Black neighborhoods of public goods.[75] Stripping

Black neighborhoods of public goods entails the mass closures of public schools and recreation centers, the demolitions of public housing (followed by resident displacement and dispersal), and the deep underfunding of public health.

One of the ultimate functions of white supremacy has been the extraction of wealth—first from Black bodies as property, then Black people as cheap labor, and finally Black neighborhoods as internal colonies.[76] While the specter of economic destruction is more readily apparent, the disruption of Black political leadership and organizing has also been a major factor. Black communities were harmed by state-sponsored entities—such as the FBI's COIN-TELPRO or the Mississippi State Sovereignty Commission—that targeted and aimed to eliminate Black leaders deemed a threat. Black political organizing has also been undermined by the destruction of Black social networks and social capital during mass uprootings. In other words, as individual Black political rights were increasing, Black neighborhoods and their inner capacity to work collectively was systematically weakened.

The Third American Whitelash

The Third American Whitelash began picking up steam after the election of President Barack Obama (2008) and the Movement for Black Lives Uprising (2014–2017). During the Obama presidency, the nation witnessed the rise in hate groups and hate crimes against marginalized populations. After the Patient Protection and Affordable Care Act was passed in 2009 and 2010, a right-wing movement called the Tea Party formed to oppose the health-care legislation in specific and President Obama in general. At Tea Party rallies, men showed up openly carrying large assault rifles; the false notion that Obama was going to confiscate Americans' guns gained a foothold. In Congress, Tea Party politics gave rise to complete resistance to any Obama legislative priorities after the GOP-Tea Party retook the House of Representatives in the 2010 elections.

White supremacist violence was also on the rise. On August 5, 2012, Wade Michael Page opened fire in a Sikh temple in Wisconsin, killing six worshippers.[77] On June 17, 2015, white supremacist Dylann Storm Roof brazenly massacred nine Black churchgoers at "Mother" Emanuel African Methodist Episcopal Church in Charleston, South Carolina.[78] That summer, I recounted the torrential stream of incidents during an excruciating period in 2015:

> In North Charleston, South Carolina, not too far from [where] the [Mother Emanuel] terrorist attack on nine Black church members took place, Walter Scott was shot several times in the back as he fled from police on foot, posing no immediate threat. In Staten Island, New York, Eric Garner was choked to death by officers as he gasped for air, exclaiming: "I can't breathe." In Barstow, California, a pregnant Black woman named Charlena Michelle Cooks was viciously thrown to the ground as she screamed and pleaded, telling the officers: "Please! I'm pregnant." Recalling the incident later, Cooks stated that officers treater her "like an animal, like a monster, like I didn't exist, like I was not human."

> In St. Louis, Missouri, protester Kristine Hendrix was walking home on the sidewalk when an officer cut off her and a male colleague and then proceeded to use a Taser on her twice as she lay on the concrete writhing and screaming in pain. . . . In McKinney, Texas, Officer Eric Casebolt verbally and physically attacked a group of Black teenagers, forcing Black boys to lie down and then violently slamming a teenager named Dajerria Becton to the ground. Officer Casebolt then put his knee on her back, placed his weight on her body, and ignored her pleas for relief.

> Then in Fairfield, Ohio . . . White police officers brutally accosted, pepper sprayed, choked, and slammed the family of Krystal Dixon

to the ground as a young white male in his swim trunks forced his forearm onto the throat of a young Black teenage male as he was already being arrested by a white cop. A White female cop grabbed a young Black girl by the back of her neck as the other white male cops viciously manhandled other Black teenage girls, so much so that a 12-year-old has her jaw broken along with 3 ribs cracked by white Fairfield police. It ended . . . with a young [Black] girl in the hospital [in a coma], with a solitary tear streaming down her face.[79]

These horrific incidents did not lead America to confront its demons of racism and white supremacy. Instead, a Republican candidate emerged and capitalized on the ascendant sentiment of whitelash. Running on the slogan Make America Great Again, the nation elected Donald Trump to become president of the United States, representing the culmination of the Third American Whitelash in late 2016.[80] Replacing the traditional GOP dog whistle with a bullhorn, Trump's election emboldened white supremacists to emerge out of the closet into full public view.

As president, Donald Trump became the champion of the Third American Whitelash in both domestic and foreign policy.[81] His anti-Muslim and anti-immigrant sentiments revealed that "making America great again" involves closing the nation's borders to refugees and asylum seekers in need, along with building physical and legal walls to keep people out, including people fleeing violence and poverty in Central America. Trump would later add fuel to the fire by derisively calling Haiti and nations in Africa "shithole countries."[82]

By 2017, emboldened white supremacist terrorists emerged with a fervor focused on keeping Confederate monuments in place. In Charlottesville, Virginia, multiple groups assembled to "Unite the Right" actions to protest the removal of the statue of Confederate General Robert E. Lee, led by white supremacist Richard Spencer (May 2017), the Ku Klux Klan (July 8, 2017), and a combined group of neo-Nazis and white supremacist sympathizers (August 11–12, 2017).[83] A white supremacist drove his car into the crowd of anti-racist protesters at full speed in Charlottesville, Virginia, killing anti-racist protester Heather Heyer. In Portland, white supremacist patriarchal group Patriot Prayer incited a riot in 2017. Later, Portland police were found to be cutting deals with Patriot Prayer members while targeting and arresting anti-fascists (Antifa) who protested their presence.[84]

In 2018, white supremacist violence again rocked the nation involving a mail bomber (Florida), a massacre at a Jewish synagogue (Pittsburgh), and another Patriot Prayer riot (Portland). Overall, hate crimes continued to escalate. In February 2019, a group of 54 white supremacists affiliated with the group New Aryan Empire were arrested in Arkansas on charges of solicitation of murder, kidnapping, maiming, and conspiracy to distribute methamphetamine.[85] A mass killer at a Muslim mosque in New Zealand even referred to Trump as a "renewed symbol of white identity" in March 2019, after which a coalition of civil rights and faith leaders called on the FBI to take the threat of white nationalist violence seriously.[86] Additionally, researchers found that hate crimes were higher in places where Trump gave speeches.[87] The threat of white supremacist violence became so apparent that FBI director Christopher Wray acknowledged the threat in a congressional hearing held on April 4, 2019.[88]

During the summer in 2019, three mass shootings in one week shook the nation with all three gunmen having either overt ties to white supremacy (El Paso, Texas, shooter) or to what the FBI labeled as "violent ideologies" (Gilroy, California, and Dayton, Ohio, shooters).[89] In particular, the back-to-back massacres in El Paso and Dayton, where gunmen killed over 30 people in two days, brought a renewed focus to white supremacy as a growing terroristic threat. Even several Republican elected officials articulated the threat of white supremacy after the El Paso shooter released a manifesto echoing the racist and nativist language used by President Trump.[90] One such Republican was Nebraska State Senator John McCollister who tweeted on August 4, 2019:

> The Republican Party is enabling white supremacy in our country. As a lifelong Republican, it pains me to say this, but it's the truth. I of course am not suggesting that all Republicans are white supremacists nor am I saying that the average Republican is even racist. What I am saying though is that the Republican Party is COMPLICIT to obvious racist and immoral activity inside our party. We have a Republican president who continually stokes racist fears in his base. He calls certain countries "shitholes," tells women of color to "go back" to where they came from and lies more than he tells the truth.

After the August 2019 massacre in El Paso, where 22 people were killed by a gunman targeting Mexicans,[91] editors of the *New York Times* admitted that America has a white nationalist terrorism problem.[92] Eddie Glaude Jr. went as far as to say on NBC's *Meet the Press* after the El Paso and Dayton massacres that America was in a cold civil war.[93] By the end of 2019, America was festering in a cold civil war because the regressive politics of whitelash arrests the nation's progress. White supremacy repeatedly sinks the nation into both a cold civil war and a hot domestic mess.

The Global Pandemic and Great Rebellion

In March 2020, American life largely came to a halt as governors ordered shutdowns to prevent the spread of the pathogen. Black Americans suffered disproportionately and died at a higher rate due to COVID-19. By late May, Black America was on the edge.

While the COVID-19 pandemic unfolded, police violence reemerged as a preexisting pandemic for Black Lives. The killings of Breonna Taylor and Ahmaud Arbery inflicted yet more trauma, and Black protestors went back to the streets in Georgia and Kentucky. When the video footage emerged of Minneapolis officer Chauvin killing George Floyd on Memorial Day, Black America had seen enough. Thunderous protests broke out in Minneapolis, where Floyd was killed. This was followed by riotous action and racial upheaval all across the country.

The Great Rebellion was covered by some national media outlets in unusually striking and blunt language. On June 1, Associated Press reporters summed up the situation in blistering terms:

> After six straight days of unrest, America headed into a new work week Monday with neighborhoods in shambles, urban streets on lockdown and political leaders struggling to control the coast-to-coast outpouring of rage over police killings of black people. Despite curfews in big cities across the U.S. and the deployment of thousands of National Guard soldiers over the past week, demonstrations descended into violence again on Sunday.

> The upheaval has unfolded amid the gloom and economic ruin caused by the coronavirus, which has killed over 100,000 Americans and sent unemployment soaring to levels not seen since the Depression. The outbreak has hit minorities especially hard, not just in infections and deaths but in job losses and economic stress. The scale of the coast-to-coast protests has rivaled the historic demonstrations of the civil rights and Vietnam War eras. At least 4,400 people have been arrested for such offenses as stealing, blocking highways and breaking curfew, according to a count compiled by The Associated Press.[94]

By June 2020, the American Reckoning had arrived. The Black forward push for freedom and three ensuing whitelashes left the nation staggered and battered in a moment of national crisis and deep reflection. The back-to-back one-two combination of CO-VID-19 and the Great Rebellion exposed America as a nation teetering on the brink. Only time will tell if America will rise to make amends and heal its wounds or whether the house divided against itself will fall.

Conclusion

America's future is linked with its past. Try as it might, the nation cannot move forward and thrive while divided. Because of its divergent histories, White America and Black America are experiencing bipolar realities. In the first half of 2020, White America largely worked to bounce back from the complications of the COVID-19 pandemic. Meanwhile, Black America lurched due to the coronavirus pandemic and ongoing historical trauma in the form of hyperpolicing and hypersegregation.

The initial earthquake of American Apartheid continues to reverberate and produce devastating aftershocks. The nation's schools are resegregating even as the nation becomes increasingly diverse.[95] Wealthy White spatial enclaves across the country are engaging in legal battles to secede from more diverse school districts and create more racially exclusive breakaway school districts.[96] President Trump pushed for a partial government shutdown in a quest to *build that wall*. American Apartheid is restructuring itself and continues to evolve.

Violence against Black people has taken many forms: from Transatlantic Slave Trade to Domestic American Slave Trade, from lynchings to breeding, from the Ku Klux Klan to the dispossession of land, and from COINTELPRO to equating Blackness with *criminal*. Violence is a central organizing principle of white supremacy in America. However, there are various forms of violence. It is relatively easy to recount the visible and overt instances of violence when force is physically inflicted against people and their bodies. Physical violence occurs relatively quickly. It might cause bleeding and leave bruises. With the right technology, physical violence can now be recorded.

But it is more difficult to call attention to the more invisible and slower forms of structural violence that have been unleashed against Black communities. No large metropolitan area can better illustrate the salience of structural violence better than Baltimore, Maryland, which gave birth to urban spatial apartheid. Baltimore reveals the sophistication of structural violence deployed in city ordinances, real estate practices, mortgage lending, code enforcement, municipal budgets, zoning laws, urban planning, urban renewal, and urban redevelopment.

Detailing how structural violence is deployed in Baltimore is necessary for healing and restoring redlined Black neighborhoods. Just as medical doctors take individual patient histories, public health practitioners must study Black communities' histories in order to facilitate healing and wholeness. *Only by taking the first step to obtain a deep understanding of how historical trauma has inflicted massive damage on Black neighborhoods can Americans have any hope of stopping ongoing historical trauma and fostering healing in Black neighborhoods* (Step 1).

The "Negro Invasion"

Today the world, north and south,
is being asked to believe
that the crux of the Negro problem
lies in keeping Black men
from buying property on your street.

W. E. B. Du Bois, *The Crisis*, May 1919

I don't know whether the real estate lobby
has anything against Black people,
but I know the real estate lobby
is keeping me in the ghetto.

James Baldwin, *The Dick Cavett Show*, 1968

Baltimore City Racial Segregation

Baltimore has long practiced racial exclusivity throughout its history.[1] From 1829 to 1867, Baltimore maintained an exclusively White public school system. Meanwhile, Baltimore's sizable free Black community was forced to establish a completely private public school system to educate Black youth. After Baltimore's Black education advocates waged a long campaign for inclusion in the public school system, Baltimore City Public Schools opened its doors to Black children on July 19, 1867, but it did so as an apartheid public school system.[2] The Baltimore City Public School System would maintain a dual system—one for White children and one for Black children—for the next 86 years until the eve of the US Supreme Court *Brown v. Board of Education* decision. Therefore, for 125 years of its history, the public school system of Baltimore City operated either a racially exclusionary or racially segregated system.

During the late 1800s, railroad, streetcar, and steamboat companies operating in Baltimore City also enforced racial segregation in public transportation in railcars, electric trolley lines, and steamboat cabins. Although Radical Republicans during Reconstruction had promised equal protection under the law in the Fourteenth Amendment, Black Baltimoreans were increasingly denied equal access to public goods or services that operated in the public arena. Baltimore was largely a Confederate-sympathizing city during the Civil War, but President Lincoln's military occupation of the city during the war had thwarted the schemes and dreams of white supremacy. With hostilities ceased and Maryland's Reconstruction on the ropes, Maryland's Democrats were hell-bent on making Baltimore a "white man's city."[3] But Black advocates such as Rev. Harvey Johnson and the Stewart sisters (Mary, Martha, Winnie, and Lucy) fought back to make the promises of the Fourteenth Amendment and Reconstruction real.[4] They organized for racial equity in schools and transit—winning key victories along the way. But white supremacists in Baltimore kept gaining strength. American Apartheid became the explicit law of the land when the Supreme Court handed down *Plessy v. Ferguson* on May 18, 1896—sanctioning separate but equal. Between 1890 and 1910, Maryland Democrats and Baltimore newspapers, such as the *Baltimore Sun*, viciously linked Black people to crime and cranked up the city's criminal justice system against Black residents.[5] Baltimore City's systems of education, transportation, and criminal justice served as the initial battlegrounds for establishing Baltimore Apartheid after the Civil War, although they would not be the last.

Home Buying While Black in the 1910s

Real estate, housing, and city neighborhoods became the next battlegrounds. Mayor John Barry Mahool (Democrat) signed the first comprehensive residential racial zoning law in the nation on December 19, 1910.[6] The legislation caught the attention of the *New York Times Magazine*, which called Baltimore's segregation ordinance "radical and far-reaching."[7] Indeed, Baltimore's radical racial zoning ordinance would be copied by cities around the nation, becoming a template for large majority White cities witnessing an influx of Southern Black migrants.[8] Baltimore City was ground zero for residential American Apartheid.

The fear of Black people moving to all-White blocks pervaded the thinking of the architects of Baltimore Apartheid. White Baltimoreans responded to their fear of a Black neighbor in a variety of ways. Baltimore attorney Milton Dashiell distilled the sequence of White flight to its essence by telling the *Times* journalist: "As soon as the Negro appears, the White man moves away."[9] Mahool also referenced this two-step sequence as the primary rationale for Baltimore City's racial zoning ordinance:

> Many blocks of housing formerly occupied exclusively by whites now have a mixture of colored—and the white and colored races cannot live in the same block in peace.

> Its sole object and intention is to protect our people in the possession of their property and to prevent the depreciation which is of necessity bound to follow when the colored family would move into a neighborhood that had hitherto been exclusively inhabited by white people.[10]

Mahool argued that enforcing racial segregation was strongly connected to protecting "our people" (i.e., White people) from the depreciating effects of simply having a Black neighbor. Why did

Mahool claim that "the white and colored races cannot live in the same block in peace" to the *Times* representative? Because the specter of a Black neighbor on a White block during the summer of that year nearly brought Baltimore City to the point of a riot.[11]

The Black person who moved into the block was none other than George W. F. McMechen—the first baccalaureate graduate of Morgan College in 1895. McMechen earned further academic distinction as a graduate of Yale University's law school in 1897. Afterward, he returned to Baltimore to practice law. In July 1910, he and his family moved into 1834 McCulloh Street.[12] Subsequently, three other Black families moved into the formerly White block.

The all-White McCulloh Street Improvement Association (MSIA) sprang into action. First, the association attempted to buy the homes back from the Black homeowners "at a fair profit," but the new homeowners refused to sell their homes. Next, the president of the MSIA (M. J. Hammen) called on a Black postal clerk (M. Z. Hamer) to encourage him to abandon his property. But Hamer would have none of it. According to the MSIA president, Hamer threatened to hit him upside the head with a chair if he broached the subject again. Dashiell recounted what happened next to the *New York Times Magazine*: "Then ensued more or less lawlessness on the part of small boys and hoodlums in the neighborhood. Window glasses of the negroes' houses were broken with stone; skylights were caved in by brick, descending bomb-like from the sky; there were muttering of plots to blow up the houses; in short, we were on the verge of riot in that neighborhood."[13]

Dashiell slickly referred to the attack in passive tense—windows were broken, skylights were caved, and plots were muttered—as if some spooky apparition of white supremacy had inadvertently caused supernatural mischief. What Dashiell failed to articulate more truthfully was that he and his compatriots sought to intimidate and terrorize the McMechens and other Black families so that they would leave the formerly all-White block. George

McMechen conveyed his side of the story to the representative from the *New York Times Magazine*:

> The first night I moved in they broke the panes in the front window and flung a brick through my skylight. No I do not know who "they" were. It was rumored that they were merely boys but it must have taken something bigger than a boy to fling a whole brick high enough to cave in the skylight in a three-story house, as this is.

> As soon as I moved in the white people in the neighborhood organized themselves into a "Improvement Association," which I have subsequently understood was particularly for the purpose of preventing negroes [from] moving into the neighborhood.[14]

McMechen disputed the narrative that "boys" were responsible, which would imply a more innocent juvenile vandalism was the motive. The adults flinging bricks meant business and wanted to send a serious message. The *St. Louis Post-Dispatch* reported on the mounting threat of white supremacist urban violence in Baltimore:

> The coming of a negro family into a white neighborhood was very often followed by a demonstration of some sort on the part of white men and boys in an effort to frighten the negroes out of their new quarters. As the negro "invasion" of the white settlements became more and more pronounced, these clashes became more frequent and in the course of time, it was believed, the only outcome would be a race war of serious proportions.[15]

The potential for a "race war of serious proportions" was a distinct possibility in the 1910s. White supremacist urban violence often provoked Black self-defense, resulting in what were commonly called "race riots." Several deadly race riots had broken out in multiple cities across the nation in previous years, including in

Wilmington, North Carolina (1898), Atlanta, Georgia (1906), Springfield, Illinois (1908), and Slocum, Texas (1910).[16] Given the outbreaks of white supremacist urban violence across the nation, the possibility for a race war in Baltimore was not farfetched. An October 8, 1910, article in the *Baltimore Sun* chronicled how White Baltimoreans in the Locust Point neighborhood threatened Black workers looking to move into the neighborhood with death.[17] The article further recalled how White residents in Locust Point had destroyed the furniture, windows, and doors of a house that a Black family attempted to move into inside the all-White enclave in 1904—causing the Black family to never return.

Baltimore's leaders knew that white supremacists might spark a race war anytime a Black homebuyer moved into a White neighborhood or block, and there was always the possibility that Black people might fight back and defend themselves. White supremacist urban violence had nearly caused Baltimore to explode in the summer of 1910. But instead of policing and prosecuting white supremacists to protect Black homebuyers, the architects of Baltimore Apartheid turned to and were influenced by various forms of media.[18] White newspapers demonized Black homebuyers and constantly denigrated them as advance scouts of an impending "Negro Invasion."[19] City officials relied heavily on the power of the law and law enforcement to criminalize Black homebuyers who attempted to move into all-White blocks.[20]

The fabricated war against the "Negro Invasion" consumed White Baltimore. Baltimore's next mayor, James H. Preston (also a Democrat), became a national champion and spokesperson in the fight for citywide, government-enforced racial segregation. Preston touted the bipartisan support for residential racial segregation and remarked on how Baltimore's White political leaders were leading the campaign for racial segregation that was in "the real interest of the city." In an interview with the *St. Louis Post-Dispatch*, Preston said:

I'll give you another example of how Baltimore is receiving segregation: William F. Broening, the District Attorney, is a Republican. I am a Democrat and the city administration is largely Democratic: but Broening is pulling right along with us in this matter of upholding segregation. He is fighting for the ordinance and every man in Baltimore with the real interest of the city at heart is fighting for it also.[21]

A headline in the August 8, 1913, *Baltimore Sun* declared "Demand for Race Segregation Measure at Once Is Becoming Insistent."[22] In September 1913, Morgan College trustees attempted to move the campus from central West Baltimore to Mount Washington, a suburban Baltimore County community. White Mount Washingtonians would have none of it. They organized in protest against the relocation of Morgan College into their community. Charles C. Homer Jr., the acting chairman of the Mount Washington Improvement Association, wrote Mayor Preston to invite him to a meeting to "protest against the invasion of established white neighborhoods by negro institutions or residents, as threatened by the contemplated establishment of Morgan College at Mount Washington."[23] Not to be outdone, the president of the Park Heights, Pimlico, and Arlington Improvement Association also wrote to Preston regarding Morgan College's potential move nearby: "Can any one conceive of a greater misfortune to this most excellent neighborhood or anything that would depreciate property values as well as the social standing of the neighborhood more than the successful consummation of this deal would?"[24]

Baltimore's spatial war to stem the "Negro Invasion" soon became a national story. Local officials across the nation kept a close eye on events in Baltimore with the aid of newspaper accounts. The *St. Louis Star-Times* covered Baltimore's efforts to craft and enact apartheid policies in an October 23, 1913, article:

Baltimore is fussed up because colored folks insist upon living next to white folks. To use a local expression, Baltimore is fussed up "right much"; several persons having been shot, more or less, heads having been dented by dornicks[25] of assorted sizes and hundreds of windows and other attached portions of real property having been smashed completely and enthusiastically.[26]

St. Louis newspapers covered Baltimore closely and reported on the threat of a race war because St. Louis was considering its own racial zoning ordinance. Baltimore had been the first city to pass a residential racial zoning ordinance in 1910. St. Louis became the first city to approve residential racial zoning through referendum in 1916. Baltimore had provided the template and served as the inspiration for St. Louis Apartheid.

Residential racial segregation was not simply a genteel action separating Black people from White people. Instituting residential racial segregation would allow an economic system to emerge that provided significant structural advantages to Whites in the real estate market based on home values and allowed public resources to be disproportionately directed to White homeowners and White communities. On February 22, 1916, in the *St. Louis Post-Dispatch*, John M. Pope, who was president of the North Baltimore Improvement Association, told the reporter:

> The best effects of segregation have been the stabilizing of the real estate market and the confidence inspired in the small home buyer. Formerly, a man didn't want to buy. He never knew when a negro would move in beside him. It was too much risk and he preferred to pay rent. The consequence was that Baltimore had no real hold upon that man, beyond his job.[27]

In other words, after segregating neighborhoods by race, the "stabilized" real estate market could confer higher housing values to White homeowners by keeping Black homebuyers out and keeping

White homeowners in the city. The assignment of home values in the private real estate market depended directly on the public government enforcement of residential racial segregation.[28] However, architects of Baltimore Apartheid would often try to obscure their rationale for residential racial segregation by shifting the blame to the Black middle-class homebuyers and highlighting supposed friendships with Black Baltimoreans. As Mayor Mahool further commented in the *New York Times Magazine* in the December 25, 1910, article:

> But it is clear that one of the first desires of a negro, after he acquires money and property, is to leave his less fortunate brethren and nose into the neighborhood of the white people. . . . [The segregation ordinance] was not passed in a spirit of race antagonism; most of us concerned in it are the best friends the colored people have; but it was passed to meet a critical condition that was crying out for a solution—and in this ordinance we think we have found that solution.[29]

Mahool would not be the only one to make note of how "friendly" the White architects of Baltimore Apartheid were toward Black Baltimoreans. The *New York Times Magazine* representative also interviewed an unidentified White woman who was "high in Baltimore's sacred circles" and she articulated the following sentiment:

> It is a most deplorable thing that even the best of the well-to-do colored people should invade our residential districts. I am sure the colored race has no better friend than I and those situated as I am. From my earliest recollection my feeling for the race has been one associated with affection; my old negro "mammy," my little nurse-girl playmate, all are among my happiest recollections.

> But the idea of their assuming to live next door to me is abhorrent. I am sure no good can come of it to them. They will be lonesome up here away from the rest of their kind. It is a sad thing and I do hope

there will be found some way to put a stop to it. I would hate at my time of life, after living so many years in such pleasant relations with the darkies, as all of my family members have, to be compelled to change my ideas upon the subject.[30]

In other words, this White "lady high in Baltimore's most sacred circles"—as described by the *New York Times Magazine*—might lose her affection for colored people if they became homeowning neighbors in her neighborhood.

Why would the White architects of Baltimore Apartheid insist on their friendship with Negroes? It is clear they are taking pains to say: "I am not like members of the Ku Klux Klan or *those* violent white supremacists." But even in their purported friendliness, Mahool and other White Baltimoreans "high in Baltimore's most sacred circles" were willing to pass and enforce deeply discriminatory Jim and Jane Crow policies that would shape the landscape of Baltimore for the next 100 or more years.[31] What could drive self-proclaimed friendly White Baltimoreans to support racial segregation and boost Jim and Jane Crow? Inflating and protecting White housing values, forestalling a race war precipitated by White violence against Black homebuyers, and guarding White neighborhood health from Negroes with infectious diseases.

On February 19, 1917, Mayor Preston convened a meeting of "150 physicians, social workers and representative citizens . . . to devise ways of improving the health of the negro element in this city," according to the *New-York Tribune*.[32] Feigning concern about the Negro death rate due to tuberculosis, Preston repeatedly turned to public health as a pretext and justification for racial segregation. The *Tribune* reported: "It is understood that the Mayor will announce a plan of partial segregation for negroes. A section of the county may be laid out along modern lines as a negro colony." Preston envisioned a plan that would result in uprooting some portion of Black Baltimore to a location outside of the city where they would be presumably out of sight, out of mind, and left to fend for themselves.[33]

Later in 1917, the community of Lauraville (still in Baltimore County at the time) was incensed at Morgan College purchasing land near its environs, fearing the establishment of Mayor Preston's suburban "negro colony." In a *Baltimore Sun* article screaming in bold font "FIGHTS NEGRO INVASION: Lauraville Is Up in Arms against Morgan College," the *Sun* representative wrote: "Lauraville has blood in its eye for any invasion of its 99 per cent, pure white community by a negro institution, colony or settlement of any kind."[34] Led by several White couples, the Lauraville Improvement Association waged a legal battle in a case called *Diggs v. Morgan*, all in the attempt to keep the Negro college out of the area. A meeting of "about 275 men and women" was convened to block Morgan College's move to Lauraville. Attendees of the Lauraville Improvement Association meeting raised "an emergency war fund" totaling $71.50 to fuel the effort.[35]

Morgan College prevailed when the case was decided by the Maryland Court of Appeals on October 30, 1918.[36] The language in the court's decision puts Lauraville's fear of a "negro colony" into sharp focus.

> The bill in this case . . . alleges that on 1st June, 1917, Morgan College, the defendant, acquired about seventy acres of land at the intersection of the Hillen road and Grindon Lane [now Cold Spring Lane]; that the amount of land so acquired was in excess of any proper and legitimate need of the defendant, and that the defendant has announced that it intends to use a portion of the tract as building lots, to establish thereon a residential negro colony.[37]

According to White Lauraville residents, Morgan College—an institution of higher learning—was a beachhead for an impending "residential negro colony," echoing Preston's rhetoric. White Lauraville's hope for victory faded on November 5, 1917, when the Supreme Court partially struck down residential racial zoning in *Buchanan v. Warley* while *Diggs v. Morgan* was still being litigated. However, the Supreme Court decision was not made to affirm the idea that Black people could live where they wished but to protect White homeowners' rights to sell to whomever they wanted.[38]

Nevertheless, *Buchanan v. Warley* was a seminal case that affirmed that Black homebuyers or institutions (like Morgan College) could not be barred from buying property in White areas. But the legal victory would only prove to be a bump in the road for pro-segregationists.[39] Mayor Preston's resolve for strengthening residential racial segregation was not diminished by the Supreme Court's ruling. But his plan for a suburban negro colony had to be abandoned due to the springtime 1918 annexation of the same area where the colony would have been located (which would have made the suburban colony a city problem once again).

No matter. By March 1918, the arch-segregationist mayor was cooking up a new scheme to prosecute the war against the "Negro Invasion." This time, Preston convened a secret conference at City Hall on March 21 where he and other leading White city leaders attempted to persuade a contingent of Black leaders to accept a voluntary and cooperative scheme of racial segregation. But by the following Saturday, reporters with the *New York Age* had gotten wind of his tactic, and the newspaper published an article on March 30, 1918, detailing his attempt to form a segregation committee.

> A conference between representative white and colored men was held in the Mayor's reception room at the City Hall on Thursday of last week, at which the whites suggested that the colored people co-operate with them in carrying out the principles of the segregation law, recently annulled by the United States Supreme Court.
>
> Finding that the colored men would not agree to the suggestion of voluntary segregation, Mayor Preston asked the newspapers not to

publish anything about the meeting. At the suggestion of Assistant Health Commissioner Howard, those present were constituted a committee to study some plan of voluntary and co-operative segregation in residential districts.[40]

Mayor Preston was soundly rebuked and rebuffed by Black leaders refusing to voluntarily segregate themselves. But the 1918 annexation of land north of Cold Spring Lane brought reinforcements. In the spring of 1918, the Maryland General Assembly passed and the governor signed annexation legislation allowing Baltimore City to add land north of Cold Spring Lane and subsume communities developed by the Roland Park Company.[41] The Roland Park Company pioneered community-wide, racially restrictive covenants in 1912 to formally stop Black people—and informally stop Jewish people—from owning homes in the four neighborhoods it would develop (Roland Park, Guilford, Homeland, and Northwood).[42]

Not to be outdone by its competitors' bigotry, the Forest Park Company in West Baltimore would follow suit and use racially restrictive covenants in their properties as well. Racist housing covenants were also deployed in other communities, including Mount Washington and Ashburton.[43] Many White homeowners in the Barclay neighborhood and the eastern edge of today's Old Goucher neighborhood also banded together under the name Home Protective Association to place restrictions on Black ownership in their home deeds.[44]

Baltimore Apartheid through Public Health and Code Enforcement

Perhaps feeling buoyed by the rise of racially restrictive covenants in so many neighborhoods, Mayor Preston pressed onward. His next idea would feature a veneer of scientific thinking as he turned to the field of public health to justify Baltimore Apartheid. According to the July 2, 1918, edition of the *Baltimore Sun*: "The Mayor . . . has conceived the idea of an ordinance based upon a municipality's police power to protect the health of its citizens, which would segregate negroes in this city because of having a much higher rate of tuberculosis among them than there is among the whites. They constitute a menace to the health of the white population."[45]

Infectious diseases such as tuberculosis were certainly at epidemic levels in the city in the 1910s, and it was clearly understood that social conditions were at the root of the epidemic among Baltimore's Negro population.[46] At the February 1917 health conference that Preston convened at city hall, a committee of public health officials, physicians, social workers, and clergymen discussed a sanitation campaign that would involve paving the remaining private alleys, treating the water, and completing the sewer system. The Preston administration and the Baltimore City Health Department understood that the lack of alley paving and sewer systems in Black living spaces were a driving force behind the tuberculosis epidemic. The city's publication of the *Baltimore Municipal Journal* on March 16, 1917, described the housing conditions concisely:

> Crowded into small houses in alleys and narrow streets, the major part of the negro population is living under conditions extremely unsanitary and unhealthful. Fresh air, sunlight and cleanliness, the essentials of correct living are distressingly absent. Living in such close contact, one member of a household falling victim to tuberculosis or some other contagious or communicable disease, endangers the life of every other member.[47]

But even as the Preston administration worked to improve the city's infrastructure—paving alleys, installing a sewer system, improving water treatment—it sought to deploy residential racial segregation to quarantine Black people in Black neighborhoods. The Preston administration's preoccupation with racial disparities in infectious disease rates did not reflect the belief that Black health matters. For Preston and his fellow Baltimoreans, it was a matter of protecting White public health.[48] Arguments regarding property value had failed in the courts so a new argument was needed. Preston decided to push a public health regime that made Black skin synonymous with disease and in keeping with treatment protocols for highly infectious diseases, the "treatment" required for the protection of White neighborhoods was quarantine. The *Baltimore Sun*'s propaganda served to help justify the race-based quarantine with a strikingly clear statement: "They [i.e., Negroes] constitute a menace to the health of the white population."[49]

In 1919, Baltimore's pro-segregation mayor visited Chicago to learn about their plan for creating and maintaining racial segregation. Mayor Preston

> borrowed from Chicago a plan to keep Negroes in their place. . . .
> City building inspectors and health department officials would
> cite for code violations those renting or selling to blacks in white
> neighborhoods. Real estate boards would sanction as unethical
> those members who violated the "color line." White property
> owners associations would encourage their members to enter into
> reciprocal covenants precluding sale or rental to Negroes.[50]

In effect, whenever Black homebuyers attempted to purchase property and move into a White neighborhood, they would be committing a violation against the white supremacist social order for the next 50-plus years. They were joined in their efforts by Baltimore City agencies and departments working together to engineer racial segregation. This included calling the police department to enforce Baltimore Apartheid. In a January 21, 1921, *Baltimore Sun* article entitled "North Baltimoreans Fear Negro Invasion," two neighborhood associations formed to maintain their all-White residential status—the Civic Improvement and Protective Association and the Maryland Avenue Association. According to the Sun, the president of the Civic Improvement and Protective Association was successful in stopping Negro tenants by means of "moral suasion," and by invoking the aid of the Building Inspector and the Health Commissioner.[51]

White Supremacist Urban Violence and Property Raids on Black Homeowners

Moving while Negro into a White neighborhood invoked a state of panic and was construed as a criminal offense, a threat to White public health, and a provocation for physical and legal attacks. Under such a pretext, a large crowd of White Baltimoreans assembled and then attacked the home of George Howe and his family on September 30, 1913. Howe returned fire on the mob with his shotgun, wounding four White youth in the crowd. Enraged, the mob nearly beat George Howe and another Black man named James Nelson to death, but both escaped alive.[52]

Other Black homebuyers also faced grave danger. In February 1919, the *Baltimore Sun* recorded another instance of white supremacist urban violence:

> Two negro families have invaded the 900 and 1000 blocks [of North Stricker Street]. . . . The trouble originated about two months ago, when a negro real estate operator tried to move into 929 North Stricker Street. He had his furniture in the house when boys of the neighborhood, forming a sort of Ku Klux Klan, raided the premises, smashed windows and doors and painted the steps a brilliant green. Placards were also placed around the house and the negro family moved.[53]

Hence, "a sort of Ku Klux Klan" was organized by White Baltimore homeowners to destroy the property of an incoming Black family, ultimately forcing them to move.[54] In another instance, White residents destroyed the home of a Black public school principal named Henry T. Pratt who attempted to move onto a "solid white" block in March 1922. A reporter described the scene at Pratt's house: "Today the front of his new house was a wreck. Every window was shattered, the front door barely hanging upon its hinges and red and blue ink spattered over the marble steps and window blinds, the result of white residents of the neighborhood storming the house early today in resentment of the negro's 'invasion.'"[55]

As with the property damage inflicted against homes occupied by the McMechens and other Black families in 1910, Black homebuyers in the 1920s faced the prospect of violence by merely moving into a White neighborhood. Property raids on Black people's homes sent a clear message that white supremacist urban violence would be deployed to block Black homeownership in streets occupied by White homeowners.

The Baltimore Sun *and the "Negro Invasion"*

In February 1923, Bolton Hill's Neighborhood Corporation sought to thwart Black homebuyers in their community. Residents of the 1200 block of Bolton Street used the circuit court to issue an injunction "against negroes moving into 1207 Bolton Street, to also cover the house at 1209 Bolton Street."[56] By publishing the exact addresses of Black homeowners, the *Sun* ensured that the White community could police, intimidate, harass, and ultimately expel the Black threat in their midst. White Baltimore's lobbying effort reached a boiling point as *Baltimore Sun* headlines repeatedly blared that the "Negro Invasion" was an imminent threat. White neighborhood associations, churches, business owners, real estate agents, and residents along with the city government's real estate and zoning boards schemed for more official means of racial segregation and the continuation of the public-private partnership to stymie potential Black homebuyers on White blocks.

The *Baltimore Sun* was the propaganda arm of white supremacy in Baltimore, helping to establish and enforce Baltimore

Apartheid. Articles on January 6 and January 17, 1924, worked to drum up support for an official committee for racial segregation as the newspaper announced that Mayor Howard Jackson would be forming a committee that would help formulate a plan for Baltimore's racial segregation. In a letter to Jackson dated January 16, 1924, the Harlem Park Protective Association representative called attention to the *Sun*'s role:

> This [Harlem Park Protective] Association was the first organization formed in Baltimore for the purpose of repelling the negro invasion of white neighborhoods. It attains its object through a private and recorded agreement of property owners in the vicinity of Harlem Park. . . . I read in this afternoon's Sun that you are contemplating the appointment of a committee to consider the segregation question.[57]

The *Sun* constantly beat the drum alarming White Baltimore about impending doom arriving in the form of a "Negro Invasion." The militant rhetoric of a "Negro Invasion" influenced the mindsets of many White Baltimoreans and neighborhood associations. Government-enforced racial segregation was not inevitable; it had to be promoted, lobbied for, and receive public support. The *Sun* had a hand in all three. Once people adopt the frame that they and their neighborhoods are being "invaded," then war is the only logical course of action.[58] In Baltimore's case, the war consisted of White homeowners securing legal sanction and police action through government systems, institutions, policies, and practices to stop Black homebuyers from buying a home and living the American Dream.

Although White homeowners clamored for Jackson to form an official committee to help institutionalize segregation, their efforts did not produce the desired results. In letters responding to pro-segregationist petitioners, Jackson explained that forming such a committee would be against the law. In a letter dated January 21,

1924, Jackson's reply to Philip Pitt shows the extent to which the city's real estate agents were working to enforce residential racial segregation:

> I acknowledge receipt of your letter dated January 19 and in reply beg to state that any impression to the effect that the Real Estate Board of Trade is trying to dominate the working out of some sort of a racial zoning plan is entirely erroneous and nothing whatever has been given out from this office which would lead anyone to such conclusion.[59]

White Baltimoreans were relentless and determined to prevent Black people from moving into their neighborhoods.[60] As George McMechen had sarcastically noted years earlier, "improvement associations" continued to magically appear whenever Black people moved into their neighborhood. On April 22, 1924, the Lafayette Square Protective Association convened a meeting at Brantly Baptist Church to discuss how they too could enforce residential racial segregation.[61] In October 1924, the Greenmount Protective Association formed to stop another "Negro Invasion."[62] On January 6, 1926, another reported "Negro Invasion" was "disclosed" by the Baltimore Sun as White Baltimoreans on Cedar Avenue, next to Gwynn Oak Park near the westernmost border of the city, discussed a possible Black homeowner moving into their community. Turns out, it was a false alarm. The Black people spotted by White lookouts were simply workers for the White family who owned the home.[63]

Clearly, the Baltimore Sun was a primary organizing tool for White protective associations. Its headlines often stoked fear and dread regarding the incoming "Negro Invasion." Sun writers also gave out the addresses of Black homebuyers to alert White neighbors of the breach of social protocol, announced meeting times and locations for meetings to stop "Negro Invasions," and used racist rhetoric to ratchet up the levels of White fear and antagonism.

White Religious Organizations and Baltimore Apartheid

White churches and religious institutions would play a central role in Baltimore's war on the "Negro Invasion." Mount Saint Agnes College—a Catholic institution located in Mount Washington—felt threatened by the potential move of Morgan College. Sister I. W. Scholastica wrote Mayor James Preston on September 23, 1913:

> My dear Mr. Preston,
>
> Allow me to approach you on a matter of grave moment—it is in reference to the sale of property in Mt. Washington as a site for the Morgan Co-educational College for Negroes. As a gentleman knowing the requirements of society, and especially as Chief Officer of our City, we ask you to use your influence with the Trustees that their decision on this subject may be changed.
>
> You are a man fair and square in your dealings; the people honor and love you as a representative Officer, therefore we feel sure your word would carry weight and help to avoid this threatening danger, for certainly if Mount Washington is converted into a negro settlement, then our property holders will be obliged to sacrifice what is justly theirs by right and title. Our college would practically be abandoned.[64]

Seeking to assuage the fears of Sister Scholastica, Preston responded on the next day:

> My dear Sister Scholastica:—
>
> I have your very kind letter of the 23rd instant.
>
> Anything in the world I can do to help you in this or any other matter I shall gladly do. I want, however, to reassure you. I do not think there is any chance of the Morgan College Trustees buying any property in Mt. Washington or any other section of the suburbs of Baltimore.[65]

This warm exchange between Preston and Sister Scholastica was but one example of the way White clergy leaned on Baltimore's government leaders to lead the fight for racial separation. White churches buttressed White protective associations in the war against the "Negro Invasion." The *Baltimore Sun* informed its readers that "many churches of the neighborhood are members of the Madison Avenue Protective and Improvement Association."[66] These same churches convened a segregation conference and typed a letter to Mayor Howard Jackson soliciting his aid by writing in the form of a church resolution:

> Whereas the Official Boards of the following churches . . . have learned with great alarm and concern of the recent invasion by the negro race on Madison Avenue and . . .

> Whereas, the properties of said Churches, and said locations, are of large financial value. Whereas, the said invasion of the negro race . . . will unquestionably, within a short period, destroy both the financial value of said Church properties, and the religious usefulness of said Churches in said communities.

> Now, therefore, be it resolved, by the Official Boards of [the five White churches] that the Real Estate Board of Baltimore City, and the proper City Authorities, be promptly informed of the danger arising by reason of said negro invasion on Madison Avenue.[67]

White supremacist religion would take other particular forms. In the nearby Harford County city of Webster, the Maryland chapter of the Ku Klux Klan started a church in 1924 with great fanfare. Also making an appearance was Mayor George Pennington of Havre de Grace. Pennington "shook the pastor's hand warmly and pledged whole-hearted support to the church and its work and to the klan." According to the *Sun*, he said: "I'll do anything I can—anything."[68]

The Klan is often viewed as an organization relegated to back-woods and rural areas, but the Second Klan (1915–1926) organized and operated in large urban areas. The Michigan Klan won the support of over 20,000 White Detroiters and supported the mayoral campaign of Charles Bowles with a Klanvocation and cross burning on the Saturday before the 1924 election. Even with the Klan's help, however, Bowles would lose.[69] Kansas City hosted a national Klanvocation in the fall of 1924.[70] The following year, hundreds of White members of the vaunted Ku Klux Klan proudly marched and paraded on Roland Avenue in Baltimore's Hampden community, sending a clear message of racial terror.[71]

Emboldened by White churches and the implied terrorism of the Klan, Baltimore's pro-segregation campaign marched on. The Mount Royal Improvement Association published a pamphlet extolling the virtues of the Bolton Hill neighborhood in June 1929 or 1930. The Bolton Hill Neighborhood Association bragged: "The greatest achievement of the Mount Royal Improvement Association has been the subjecting of the property in its area to a restriction for white occupancy only."[72] William L. Marbury Sr.—arch-segregationist and the president of the association—urged Bolton Hill's White homeowners' participation in the effort.[73] In a letter to Bolton Hill's homeowners announcing a meeting held at Associate Congregational Church, Marbury sought to give religious sanction to racial segregation, making sure to highlight the endorsement of White churches:

> When the present officers of the Mount Royal Improvement
> Association assumed office, assurances were given that plans would
> be presented for the maintenance of this district as the most
> beautiful and most desirable urban section of Baltimore, but that
> this could be done only after the property owners had made the
> district safe for white occupancy by the execution of a sufficient

number of the association's protective agreements. . . . This work has the endorsement of practically every church in the district.[74]

Armed with racially restrictive covenants and cover provided by the pro-segregationist propaganda of the *Baltimore Sun*, White neighborhood associations, churches, attorneys, real estate brokers, public health officials, and city government officials worked in unison to sustain the residential and neighborhood manifestation of Baltimore Apartheid.[75] The same racist strategies deployed in Baltimore City were exported to and deployed by other cities, giving rise to urban apartheid across the nation. In the war against the "Negro Invasion," no racist tactic was beyond the pale for White Baltimoreans, and with White clergy at the helm, the implication was that God was on pro-segregationists' side.

The Federal Government and the Housing Authority of Baltimore City

It was not long before urban pro-segregationists in cities across the nation had a powerful federal partner in their effort to exclude Black homebuyers from White neighborhoods. In 1933, the federal government's Home Owners' Loan Corporation (HOLC) began drawing Residential Security Maps, which systematically redlined neighborhoods with higher percentages of Black people and structurally greenlined neighborhoods that were exclusively White due to the various policies and practices previously highlighted. Baltimore's Residential Security Map was drawn in 1937 with local Baltimore's real estate brokers, real estate companies, a store cashier, a Goucher professor, and federal and state HOLC and FHA (Federal Housing Administration) employees.[76] Ever the team player, the City of Baltimore's Bureau of Plans and Surveys provided HOLC (which later became the FHA) with city data to help create Baltimore's Residential Security Map.[77]

After the Housing Authority of Baltimore City (HABC) formed in 1937, it also enforced a policy of segregating public housing in the city by race. In fact, HABC would become the most powerful city government enforcer of residential racial segregation in Baltimore City's history. Although HABC was a locally run agency, it was funded by the federal government. In the late 1930s and early 1940s, HABC started out by segregating its public housing developments by race (during the last of Mayor Howard Jackson's four terms in office). HABC designated Douglass, McCulloh, and Poe as Black public housing sites while making Perkins and Latrobe White public housing sites.[78]

While World War II raged across the oceans, White Baltimoreans organized a campaign of desegregation resistance to keep the federal government from building wartime public housing in 1943 near Armistead Gardens, near the easternmost border of the city between Moore's Run and Herring Run Park.[79] The *Baltimore Afro-American* newspaper covered a testy hearing regarding where temporary Negro public housing would be located on July 17, 1943. In a meeting attended by Mayor Theodore McKeldin, a large group of 800 White Baltimoreans showed up to protest the war housing project near Herring Run Park. Once again, White clergy served as spokespersons for the "Negro Invasion" resistance group.[80] After attempting to mollify the concerns of angry White residents who were heckling him as he spoke, McKeldin buckled and revealed his true feelings: "I am as much opposed to in-migrant colored people coming here as you are." At that point, White pro-segregationists protesting wartime housing for Black soldiers burst into applause.[81]

While Black soldiers shed their blood to halt the advance of Nazis in the European theater of war, they were also forced to fight in the spatial war to stop the "Negro Invasion" at home. Black homebuyers—many of them American soldiers and war veterans—were confronted with white supremacist mob violence if they tried to move into White neighborhoods. The racial integration of far east Baltimore would have to wait until another day.

In South Baltimore, White communities assembled to oppose federal wartime public housing for Black soldiers as well. Representatives from Lakeland, Morrell Park, Dorchester Heights, Westport, English Consul, and Highland Park organized at the Lakeland Presbyterian Church as they planned to send a delegation to Washington, DC, to protest the potential siting of public housing for Black soldiers in Mount Winans.[82] Because of this organized protest and the possibility of white supremacist violence, the Federal Public Housing Authority acceded to the recommendation of the HABC and Mayor McKeldin who urged the federal government to keep Baltimore Apartheid alive.[83] On October 26, 1943, the *Baltimore Sun* reported that public housing units for Black soldiers and their families were moved to four areas near heavy industrial activity—Cherry Hill, Sparrows Point, Southeast Baltimore (along Holabird Avenue), and Turner's Station (in Baltimore County).[84]

Throughout the 1940s and 1950s, the HABC maintained an explicit system of racially segregated public housing. Although HABC began a process of controlled desegregation of its public housing developments in the mid-1950s, the housing authority had strategically placed public housing developments either in already redlined neighborhoods or in undesirable industrial areas that were not attractive to higher-income White Baltimoreans. When HABC began developing scatter site units in the 1970s, it placed nearly all of its scatter site units in neighborhoods that were being occupied by African Americans.[85] Even in the putative age of desegregation (1970–1995), HABC intentionally concentrated lower-income Black public housing residents into redlined or yellowlined neighborhoods.

White desegregation resistance and flight would mean that many formerly White neighborhoods would become virtually all Black in a span of just 20 years or so. HABC deftly avoided placing units in neighborhoods that were wealthier and maintained a majority White status through its controlled desegregation strategy. HABC's actions solidified and concretized the hypersegregation that haunts the city, giving rise to the White L and the Black Butterfly—Baltimore's currently identifiable pattern of racial segregation.[86] In this way, HABC helped further reinforce racial segregation and concentrate lower-income African Americans into already redlined Black neighborhoods.[87]

Maintaining Baltimore Apartheid

In 1959, residents from the Baltimore neighborhood Mount Washington loaded buses to pursue a zoning ordinance to secure its status as a racially and economically exclusive community. The Mount Washington Improvement Association—raising $2,000 to secure a land and zoning expert with 400 families paying $5 each—produced a report giving them critical insights into the zoning ordinance they sought to keep lower-income residents from moving to the neighborhood, effectively barring most Black residents. Mount Washington residents were able to convince the mayor to sign an ordinance limiting future residential units to no more than six families per acre. This effectively blocked any new apartments or denser developments that would allow lower-income residents to afford to live in the neighborhood. When the comprehensive rezoning ordinance was drafted in 1971, residents of Mount Washington were able to retain the provision won in 1959, keeping their sophisticated race/class zoning provision in place.[88]

Racial segregation has also been maintained by real estate agents engaging in *racial steering*. Racial steering is when Black homebuyers are steered away from majority White neighborhoods and White homebuyers are steered away from majority Black neighborhoods. Real estate agents may not show Black homebuyers properties in majority White neighborhoods or show White homebuyers homes in majority Black neighborhoods. This illegal practice (since 1968) maintains racial segregation. The fair housing advocacy group Baltimore Neighborhoods Incorporated won a lawsuit against a real estate firm in 1992 due to its racial steering practices.[89] Thus, racial steering by real estate agents and firms are another way Baltimore Apartheid has been maintained.

More recently, government-enforced racial segregation is maintained through Baltimore City's noncompliance with the 1968 Fair Housing Act's mandate to "affirmatively further fair housing." By willfully leaving segregation intact when there are opportunities to implement desegregation policies and practices, Baltimore's public officials maintain Baltimore Apartheid. For instance, by continually approving zoning codes—such as Trans-Form Baltimore—that prevent affordable housing from being built in neighborhoods such as Mount Washington, city officials ensure the same neighborhood that resisted "the invasion of established white neighborhoods by negro institutions or residents" in 1913 and organized an exclusionary zoning campaign in 1959 can remain a supermajority White neighborhood. By approving the massive Port Covington development in 2016 without strong accompanying inclusionary upzoning legislation or requiring that at least 10% of total housing would be built inside Port Covington for public housing residents, the City of Baltimore allowed new residential development to be constructed that will be supermajority White in population.

Baltimore City's Repeated Uprootings

Racial segregation has been only one way White Baltimoreans have dealt with the unwanted presence of Black people. The war against the "Negro Invasion" was also waged via repeated forced relocation and uprootings. Many of Baltimore's Black residents had involuntarily migrated—or fled—from the Deep South during the Great Migration between 1910 and 1970 to escape over 4,000-

plus racial terror lynchings and the 300 or so instances of white supremacist mob violence, pogroms, and coup d'états prosecuted in Black independent cities, neighborhoods, or economic districts in the Deep South. In addition, many Black people were also forced out of smaller rural sundown towns during expulsive campaigns of racial cleansing.

Therefore, many African Americans arrived in Baltimore seeking fair housing and economic opportunities. But they unwittingly arrived in the midst of White Baltimore's war against the "Negro Invasion," where city officials and residents colluded to weaponize policies, practices, systems, and budgets that enforced racial segregation and enacted serial forced displacement. Throughout Baltimore's history, there have been at least 14 different waves of displacement of Black communities and institutions in Baltimore's history.[90] These successive waves of forced displacement wreaked tremendous havoc on the stability of Black Baltimore.

The Baltimore to New Orleans Slave Trade

In the early portion of Baltimore City's history, thousands of enslaved Black people would arrive in Baltimore due to the Trans-Atlantic Slave Trade and nearly 30,000 enslaved Black people would pass through Baltimore to be shipped to the Deep South as cotton became a dominant cash crop for White Southern plantation owners.[91] Lest the Domestic American Slave Trade is sanitized of its gut-wrenching horrors, Frederick Douglass provided a firsthand account of Baltimore's slave trading in the area known today as the Inner Harbor.

> I was born amid such sights and scenes. To me the American
> slave-trade is a terrible reality. When a child, my soul was often
> pierced with a sense of its horrors. I lived on Philpot Street, Fells
> Point, Baltimore, and have watched from the wharves, the slave
> ships in the Basin, anchored from the shore, with their cargoes of

human flesh, waiting for favorable winds to waft them down the Chesapeake. There was, at that time, a grand slave mart kept at the head of Pratt Street, by Austin Woldfolk. His agents were sent into every town and county in Maryland, announcing their arrival, through the papers, and on flaming "hand-bills," headed CASH FOR NEGROES. These men were generally well dressed men, and very captivating in their manners. Ever ready to drink, to treat, and to gamble. The fate of many a slave has depended upon the turn of a single card; and many a child has been snatched from the arms of its mother by bargains arranged in a state of brutal drunkenness.

The flesh-mongers gather up their victims by dozens, and drive them, chained, to the general depot at Baltimore. When a sufficient number have been collected here, a ship is chartered, for the purpose of conveying the forlorn crew to Mobile, or to New Orleans. From the slave prison to the ship, they are usually driven in the darkness of night.[92]

As Douglass's harrowing description makes clear, Baltimore was deeply enmeshed in the infernal workings of the American Domestic Slave Trade as Black people were placed on boats to be shipped as property to slave masters in Mobile, Alabama, or New Orleans, Louisiana. In Baltimore, especially in and around the Inner Harbor, Black Lives were constantly destroyed. Black families were split apart.[93] Black people were placed in slave jails or slave pens by slave traders and slave masters.[94] Slave trading in Baltimore provided fuel for the city's economy.[95] In antebellum Baltimore, the city government was a complicit partner in the auctioning and trading of Black people and the splitting apart of Black families.

Uprooting Black Baltimore Neighborhoods

Black neighborhood displacement in Baltimore would begin in the late 1800s when around a hundred Black families were uprooted in the Pigtown community by the Baltimore and Ohio Railroad.[96] The next Black community uprooting was enacted by Mayor Preston in 1917. Just as he had distinguished himself by being a chief architect of racial segregation in Baltimore, he enforced the displacement of a historic enclave of Black residents and churches along St. Paul Street called Gallows Hill.[97] The neighborhood was the home of the great Black lawyer-activist William Ashbie Hawkins as well as several prominent Black churches, such as Union Baptist Church and Bethel AME. In its stead, Baltimore City placed a park where the Black enclave Gallows Hill once stood and called it Preston Gardens, located on St. Paul Street across the street from Mercy Hospital.[98]

Just as racial segregation was called "radical and far-reaching," the forced displacement of the Gallows Hill community was also described as a "radical measure" by the *Baltimore Municipal Journal*, an official city publication.

> One of the radical measures which would seem advisable in dealing with this situation is the elimination of congested sections, populated by negroes, in which has been noted a very high percentage of death from this and other communicable diseases. The remedy suggested is the tearing down of these pest holes and converting them into parks. Through the activities of Mayor Preston's Commission on Housing Conditions, one of the worst infected blocks of the city is to be converted in this manner, the cost to be privately financed.[99]

The Preston administration leaned heavily on the field of public health for justifying the uprooting of the historic Black cluster of residents and churches. As mentioned earlier, the Preston administration was planning for the resettlement of a number of Black city residents to Baltimore County in 1917, which is what helped alarm White residents of Lauraville when Morgan College relocated to the area. The *Baltimore Municipal Journal* outlined the rationale embedded in the proposed plan: "The withdrawal of several hundred Negro families from the congested districts to the suburban settlements will undoubtedly make more room for those left behind."[100] Although the Preston plan for Black suburban resettlement would not take place (due to the city's expansion in 1918), displacing Black people and uprooting Black neighborhoods were both considered legitimate public health strategies.

The *Baltimore Municipal Journal* described areas such as the Gallows Hill community as "pest holes" and "infected blocks" that needed to be torn down. A century later, President Donald Trump (a real estate developer) would invoke the same imagery with his description of Baltimore as "a disgusting, rat and rodent infested mess" where "no human being would want to live."[101] The lurid logic of uprooting Black neighborhoods is revealed in the rat/rodent metaphor deployed by elected officials. If Black neighborhoods are viewed by government leaders as "pest holes" where "no human being would want to live," this would provide ample justification for the eradication of those "pest holes."

Preston's plan touted demolishing "one of the worst infected blocks of the city" and putting a lush park in its place so people could be afforded fresh air and sunlight. Who would argue against the need for more parks and green space? The problem was twofold however—the demolition of Gallows Hills took place without the Black community's consent, and residents were forced to move from downtown, eventually migrating to West Baltimore near Pennsylvania Avenue. Gallows Hill residents were not around to experience the fresh air and sunlight afforded by Preston Gardens.

Beginning in the 1940s, various Baltimore City government agencies would each play a significant role in leading the implementation of urban renewal and forced displacement citywide. On March 6, 1941, an ordinance was passed that gave the Baltimore City Health Department expanded code enforcement powers and established a new Division of Housing.[102] Code enforcement by local public health departments declared various dwellings "blighted" and in need of demolition. Code enforcement would later become a vital component of urban renewal.[103]

When the HABC built its first five public housing communities, it prosecuted its program known as "slum clearance." HABC displaced 1,863 Black families to do so, but only made 1,125 living units available to Black families in their segregated public housing developments. This is a reduction of 738 housing units, which made overcrowding in Black neighborhoods even more severe than it already was. By comparison, only 870 White families were displaced and 1,389 public housing units were available for White tenants. Hence, Black Baltimore was left with a devastating housing deficit while White Baltimore reaped a tremendous housing surplus.[104]

Between 1951 and 1971, the Baltimore Urban Renewal and Housing Agency (BURHA), displaced tens of thousands of Black Baltimoreans during the mayoralties of Theodore McKeldin, Thomas D'Alesandro Jr., Joseph Harold Gray, Philip Goodman, and Thomas D'Alesandro III. Thirteen urban renewal projects took place in Baltimore and were heavily funded by the federal Urban Renewal Administration. BURHA would later become the Department of Housing and Community Development in the late 1960s. HABC also displaced several thousand families through slum clearance to build public housing in the 1940s and then again through the demolition of large public housing developments in the 1990s to 2000s as a part of federal HOPE VI implementation.[105] HOPE VI resulted in the displacement and dispersion of thousands of Black families from public housing communities, such as Lexington Terrace, Hollander Ridge, Murphy Homes, Flag House, Broadway Overlook, and Julian Gardens.[106]

Taking place alongside HOPE VI was President Bill Clinton's Empowerment Zone initiative. Baltimore's Empowerment Zone was led by the Empower Baltimore Management Corporation

(EBMC), funded with a $100 million federal grant and implemented by the administration of Mayor Kurt Schmoke. Empowerment Zones were designed to promote, foster, and create job growth, business development, and livable communities in urban areas that were distressed. However, Baltimore's population in its six Empowerment Zones decreased by 17,988 between 1990 and 2000, including an estimated 13,940 Black residents.[107] Much of this Black depopulation was likely due to HABC's demolition of public housing in Empowerment Zone communities.

But Black depopulation was also facilitated by private housing market action. In a report of residential home sales in Baltimore's six Empowerment Zone areas, AB Associates found that 68% of the home sales were directed to investors while only 31% of the home sales went to owner occupants.[108] HABC's public housing demolition and disproportionate private home sales to investors reveal the actual result of Baltimore's Empowerment Zone initiative: facilitation for gentrification and more displacement of Black residents. Since 1990, neighborhoods such as Poppleton, Pigtown, Middle East, Madison Park, Fells Point, and Inner Harbor East have experienced significant growth in White population and turnover consistent with gentrification.[109]

After winning election in 1999, Mayor Martin O'Malley would also play a major role in the uprooting of Black residents. In the 2000s, O'Malley steered the creation of East Baltimore Development Incorporated (EBDI) to lead the redevelopment of the area near the Johns Hopkins medical campus in East Baltimore.[110] In the 1950s, Johns Hopkins University partnered with the city government in one of the city's urban renewal projects to displace over 1,335 Black households.[111] EBDI would be the second time a mass uprooting of Black people occurred at the behest of Johns Hopkins Medical Institutions—this time displacing 742 Black households.[112] Interestingly, a June 2004 planning document from the O'Malley administration revealed that both Poppleton and Reservoir Hill were listed as "upcoming major development opportunities" by city officials.[113] Both communities would become home to large-scale redevelopment projects: the University of Maryland BioPark in Poppleton and Innovation Village in Reservoir Hill.

The Scope of Baltimore City's Forced Displacement

Relatively little attention has been paid to the full scale and scope of serial forced displacement in Baltimore City. Hence, little thought has been given to the social impacts of constantly displacing and uprooting Black communities and forcibly relocating Black Baltimoreans. However, the number of Black families forcibly uprooted by city government policies and practices can be enumerated with tremendous specificity:

- 1,863 Black families displaced by slum clearance[114]
- 8,091 Black families displaced by urban renewal[115]
- 3,055 Black families displaced by code enforcement[116]
- 313 Black families displaced by the city to build public schools[117]
- 2,508 Black families displaced for new public housing construction between 1951 and 1971[118]
- 4,051 Black families displaced by HABC public housing demolition in 1987 and 1995–2001[119]
- 965 Black families displaced by the construction of I-70 or Route US-40[120]
- 742 Black families displaced by EBDI[121]

A combined total of 21,588 Black households have been displaced by large-scale displacement projects between 1940 and 2010.[122] Using a conservative estimate of three persons per household, this calculation likely involves an estimated 64,764 Black people who have been displaced by large-scale displacement projects—a staggering amount. If the approximately 35,000 or so Black people shipped to or from Baltimore during the period of American slavery were added, then a sum of nearly 100,000 or more Black people have been forcibly uprooted and displaced throughout Baltimore's history.[123]

The cumulative toll of this uprooting and displacement is staggering when the impact on Black families and Black communities is considered. Multiple Black communities have been partially or completely uprooted in Baltimore City's history:

- Pigtown (by the Baltimore and Ohio Railroad)
- Gallows Hill (by the Preston administration for a park named Preston Gardens)[124]
- Waverly, Madison Park, Harlem Park, Broadway East, and other communities (by the Baltimore Urban Renewal and Housing Agency)
- Multiple communities in central West Baltimore along a nearly two-mile stretch of the Franklin-Mulberry corridor (due to US-40 highway construction)
- Cross Keys Village (due to I-83 exchange)[125]
- Middle East (by Johns Hopkins Medical Institutions and EBDI for a planned biotechnology park)[126]
- Poppleton (due to expansion by the University of Maryland, particularly the UM BioPark)
- Multiple public housing communities (by HABC due to HOPE VI)

In the process of these uprootings and forced displacements, an unknown number of Black churches, small businesses, and cultural institutions were also decimated.

Baltimore County Racial Segregation

Baltimore County has also contributed to Baltimore City's war against the "Negro Invasion." When racially restrictive covenants were created in 1912 by the Roland Park Company's general manager Edward Bouton, the land being developed was a part of Baltimore County. Over a century later, residents of Rodgers Forge in Towson—a city in Baltimore County just to the north of Roland Park—were shocked to find racially restrictive covenants in the property deeds for homes developed by the James Keelty Company.[127]

Baltimore County would serve as the main place where Whites in Baltimore City fled in order to escape racial integration.[128] As discussed in Track 2, the federal government helped to subsidize White flight and suburban exclusivity. Baltimore County would benefit from white affirmative action. The FHA helped finance home mortgages for Whites while the Federal Highway Administration financed highways that would facilitate White Baltimoreans leaving the city to live in Baltimore County and commute to city jobs. During the 1950s—as Baltimore City's schools began to integrate—Baltimore City's Black population swelled by nearly 100,000 while the White population in the city shrank by approximately 100,000. Many White residents departed Baltimore City so that they would not have to send their children to schools with Black children. Between 1950 and 2010, White Baltimore's population would fall from a high of 700,000 to less than 200,000—a massive decline of over half a million people. As such, Baltimore County became a haven for Baltimore City residents opposed to desegregation.

Baltimore County also threatened the viability of its Black communities through discriminatory zoning.[129] In addition, Baltimore County has never built public housing developments, unlike the HABC, which meant that many residents who needed public housing would end up in Baltimore City. According to the Maryland American Civil Liberties Union, "Baltimore County has never had any public housing and currently has fewer than 1,400 privately owned subsidized housing units open to families, despite a voucher waiting list of over 15,000 households. In contrast, the County has actively used federal and state housing funds to build elderly housing, which in Baltimore County is mostly occupied by whites."[130]

In 1964, Baltimore Mayor Theodore McKeldin attempted to work with Baltimore County Executive Spiro Agnew to create a desegregation plan, but Agnew would oppose the plan. In 1972, Dale Anderson, Agnew's successor as Baltimore County Executive, openly defied the Fair Housing Act, claiming that it would "bring hordes of migrants" to the county.[131] This is how Baltimore County waged its war against the "Negro Invasion," or the "hordes of migrants."

In 2016, the Baltimore County Commission continued to oppose fair housing. In a 6–1 vote, the commission rejected voting for the Housing Opportunities Made Equal, or HOME Act, which was designed to stop discrimination based on the source of income—particularly against people with Housing Choice Vouchers—as part of a conciliation agreement with the US Department of Housing and Urban Development.[132] During the 2018 election season, Al Redmer, the Republican candidate for county executive, actively campaigned on preventing more people with Section 8 vouchers from moving into Baltimore County.[133] He lost the election but garnered 43% of the vote with a tally of 119,856 supporters.[134]

In 2019, both Baltimore City and Baltimore County finally passed the HOME Act—over 50 years after the passage of the 1968 Fair Housing Act. The Baltimore City version featured a cap mechanism that weakened the legislation, while the Baltimore County Council passed a more robust HOME Act by a slim 4–3 margin. Baltimore County opponents called the HOME Act a "forced Section 8 Bill" and Councilwoman Cathy Bevins received threats requiring police protection.[135] According to former Baltimore County Executive Don Mohler, HOME Act opponents "demonized some of the most vulnerable people in our community."[136]

Between 1910 and 1930, the *Baltimore Sun* provided propagandistic support for pro-segregationists to halt the "Negro Invasion." In a move eerily consistent with its actions a century ago, the *Baltimore Sun* surreptitiously published a front-page article on the 52% rise in homicides in Baltimore County on the exact day the County Council convened to vote on the HOME Act.[137] Although the HOME Act passed, the same playbook was deployed to halt desegregation, including the threat of violence and the demonization of Black people. Given this, implementation of the HOME Act is likely to face many challenges. The laws may have changed, but it remains to be seen whether desegregation will be rigorously enforced to make desegregation a reality in Baltimore County.

Conclusion

Although the Civil War formally ended in 1865, America's struggle to protect the humanity of Black people continues. America's propensity to whitelash has produced a series of wars—a war to roll back Black Reconstruction and enforce Jim and Jane Crow, a war to block the "Negro Invasion" and enforce racial segregation in urban areas, and a war on Black communities under the guise of the War on Drugs that featured hyperpolicing. Each war was accompanied by violence: terrorism, mob violence, lynchings, and rape (to roll back Black Reconstruction), white supremacist urban violence to force out Black homebuyers in White neighborhoods (to block the "Negro Invasion"), and the militarization of police forces and police killings of unarmed Black people (to control Black communities).

When Baltimore City Solicitor S. S. Fields spoke to *St. Louis Post-Dispatch* reporters in 1916, he spoke forthrightly regarding the aims of passing government-enforced racial segregation:

The encroachments of the negro upon white settlements were daily becoming more pronounced and in a short time a race war, started by the whites, might have ensued. In a city with the heavy negro population of Baltimore, this was an outcome devoutly to be avoided and in our effort to avoid it, we framed the segregation ordinance.[138]

Little did Fields realize that a war was in fact "started by the whites." At its core, both white supremacist urban violence and hyperpolicing were tactics of a broader spatial war that dictated the differential levels of resources and opportunities that flow into various city neighborhoods. At the onset, this war was more often waged with physical violence or property destruction, but as the decades passed, invisible structural violence would take prominence. Government-enforced racial segregation and serial forced displacement would become two of the most devastating forms of structural violence in the spatial war. America retains a fear of the "Negro Invasion" as revealed by ongoing resistance to legal mandates for desegregation in the Baltimore metropolitan area and beyond.

After the 1980s, national progress on desegregation stalled and research shows that many White Americans were striving to make America segregated again.[139] Why is White America choosing to keep racial segregation alive? Brian Resnick highlights the research of psychologist Jennifer Richeson. Resnick writes:

Richeson's studies on interracial interactions had taught her that when people are in the majority, the sense of their race is dormant. But the prospect of being in the minority can suddenly make white identity—and all the historical privilege that comes with it—salient. And, she guessed, the prospect of losing majority status was likely to make people (perhaps unconsciously) uneasy.[140]

Hence, White Americans' possessive investment in whiteness, especially "all the historical privilege that comes with it" (i.e., in-

creased wealth derived from higher home values, increased resources for neighborhoods and schools, lower interest rates from
banks), includes too many benefits for White America to abandon.
Loss of these benefits animates the fear of a rainbow nation and
resistance to demographic transition (i.e., losing majority status).
As a result, American Apartheid lives on in public and private institutions, budgets, systems, policies, and practices.

America and its hypersegregated cities cannot move forward
without acknowledging the fundamental aspects of spatial war that
characterized how Black people and Black communities would
be treated according to the law. A race war is what government-
enforced racial segregation and repeated uprootings were designed
to avoid (by keeping races separate), but it would only plant the
seeds for future racial conflicts as urban Black neighborhoods fell
deeper and deeper into despair. To paraphrase poet laureate Langston Hughes, when dreams are deferred, do they simply dry up? Or,
at some point, do they explode?

Ongoing Historical Trauma

They use the TV to chain us and tell us Blacks are so dangerous
They gave us lead in our homes and wonder why we go brainless.
Martina Lynch, "Concrete"

And it's no need of running and no need of saying,
"Honey, I'm not going to get in the mess,"
because if you were born in America with a black face,
you were born in the mess.
Fannie Lou Hamer, "We're on Our Way"

American Apartheid and Historical Trauma

On July 27, 2019, at 7:14 a.m., the president of the United States attacked Maryland Congressman Elijah Cummings on Twitter using Baltimore as the justification for his excoriation. Calling Baltimore a "disgusting, rat and rodent infested mess," President Trump continued insulting residents: "No human being would want to live there."[1] Conveniently ignoring the fact that Baltimore is an American city—a place for which American presidents also shoulder responsibility—Trump sought to demonize an entire city for the purpose of diverting national media attention away from his policies at the Southern border.[2] Lost in the political firestorm was a substantive discussion about why the conditions in Baltimore exist, particularly in redlined Black neighborhoods. Also missing was a discussion of who passed the policies and enacted the practices that gave rise to such conditions.

The historical record is clear: apartheid policies, practices, systems, and budgets devastated redlined Black neighborhoods in Baltimore City. In the 1900s, war was upon Baltimore as White residents waged a block-by-block war against the "Negro Invasion." Initially, white supremacists lobbed rocks and bricks or conducted property raids to intimidate and scare Black homebuyers. But over time, with increasing frequency, White Baltimoreans turned to structural forms of violence—using institutional policies, practices, systems, and budgets—to erect and enforce a regime of urban apartheid.[3] After losing the war against the "Negro Invasion" in the mid-1970s, Baltimore City's government shifted strategies and turned to a spatial war on Black neighborhoods giving rise to a hypersegregated city. An examination of a racial dot map of Baltimore City reveals the city's spatial and racial geography in the form of a White L and a Black Butterfly.

The long legacy of American Apartheid collectively constitutes *historical trauma*.[4] Historical trauma is a conceptual framework first developed by Lakota scholar Maria Yellow Horse Brave Heart. Trauma occurs when an external force inflicts tremendous damage on the affected entity, thereby threatening its health and viability. According to Brave Heart, the social, economic, and emotional wounding—resulting from damage inflicted by powerful groups onto vulnerable groups—can be passed down from one generation to the next.[5] Research in the field of epigenetics reveals how trauma can be passed intergenerationally from parents to their offspring.[6]

American Apartheid is the primary spatial construct through which ongoing historical trauma is transmitted in Black spaces and neighborhoods. American Apartheid is most devastating in large hypersegregated cities, such as Baltimore, Chicago, Detroit, Flint, St. Louis, Cleveland, Birmingham, Milwaukee, Philadelphia,

New York, Dayton, Kansas City, Boston, Hartford, and Rochester. In these and other urban areas, municipalities and banks continue to redline and subprime the spaces and places where Black people live, work, play, pray, earn, and learn. But apartheid practices have also been visited upon Black people living in rural areas through lynchings, sundown towns, and the dispossession of waterfront and farmland properties.

Urban Black neighborhoods and rural Black communities have never been repaired or allowed to heal in any substantive and intentional way from these historically traumatic actions. White supremacist institutions, systems, policies, practices, and budgetary decisions that harmed Black neighborhoods in the past are still inflicting harm and causing damage in Black neighborhoods today. The mentality that informed America's war against the "Negro Invasion" thoroughly warped the real estate market to the extent that real estate values of homes today are strongly determined by the racial composition of people living in neighborhoods.[7]

Although there were attempts by the federal government to desegregate schools and neighborhoods during the 1950s–1970s, these attempts were undermined by militant White desegregation resistance, including strategies such as mobs harassing Black students integrating schools or bombing the homes of Black homebuyers in White areas.[8] Overt resistance was accompanied by more covert "White flight" away from center cities to surrounding sundown suburbs. This Second American Whitelash was subsidized by the federal government through the insurance of suburban home mortgages and building of highways to those suburbs.[9] As a result, the spatial contours of American Apartheid merely reconstituted itself as many large urban areas morphed into what Parliament-Funkadelic mastermind George Clinton dubbed "Chocolate Cities" surrounded by "Vanilla Suburbs" in the mid-1970s—majority Black cities flanked by supermajority White suburbs.

The promise of a racially integrated nation remains unfulfilled 50 years after the passage of the seminal 1968 Fair Housing Act. The Fair Housing Act itself had no enforcement mechanism until 1988. Perhaps this is what led the legendary soul and jazz singer Nina Simone to quip: "Desegregation is a joke."[10] American policies and strategies for desegregation have typically involved mixing people from different racial backgrounds (particularly in schools), but little has been done to restore the resources and wealth of Black neighborhoods and small towns harmed by exploitation and extraction. Wealth is still disproportionately concentrated firmly in the hands of White-owned corporations, institutions, and philanthropic organizations while the racial wealth gap has widened. Desegregating people while leaving racial disparities in wealth intact does little to address the damage caused by ongoing historical trauma.[11] What redlined Black neighborhoods have needed for restoration, but what they have never received, is the authentic desegregation of power, resources, and wealth.

Ongoing Historical Trauma

Historical trauma is not a bygone novelty. It is an ongoing reality. Starting after 1900 in Baltimore City, White Baltimoreans waged a war against the "Negro Invasion" and then a war against Black neighborhoods. As a result, Black neighborhoods were redlined by both their own city government and private banks. Black home-buyers received subprime loans from banks and predatory lenders known as blockbusters. Because of capital denied and wealth extracted, urban apartheid continues to damage Black neighborhoods and diminish Black Lives. To unpack the precise nature of the harms inflicted, the following elements of ongoing historical trauma will be examined: hypersegregation, resource removal, forced uprootings, hyperpolicing, economic destruction, and wealth extraction.

Hypersegregation Today

Today, in the Baltimore metropolitan area, hypersegregation is primarily manifested through spatial residential patterns that form the White L and the Black Butterfly.[12] Over the past 110 years, government-enforced racial segregation has constituted the platform from which structural weapons of environmental and economic destruction have been launched against Black neighborhoods. Such weapons have included private bank redlining, inequitable allocations of public goods, underfunded public school systems, and the proximate location of toxic environmental facilities or disamenities.

Elevated levels of residential racial segregation result in greater levels of economic extraction or what education scholar Noliwe Rooks calls *segrenomics*. Rooks defined segrenomics as "the business of profiting specifically from levels of racial and economic segregation."[13] She coined the term to discuss how corporations profit from segregation in the education system, but it is clear that segrenomics operates in multiple systems, including criminal justice, finance, community development, real estate, housing, food, transportation, and other systems. Building on Rooks's terminology, I offer the friendly amendment that segrenomics in its totality is the economic weaponization of racial segregation. Segrenomics allows landlords, corporations, and wealthy entities to extract additional profits from redlined Black neighborhoods through predatory mortgages and rents, subprime auto insurance, and discriminatory taxation.

One of the most recent examples of segrenomics involves the rise of reverse mortgages, where financial institutions offer lines of credit to elderly homeowners based on their home mortgages. When the elderly homeowner dies, the financial institution can claim possession of the home if family members are unable to pay a large lump sum. This means the primary source of wealth for most Americans—their homes—is not transferred intergenerationally so that wealth accrued by parents cannot be handed down to their children. A *USA Today* analysis of 1.3 million home loans found that nearly 100,000 reverse mortgages have ended in foreclosure (between 2013 and 2017) and that reverse mortgage foreclosures were six times more likely to take place in Black neighborhoods compared to neighborhoods that were 80% White.[14] Baltimore was among the cities hardest hit along with other hypersegregated cities, including Chicago, Detroit, and Philadelphia.

When metropolitan areas are hypersegregated, Black neighborhoods can be easily identified. Once Black neighborhoods are identified, they can be targeted for wealth extraction while being denied private capital and public goods. In Baltimore, segrenomics results in White L neighborhoods being able to hoard resources and opportunity while simultaneously extracting wealth from and denying capital access to Black Butterfly neighborhoods. Segrenomics, therefore, is economic and structural violence. The smooth functioning of segrenomics relies on the continued government enforcement of racial segregation and governments' studied disregard for dismantling American Apartheid.

The ongoing effects of American Apartheid are devastating, escalating economic exploitation and proliferating poverty. Because public policy was never designed to dismantle America's spatial apartheid in any serious way, it has metastasized into a social cancer and resulted in a destructive hypersegregation—a spatial matrix that damages Black Lives and devastates Black neighborhoods. The racial segregation of Black communities is actively maintained through the existence of racially discriminatory practices, such as exclusionary zoning ordinances that restrict the building of multifamily apartments, government refusal to mandate inclusionary and fair housing in new developments, and the brazen lack of government enforcement of the 1968 Fair Housing Act's mandate to affirmatively further fair housing.[15]

In Baltimore, the active maintenance of racial segregation plays out in striking ways. The Housing Authority of Baltimore City (HABC) deserves scrutiny as the primary purveyor of residential racial segregation in Baltimore. As Karl Taeuber and Arnold Hirsch highlighted in their research for plaintiffs in the *Thompson v. HUD* court case, HABC not only racially segregated its public housing but also concentrated most of its public housing developments in Black neighborhoods or environmentally oppressed communities. HABC located virtually all of its scatter sites in Black neighborhoods after 1970—during the time of supposed desegregation.[16] On top of this, a vast majority of Baltimore's residents with Housing Choice Vouchers (formerly known as Section 8) reside in the Black Butterfly.[17] Despite its pivotal role in intensifying racial segregation, HABC does next to nothing to actively desegregate Baltimore City unless compelled by the judicial system. Baltimore is not alone in this regard. The same pattern of public housing authorities maintaining racial segregation with Housing Choice Vouchers exists nationwide.[18]

It is important to remember America's housing history and recall that the architects of American Apartheid intentionally placed public housing developments in already impoverished and redlined neighborhoods. This critical history runs counter to how people in government, in development, and in academia often talk about "concentrated poverty" today. Concentrated poverty is discussed as though people with lower incomes randomly decided to live together in redlined and environmentally oppressed neighborhoods. When used in a noncritical way, the phrase *concentrated poverty* obscures ongoing historical trauma and overlooks key questions that demand an answer. Who concentrated people living in poverty into redlined neighborhoods? Who maintains spatial racism? Who benefits from urban apartheid?

Without critical historical context, the phrase *concentrated poverty* keeps people from going to the root of the problem:

government-enforced racial segregation and discriminatory site placement by local public housing authorities. Intentional govern-ment policies and practices concentrated lower-income Black families in redlined and environmentally oppressed neighbor-hoods. Concentrated poverty is ultimately profitable for banks, slumlords, industries, police, and the criminal justice system. It also props up philanthropies and large nonprofits that gain fund-ing under the guise of helping Black people while leaving apart-heid systems intact.

The flip side of concentrated poverty is concentrated wealth, which leads to disproportionate structural advantage. For exam-ple, in Baltimore City's White L neighborhoods, residents are able to benefit from special benefits districts (often called community benefits districts). Residents in the city's special benefits districts are able to secure additional resources for city residents through an additional tax assessment. While paying more for more ser-vices may seem fair on the surface, White L corporations and residents are often already beneficiaries of significant tax savings as recipients of tax breaks (White L corporations) or historic tax credits (White L residents).[19] Therefore, White L neighborhoods are often able to avoid paying taxes—that would go into the Gen-eral Fund for the benefit of the entire city—and then use those tax savings to pay for resources that stay in their neighborhoods. This discriminatory taxation scheme rests on the foundation of hypersegregation and constitutes municipal segrenomics.

Baltimore City, Baltimore County, and the State of Maryland each allow and enforce racial segregation in ways that structurally advantage wealthier and demographically whiter neighborhoods. Baltimore City maintains racial segregation by allowing neighbor-hoods such as Mount Washington, Roland Park, Guilford, and Homeland to keep exclusionary zoning codes that restrict where multifamily apartments can be built for families with lower in-comes. Baltimore City proliferates transit inequity by selectively placing transit resources such as the Charm City Circulator, Bike Share stations (now defunct), and bike infrastructure (such as protected bike lanes and bike racks) in the White L. Baltimore County maintained racial segregation by rejecting fair housing agreements with the US Department of Housing and Urban Development (HUD) until November 2019. The State of Maryland played a role by building a north-south rapid rail system through the White L, but rejecting an east-west rapid rail line that would run through the Black Butterfly.

Lack of affordable and diverse modes of quality transit options leave Black Baltimoreans disadvantaged in the labor force. Black Butterfly residents without vehicles have a harder time accessing critical areas where jobs are available. Samuel Jordan of the Baltimore Transit Equity Coalition makes the argument that when people have a commute time longer than 45 minutes, it should be considered "transit detention." Baltimore Neighborhood Indicator Alliance maps reveal that White L neighborhoods have the highest percentage of people that can commute to work in 15 minutes or less. For many Black residents, the lack of rapid transit in Black neighborhoods means they disproportionately experience transit detention. Hence, hypersegregation affects access to healthy housing and food, well-resourced schools, efficient transit systems, bank capital, and public goods.

Contemporary Resource Removal and Forced Uprootings

Public goods are increasingly stripped from Black neighborhoods in Baltimore, and Black residents are continually uprooted. These processes facilitate the destabilization of Black communities—often for the benefit of private corporations and incoming wealthier and demographically whiter residents. In Baltimore, city leaders have permanently closed scores of recreation centers and public schools. Baltimore City has permanently closed nearly 90 recreation centers since the late 1970s. The Baltimore City Public

School System (BCPSS) permanently closed 84 public schools since 2000, nearly all in Black neighborhoods.[20] Unsurprisingly, school closures disproportionately affect Black youth. For example, since 2013, Black students have been roughly 80% of the BCPSS student population, but the average student body of the students in schools permanently closed has been 95% Black.[21]

Under former BCPSS CEO Andrés Alonso, many schools were closed under his Expanding Great Options initiative. The main reasons for school closures were low academic performance and low enrollment.[22] The Baltimore City Public Schools Construction and Revitalization Act of 2013—passed by the state legislature and signed by Governor Martin O'Malley—required the closure of another 26 schools in order for BCPSS to receive $1.1 billion in funds from the State of Maryland.[23] The permanent closures of 84 public schools has had a disruptive effect on multiple neighborhoods already teetering in a state of instability.[24]

In a national empirical analysis of the effects of school closures on neighborhood home values, Noli Brazil found evidence that school closures were more clustered in majority Black neighborhoods. School closures were also statistically associated with subsequent declines in median home values nationally, but most acutely in Black neighborhoods. Brazil also explained how school closures might have such a devastating impact on Black neighborhood stability:

> The results also show that school closures have greater negative effects in neighborhoods with larger percentages of Black residents. This result may be explained by the greater dependency of Black neighborhoods on local schools for community services. Moreover, neighborhoods with larger percentages of Black residents tend to be more disadvantaged and segregated, and experienced declining socioeconomic status between 2000 and 2010. Given this compounding effect of baseline disadvantage and

trending decline, a school closure may act as a tipping point for these neighborhoods such that the preceding decline may accelerate and be difficult to reverse.[25]

In other words, when school boards and districts permanently close schools in Black neighborhoods, they are contributing to accelerating neighborhood decline in areas that have already been redlined and subprimed. As Baltimore parent Michael Johnson articulated: "When you are dismantling the schools you dismantle the neighborhoods."[26] School closures also disrupt the community's sense of identity and levels of democratic participation, inducing what sociologist Eve Ewing calls "institutional mourning"—a collective grieving over the loss of a historically and spatially significant community resource. In many Black communities, Ewing writes, social bonds "are defined by a shared sense of participation and ownership—a sense that *this place is ours.*"[27]

This shared sense of participation and ownership enhances the fact the affected schools are *public* institutions. Public facilities—whether they are schools, recreation or neighborhood centers, or housing developments—are often the nexus of democracy and inclusion for many Black residents. In many Black neighborhoods, public facilities amplify community identity and enshrine Black history. Public facilities in Black neighborhoods are often named after historical Black figures such as W. E. B. Du Bois or Harriet Tubman. Hence, the closures of recreation centers, public schools, and public housing developments decrease Black resident participation and ownership, disrupt community identity, and destroy Black history.

Black Teacher Displacement

The BCPSS teaching workforce has undergone a tremendous demographic shift. Black teachers have declined from being 63.2% of the BCPSS workforce in 2005 to just 38.4% of the BCPSS workforce in 2014—a 39.2% decline and a drop from a majority to a minority of the teacher workforce in less than 10 years. This has caused a widening gap in teacher-student racial concordance as the BCPSS student population remains over 80% Black.

Black teacher displacement is significant when one considers the battle for Black education in Baltimore after the Civil War. Regarding the fight for Black teachers being able to teach Black students in BCPSS's segregated schools, David Armenti wrote:

> Black leaders still had to battle for control of the Colored Schools, which were initially staffed exclusively by white teachers. Prominent lawyer Everett J. Waring and the Reverend Harvey Johnson led efforts to gain employment for black teachers, while also lobbying for better facilities and more advanced programs for students. The first "Colored High School," which would later become Frederick Douglass High School, was established in 1882. Black teachers were hired as early as 1889, and by 1907 the student body and faculty was completely segregated.[28]

Armenti characterizes the hiring of Black teachers to teach Black students as "completely segregated," but this elides an important point. When Baltimore's public schools first opened to Black students in 1867, Black students were not allowed to be taught by Black teachers. Baltimore's Black community understood that excluding Black teachers and only hiring White teachers to instruct Black children was not racial integration, but racial domination. Given the social fabrication of Black inferiority, Black children needed to see living examples of their future selves and receive culturally enriched instruction from Black teachers in order to survive and navigate the threats to Black life.

Since Black teachers were not allowed to teach Black children from 1867 to 1889, White teachers in Baltimore completely controlled the education of Black children for a period of roughly 22 years. In essence then, what Black activists were fighting for was the right to offer racially and culturally congruent education to Black children. This history is largely forgotten as the numbers of Black teachers drastically dropped in the BCPSS workforce after 2005 at the same time more stringent requirements for teacher certification were rolled out, public school conversions to charter schools escalated, and the numbers of permanent closures of Black public schools mounted. Issues with Black teacher retention are also implicated. It is likely that the combination of these factors resulted in the tremendous decline in the numbers of Black teachers in Baltimore's public schools.

The fight for culturally congruent and racially concordant education for Black students is deeply rooted in Black Baltimore's fight for equitable access to public education. The Black teacher workforce has been decimated once before, when Black Baltimore's private education system was shut down in 1867 once Black children were allowed to enroll in Baltimore City public schools.[29] Although some measure of desegregation was implemented in the city's public schools after *Brown v. Board of Education* was decided in 1954, the need for Black teachers remains as high as ever. Research indicates increased learning outcomes when Black children are taught by Black teachers.[30] In addition, research by Philip Goff and colleagues demonstrates that many White authority figures—including teachers—harbor racist views of Black children that cause them to overestimate the ages of Black children and leads to the loss of presumed innocence.[31] Racial bias and the loss of presumed innocence both help explain why many Black children experience disproportionate levels of corporal punishment, suspensions, expulsions, criminal justice contact, and arrests by school or city police in school systems across America compared to their White counterparts.

In short, Black teachers matter. But as school districts across the country turn increasingly to private charters, public education increasingly becomes a profit center. In this environment of standardized testing, the value of Black teachers who come from the communities of the students they teach has been ignored. The trend of Black teacher labor displacement in Baltimore mirrors what is taking place in cities across the nation. Between 2002 and 2012, Black teachers have declined precipitously in cities across the nation in Boston (down 18.3%), Chicago (down 39.2%), Cleveland (down 33.9%), Los Angeles (down 33.2%), New Orleans (down 62.3%), and San Francisco (down 32.4%).[32]

Black Public Housing Displacement and Housing Instability

In addition to public education, public housing is another area where forced displacement and resource withdrawal takes place. In Baltimore, the dismantling of public housing has occurred at a rapid pace. HABC is in the process of dismantling project-based public housing through demolition and selling the buildings to private entities. HABC has reduced the number of public housing units "from 16,525 units in 1992 to 9,625 in the spring of 2007," according to a 2007 report by Joan Jacobson.[33] Several large public housing communities were demolished in the 1990s and 2000s under the federal HOPE VI policy—Lafayette Courts, Lexington Terrace, Murphy Homes, and Flag House Courts.

In the private market, Black housing instability and forced displacement is at emergency levels. In the investigative series "Dismissed," *Baltimore Sun* reporters Doug Donavan and Jean Marbella found that Baltimore leads the nation in rental evictions per capita.[34] *Baltimore Business Journal* reporter Melody Simmons found that the Baltimore area was fourth nationally in metro area foreclosure filings in 2015.[35] Data indicate that Baltimore City is averaging nearly 4,000 foreclosure filings largely targeting Black homeowners and about 7,000 rental evictions largely affecting Black renters each year.[36]

In other words, Baltimore City landlords, banks, and courts are exceedingly efficient at kicking people out of their homes. High rental evictions and mortgage foreclosure threats make sense in light of other data indicating that 59.3% of Black renters and 45% of Black homeowners in Baltimore pay more than 30% of their income for housing.[37] Given that the median annual household income for Black Baltimoreans is only $38,688, over half of all Black Baltimore households are living in dire economic conditions and struggle to pay their rent or mortgage. This catalyzes a catastrophic chain reaction as low incomes fuel housing instability and place Black residents at high risk for rental evictions and mortgage foreclosures.

The city's historically segregating universities have repeatedly uprooted Black neighborhoods and residents. Johns Hopkins Medical Institutions (JHMI) engaged in the massive displacement of the Middle East community near its medical campus in East Baltimore in the 2000s.[38] Its proxy organization—the East Baltimore Development Incorporated (EBDI)—renamed (i.e., rebranded) the community Eager Park. In the city's center, historically Black neighborhoods such as Sharp Leadenhall and Hoes Heights are threatened by development and uprooting. On the city's west side, the city purchased homes and businesses in the area around the University of Maryland BioPark, displacing West Baltimore residents.[39] The city's redevelopment strategy helped spur rapid gentrification in the Poppleton community. A real estate agent unwittingly revealed the exact logic of gentrification underway in Poppleton in 2008:

> Housing is going to be an issue once biotech really gets moving. People are feeling better about the neighborhood, thinking that there will be *better people* [emphasis mine] over there. . . . Everyone's still a little nervous with the market, but the word "biotech" is helping turn things around. A lot of people who come to me say they're looking for a 10-year investment, and that's smart.[40]

The decline in Baltimore's Black population is also a concern although it may not all be due to forced displacement. Between

1990 and 2016, Baltimore saw a decline of Black population of 48,137 people.[41] Although some of this Black decline in population may be due to reverse migration back to the Deep South or a disproportionate number of early Black deaths,[42] another portion of depopulation is due to the housing mobility victory won by Black public housing residents in the *Thompson v. HUD* consent decree that resulted in 3,500 or so Black families being given vouchers to live in the counties surrounding Baltimore City.[43] While the exact numbers are not clear, the loss of Black population has contributed to the declining student populations of Black public schools. As noted earlier, low student population is used as one of the main rationales to permanently close Black public schools.

Black Depopulation and Gentrification

On the flip side of Black depopulation and displacement, Baltimore City subsidizes wealthier and demographically whiter populations to live in the city. One of the major ways gentrification is incentivized is through public-private city and employer grant programs such as Live Near Your Work (LNYW).[44] Baltimore's historically segregating universities have been especially prolific in using gentrification grants. JHMI has offered grants of up to $36,000 for its professional (i.e., full-time, benefits earning) employees.[45] By comparison, JHMI's nonprofessional employees who are subcontracted through a separate entity—named Broadway Services—are only eligible to obtain grants up to $5,000 to move into East Baltimore and Central Baltimore neighborhoods.[46] In January 2018, the University of Maryland Baltimore announced it was offering LNYW grants of up to $16,000 for its employees to move to its surrounding West Baltimore communities—Barre Circle, Franklin Square, Hollins Market, Pigtown, Poppleton, Mount Clare, and Union Square.[47]

Homer Favor, a renowned economist and urban scholar who taught at Morgan State University, was prescient about the return of Whites to the city after many had been fleeing since the desegregation of schools after the Supreme Court handed down *Brown v. Board of Education* in 1954. In a seminal 1978 interview in the *Baltimore Afro-American*, he commented: "There is some question about who the city is being revitalized for. . . . It seems to me that the city has indicated that it will attempt to solve the city's problems by bringing in middle class and upper middle class privileged— basically whites and dislocating the blacks who are here and then viewing this transformation as a major accomplishment."[48]

Favor's assessment would prove prophetic. A March 2019 study found Baltimore ranked sixth nationally in intensity of gentrification (measured by percentage of eligible census tracts gentrified) and seventh nationally in average Black population loss in census tracts experiencing gentrification between 2000 and 2010.[49] Study maps show gentrification taking place in Station North and Greenmount West in Central Baltimore near the Maryland Institute College of Art and in McElderry Park, Patterson Place, and CARE in East Baltimore.[50] However, other communities, such as Remington in the city center, have also experienced rapid development that threatens the housing stability of existing lower-income Black residents. Since 2000, Remington has witnessed an influx of capital and investments funding new businesses such Johns Hopkins Homewood Physicians, Howard Bank, and R House. But as new development raised the neighborhood's fortunes, Remington's Black population declined 11.4% between 2000 and 2010 while all other racial and ethnic groups saw increases in population.[51]

The Five Stages of Publicly Subsidized Gentrification

The public funding of gentrification policies—through mechanisms such Live Near Your Work or tax breaks for Arts and Entertainment Districts—amounts to a subsidy for a wealthier and demographically whiter group of residents to move into these communities. Data show that gentrification can take place with

Black residents in the White L (e.g., Remington) or in neighborhoods in the Black Butterfly. When gentrification in the form of neighborhood turnover hits redlined Black communities, it is part of a five-stage process:

- Stage 1: governments redline Black communities and deprive them of critical economic resources
- Stage 2: redlined communities fall into disrepair and crime and violence rise due to lack of resources
- Stage 3: the communities are declared "blighted" and residents "diseased" with no hope for a turnaround, requiring and justifying a "reset" involving the demolition of the community and the uprooting of the residents (paid for with public dollars)
- Stage 4: public governments create subsidies for developers and incentives for wealthier and demographically whiter residents to move in
- Stage 5: outside developers "revitalize" the neighborhood with the former residents out of the way, accelerating the pace of displacement, rebrand or rename the neighborhood, and erase the historical legacy of the previous residents

Hence, gentrification is not simply "the private market at work." Gentrification is the culmination of public policies and practices, including government-sanctioned redlining on the front end, government-financed demolition and displacement in the middle, and government-subsidized incentives and grants for incoming corporations and people at the end. This is also why gentrification does not amount to desegregation. Pushing out lower-income Black people for "better people" does not result in a community where resources have been desegregated and everyone has opportunity. Instead, gentrification is the latest manifestation of serial forced displacement, one that ends with rebranding Black communities and erasing Black history.[52]

White L communities are more consistently able to operate with sufficient capital flows. They are rarely subjected to the economic deprivation and policy prescriptions of stages 1, 2, and 3. Meanwhile, most Black Butterfly communities are often stuck in stages 1 and 2, with the only prescription for solutions being stages 3–5. They are denied capital and resources that restrict their ability to develop their community and address community issues. When stage 3 arrives, it is disruptive, and residents are not involved in making decisions that impact the communities they live in.

In the Fulton Heights community in West Baltimore, Black residents organized and planted yard signs on Payson Street that read "Stop Demolishing and Rebuild Our Neighborhoods" and "We Need Our Homes Not Unsightly Trashed Green Spaces" in a direct rebuke to the way that vacant homes were demolished by the City of Baltimore.[53] Residents in the Fulton Heights Community Association clearly understand that they are on the verge of entering stage 3, where their neighborhood will be demolished and they will be uprooted. If and when development comes, they will not be around to benefit from it.

The path from redlining to gentrification can be seen more clearly once all the dots are connected in sequence. In redlined Black neighborhoods, publicly owned or publicly subsidized properties are often kept in a state of disrepair by government agencies such as the HABC or HUD as their properties do not receive the proper maintenance funds from Congress to keep the developments up to par. The neighborhoods surrounding HABC or HUD properties are redlined by both private banks and city government leading to scarce resources and limited opportunity. Eventually, this contributes to the escalation of crime and violence as people trapped in these dynamics struggle to make ends meet.

After decades of economic deprivation, HABC announces that public dollars will be used to demolish residential units in these areas, often citing crime, violence, and blighted conditions as the reason entire units must be torn down. Examples of this include public housing developments such as Somerset Court in the Oldtown neighborhood or apartments such as Pall Mall in Park Heights and Madison Park North in Reservoir Hill. Lower-income Black residents are uprooted as these properties are torn down.[54]

Following the clearing of the land and the uprooting of lower-income people, suddenly new developments are announced that will "revitalize" the now empty area. Private developers are able to swoop in and purchase the land—often with public subsidies or tax breaks such as tax increment financing (TIFs) or payments in lieu of taxes (PILOTs). In the Oldtown neighborhood, Beatty Development Group is leading a group of developers executing the Oldtown Mall Redevelopment project adjacent to where the Somerset public housing residents once lived. In the area where Pall Mall Apartments once stood, Park Heights Renaissance will soon identify a developer to revitalize that community. On the plot where Madison Park North apartments once stood in Reservoir Hill, the $100 million Innovation Village development was announced led by MCB Real Estate.[55] In the Inner Harbor community, the $900 million Perkins Somerset Oldtown (PSO) Redevelopment project will also be co-led by the Beatty Development Group. Residents currently living in the Perkins Homes public housing community near the Inner Harbor face potential displacement, depending on whether the one-for-one unit replacement mandate of the federal Choice Neighborhoods grant is honored by HABC and HUD.[56]

Every completion of the five-stage cycle of publicly subsidized gentrification pulls the rug out from under Black families already struggling to make it. Often, publicly funded gentrification destabilizes Black neighborhoods and accelerates the spread of chaos and despair rooted in the feeling that the economic and political forces affecting their lives are beyond their control. Repeatedly uprooting people against their will only results in shuffling lower-income people between struggling redlined communities instead of addressing the segrenomics and spatial inequity at the root.

Hyperpolicing the Black Butterfly

Much of the physical and psychological violence affecting Black communities comes from hyperpolicing. From 1992 to 2002, Baltimore Police Department (BPD) officers killed 127 city residents.[57] BPD also inflicted other less deadly but impactful forms of violence. On September 28, 2014, Mark Puente published a powerful investigative series entitled "Undue Force" that outlined the multiple violent abuses by BPD officers against Black residents in the city.[58] On April 23, 2015—as mass protests shook the city after Freddie Gray's death—*Baltimore Sun* reporters Doug Donavan and Mark Puente published another story outlining multiple instances of Baltimoreans seriously harmed by "rough rides" in the back of BPD police vehicles after detainment.[59] On May 9, 2015, reporters Mark Puente and Meredith Cohn documented BPD's denial of medical care for suspects who needed medical intake before being taken to Central Booking.[60]

BPD had also implemented a widespread stop-and-frisk regime under Mayors Kurt Schmoke, Martin O'Malley, Sheila Dixon, and Stephanie Rawlings-Blake. Over a 25-year period between 1980 and 2014, BPD made 536,005 total drug arrests as a part of Baltimore's War on Drugs. Black residents were slightly less than two-thirds of the city population, but nearly 90% of drug arrests during that time.[61] In effect, BPD's actions were less of a generalized War on Drugs and more of a war on redlined Black communities. These arrests often tied up Black residents in the criminal justice system, preventing them from obtaining jobs once background checks were performed.

Beyond lethal violence and drug arrests, BPD operated a large-scale technological surveillance apparatus aimed at tracking protesters and residents. BPD partnered with a social media firm called ZeroFOX to track the social media activities of Baltimore's activists who were calling for police accountability and reform—especially groups like Baltimore Bloc and activist DeRay Mckesson.[62] BPD also used military technology and a variety of social media platforms to continue tracking police accountability activists.[63] Additional investigative reporting uncovered BPD's illegal use of tracking technology called Stingray to intercept cell phone signals for entire areas where the device was deployed.[64] A Texas billionaire even funneled money through the Baltimore Community Foundation to conduct secret aerial surveillance for BPD without revealing the program to elected officials or to the general public.[65]

Perhaps the strongest documentation of BPD's abusive policing would come from the August 2016 US Department of Justice's (DOJ) *Investigation of the Baltimore City Police Department*. In the 163-page report, DOJ officials in the Obama administration found that the BPD engaged in an unconstitutional pattern or practice of policing, targeting African Americans in the city using discriminatory enforcement strategies and excessive force.[66] The DOJ also concluded that the BPD mistreated victims of sexual assault and mishandled people with mental illnesses. Much of this mistreatment is an outgrowth of the thinking BPD adopted—a mindset that it is at war with residents in the Black Butterfly. As evidence of this, BPD maintains what the police commissioner calls a "war room" and officers' shifts are called a "tour of duty."[67]

To top it all off, a unit within the police department operated as a criminal gang for nearly 10 years.[68] In 2018, eight convicted police officers in the Gun Trace Task Force (GTTF) were caught selling drugs they had looted from looters and stealing money from people who were selling drugs. The officers also pleaded guilty to stealing money from Baltimore City by using false overtime claims, committing wire fraud, and engaging in racketeering.[69] In 2019, another officer, who assisted GTTF in its brazen acts of criminality, was indicted revealing an even wider scope of complicity in criminal behavior by Baltimore police officers.[70]

The sprawling constellation of deadly excessive force, expansive stop-and-frisk, sweeping surveillance, the pattern and practice of racist policing, and the GTTF gang enterprise has destroyed the public trust in the BPD for many people living in redlined Black neighborhoods. While White neighborhoods have been afforded constitutional policing, Black neighborhoods have been subjected to hyperpolicing. The DOJ summed up many people's view of BPD:

> Central to this divide is the perception that there are "two Baltimores" receiving dissimilar policing services. One is affluent and predominately white, while the other is impoverished and largely black. The notion that residents in more affluent neighborhoods receive better policing services than residents in poor neighborhoods was evident in many of our conversations with community members. The disparities described to us go beyond aggressive behavior and misconduct; some residents spoke about a police non-response to poor, minority areas as well as a lack of thorough investigation into crimes committed in these communities.[71]

As the DOJ's findings highlighted, many Black residents not only feel overpoliced but also underprotected. This is a quintessential paradox of Black life in redlined Black communities that undermines the right to equitable public safety. Most residents want BPD officers to apprehend the people who have killed their loved ones or committed sexual violence. But without the ability to turn to BPD for thorough and fair investigations, many residents feel profoundly unprotected and left without a sense that justice has been served. The lack of accountability and community control of police severely damages the ability of people in redlined Black communities to experience quality public safety.

Hyperpolicing Black Neighborhoods Nationwide

The hyperpolicing deployed in Baltimore is not an anomaly. It occurs nationwide, particularly in deeply redlined Black neighborhoods. In 1968, the scholars who wrote the Kerner Commission report predicted the rise of hyperpolicing and oversurveillance in hypersegregated cities. They understood that hypersegregation would lead to hyperpolicing and urban uprisings would lead to whitelash, which is in many ways exactly what happened. They wrote:

> If the Negro population as a whole developed even stronger feelings of being wrongly "penned in" and discriminated against, many of its members might come to support not only riots, but the rebellion now being preached by only a handful. Large-scale violence, followed by white retaliation could follow. This spiral could quite conceivably lead to a kind of urban apartheid with semi-martial law in many major cities, enforced residence of Negroes in segregated areas, and a drastic reduction in personal freedom for all Americans, particularly Negroes.[72]

During the first wave of the Great Rebellion, "urban apartheid with semi-martial law" would be enforced against "Negroes in segregated areas" in cities such as Ferguson (2014), Baltimore (2015), Minneapolis (2016), Baton Rouge (2016), Charlotte (2016), Milwaukee (2017), and St. Louis (2017). City officials deployed semi-martial law to quell direct actions and disruptive shutdowns in the aftermath of police officers shooting and killing Black people or in the wake of police officers responsible for these shootings not being indicted or convicted. The Movement for Black Lives and Black Lives Matter emerged as responses to ongoing hyperpolicing of Black communities and traumatic police violence.

How did militarized hyperpolicing in Black neighborhoods become so entrenched in America? The legal framework did not spring out of thin air. While most people have associated the rise of hyperpolicing with President Richard Nixon and the War on Drugs, the groundwork was laid by President Lyndon Johnson. During the Great Uprising (1963–1971), Johnson signed two of the most sweeping pieces of legislation that strengthened and bolstered policing in urban areas—the Law Enforcement Assistance Act of 1965 and the Omnibus Crime Control and Safe Streets Act of 1968. Those acts helped to create a state of semi-martial law and hyperpolicing in large cities across the nation.[73]

In addition to federal legislation, Supreme Court case law laid the ground for discriminatory and aggressive policing in redlined Black neighborhoods. Discriminatory Supreme Court case law means that Black neighborhoods are hyperpoliced precisely because they are hypersegregated even while they are redlined and subprimed. Starting in 1968, the Supreme Court decided cases that authorized stop-and-frisk, ignored racial biases in police shootings, legalized differential policing, and supported the use of evidence obtained from unconstitutional policing.

- *Terry v. Ohio* (1968) held that the Fourth Amendment prohibition on unreasonable searches and seizures is not violated when a police officer stops a suspect on the street and frisks him or her without probable cause to arrest, if the police officer has a reasonable suspicion that the person has committed, is committing, or is about to commit a crime and has a reasonable belief that the person "may be armed and presently dangerous."[74]
- *Graham v. Connor* (1989) applies the "objective reasonableness" standard to determine whether an officer is in fear of their lives when a police officer shoots a person in the line of duty.[75]
- *Illinois v. Wardlow* (2000) allows differential policing when an area is designated as a "high crime area" where "unprovoked flight" becomes the basis for reasonable suspicion.[76]

- *Utah v. Strieff* (2016) allows that unconstitutional stops can still produce evidence to be used in court.[77]

These pivotal Supreme Court case laws would be paired with Johnson's law enforcement bills (1965 and 1968), followed by Nixon's executive orders authorizing the War on Drugs (early 1970s), and capped by President Bill Clinton's Violent Crime Control and Law Enforcement Act of 1994 that together would coalesce and congeal into a legal nationwide system of hyperpolicing Black neighborhoods. The icing on the cake was militarizing police departments nationwide with the little known but heavily used 1033 Program, [78] which allows the US Department of Defense to pass on surplus military equipment to police departments around the nation. During the 2014 Ferguson Insurrection and the 2015 Baltimore Uprising, protesters were greeted with tanks and heavy artillery supplied through the 1033 Program.

Hyperpolicing and hypersegregation go hand-in-hand. The intensity of policing often reflects the intensity of government-enforced racial segregation. Research shows that areas with higher levels of racism and racial segregation feature higher levels of police violence. Mesic and colleagues found greater disparity in the rates of police shooting Black versus White people when a state's racism index is elevated.[79] The higher a state's racism index, the greater the likelihood that police will shoot Black people compared to White people. This is consistent with another study by Brad Smith and Malcolm Holmes who found more sustained excessive force complaints from residents who live in cities with higher levels of residential racial segregation.[80] A 2019 study examining fatal police shootings of Black people in the 75 largest cities in America between 2013 and 2017 found that police violence increases as racial segregation rises, resulting in more police killings in hypersegregated cities compared with cities with lower levels of racial segregation.[81]

Hypersegregated cities would not be the only ones to experience hyperpolicing. Following the police lynching of George Floyd, the vast apparatus of militarized hyperpolicing in America was unveiled. Police and military forces were deployed in massive numbers by the end of the first week after protests and uprisings started. According to the *Washington Post*:

> Nationwide, more than 60 million people were under curfews as a result of the protests, in 200 cities and 27 states. . . . At least 17,000 National Guard troops have been activated in response. In Washington—where peaceful protests and looting rampages have both occurred in recent days—downtown streets were full of Army trucks and federal agents on Tuesday.
>
> On Monday night, Army helicopters had flown low over protesters in Washington, blasting them with high wind from the rotors—a dangerous maneuver used to intimidate enemies on overseas battlefields. It was a moment unlike any in recent American history, as hundreds of cities already beset by the coronavirus pandemic faced a historic wave of protests.[82]

After a week of unrelenting and peaceful protests punctuated by riotous upheaval, President Trump became frustrated with the nation's governors. The president deployed federal law enforcement and activated military personnel to crush the Great Rebellion.[83] Flustered by the vastness of the nationwide uprisings and militant protests, Trump excoriated governors in a blistering phone conference on June 1. According to CNN transcripts, he encouraged a plan of action:

> You have to dominate. If you don't dominate, you're wasting your time. They're going to run all over you, you'll look like a bunch of jerks. You have to dominate, and you have to arrest people, and you have to try people and they have to go to jail for long periods of time. . . .

This is a movement. . . . This is like Occupy Wall Street. It was a disaster until one day, somebody said, that's enough and they just went in and wiped them out and that's the last time we ever heard the name Occupy Wall Street . . . [84]

As protestors decried the use of excessive force, police responded with even more force against journalists, bystanders, and protest participants.[85] Democrats and Republicans rushed to put together federal legislation to curb the power and abuse of police as a response to public outcry. Congressional Democrats proposed the Justice in Policing Act, but the bill faced an uphill battle with an obstinate GOP controlling the Senate and President Trump in the White House.[86]

Economic Destruction and Wealth Extraction Today

Black neighborhoods have consistently weathered withering economic attacks across America. Government-enforced racial segregation and repeated uprootings have resulted in capital denial in and wealth extraction from Black communities—whether through redlining, subpriming, or demolishing and dispossessing Black land, homes, businesses, churches, schools, and institutions. Black wealth is also decimated when forcible relocation summarily severs Black social networks and bonds. Collectively, the multiple forms of wealth extraction and capital denial result in the economic underdevelopment of Black neighborhoods.

Research shows that the federal Residential Security Maps, initially drawn in the 1930s, have an enduring effect on housing values today. Bruce Mitchell and Juan Franco found that 75% of the communities that were officially redlined by the federal Home Owners' Loan Corporation in the 1930s are still damaged today.[87] Sarah Mikhitarian's work reveals that home values in red color-coded communities are still below the value of homes built in green, blue, and yellow color-coded communities with precise figures.[88] Andre Perry and colleagues found that Black homeowners' homes are worth $48,000 less than their White counterparts, due to the devaluation of homes in Black neighborhoods.[89]

Black homebuyers in Baltimore are still denied fair access to capital for home mortgages and small businesses. The National Community Reinvestment Coalition (NCRC) documented ongoing redlining by private banks in Baltimore City between 2011 and 2013.[90] NCRC also found ongoing redlining in other Category 5 hypersegregated cities, such as Milwaukee and St. Louis along with Minneapolis and St. Paul between 2012 and 2016.[91] A 2019 analysis by S&P Global Market Intelligence authors found that bank closures were disproportionately clustered in Black neighborhoods.[92]

On the flip side of redlining, however, is subpriming, or predatory lending, where Black homebuyers are charged a higher interest rate compared to their White counterparts. Advocates such as Walter P. Carter and Activists for Fair Housing Inc. documented and challenged the devastation wrought by contract lenders in the 1960s and early 1970s.[93] Because of bank redlining, Black homebuyers were often forced to rely on White contract lenders who financed "blockbusting" and charged Black homebuyers a severe surcharge.[94] In their report, Activists for Fair Housing referred to this financially punitive arrangement as the "Black Tax."

More recently, national and regional banks such as Wells Fargo, JP Morgan Chase, Bank of America, M&T, PNC, and BB&T all engaged in predatory mortgage lending in Black neighborhoods in Baltimore and other urban areas, particularly in the period leading up to the housing bubble and Great Recession in 2007 and 2008.[95] Because of rampant subprime lending, buying a home while Black has subjected Black homebuyers to paying a racist financial surcharge that White homebuyers do not pay.

The process for banks initiating subprime mortgages was quite devious in Baltimore City. Jacob Rugh and colleagues calculated the Black Tax for Black homebuyers in Black neighborhoods in Baltimore who received subprime loans from Wells Fargo. They found that Black homebuyers with Wells Fargo paid $14,904 more than their White counterparts.[96] They also found that bankers often coercively engaged trusted Black leaders to carry out their subprime scheme:

> Loan originators also reported targeting church leaders in order to gain access to congregants through trusted intermediaries, with the originators often providing a donation to a nonprofit of the borrower or intermediary's choice for each new loan, further cementing the relationship between mortgage lenders and local religious and civic leaders. . . . Solicitations for high-cost subprime loans in predominantly black communities were promoted through "wealth building seminars" held in churches and community centers at which "alternative lending" was discussed. No such solicitations were made in predominantly white neighborhoods or churches.[97]

While Black religious and civic leaders thought they were engaging in wealth building, Wells Fargo was engaged in wealth extraction. While much of the blame belongs to banks that engaged in such practices, some attention must also be directed at the quid pro quo arrangements that benefited Black religious and civic leaders while their followers suffered.

Baltimore's economic development triumvirate—led by elected officials, the corporate lobbying group Greater Baltimore Committee (GBC), and the quasi-public economic development agency Baltimore Development Corporation (BDC)—has historically concentrated its efforts to stimulate economic activity in the White L. Between 1940 and 2010, Baltimore's mayors and the GBC vigorously supported urban renewal or urban redevelopment, decimating many Black neighborhoods in Central Baltimore and uprooting over 21,500 Black families. Since the mid-1960s, nearly $3 billion in public subsidies have been allocated to the White L—with nearly

$2 billion by the year 2000 and another $1 billion since then.[98] Much of it has been allocated near the waterfront, or harbor area, in the city.

TIFs and PILOTs have increasingly become the primary tax policy tools intensifying racial inequity as investments are clustered almost exclusively in the White L and absent from the Black Butterfly.[99] The inordinate focus of the BDC and GBC has been tourist-oriented development in the Inner Harbor and commercial activity expansion in Harbor East. White L corporations receive tremendous government support as well as access to public resources to ensure their welfare and success.

Meanwhile, Baltimore's lower-income workers did not receive the same amount of concern for their development or success. In the wake of the April 27, 2015, uprising, Baltimore's large corporations started workforce development programs called BLocal and HopkinsLocal to train and hire workers for jobs. However, the corporations operating BLocal and HopkinsLocal often do not pay their workers a living wage. BLocal and HopkinsLocal would garner positive press for affiliated corporations after the April 2015 uprising, but the same corporations involved in BLocal and HopkinsLocal supported a letter written by GBC Executive Director Donald Fry calling for Mayor Catherine Pugh to veto the $15 an hour minimum wage bill.[100]

HopkinsLocal in particular falls short as the effort's progenitor—JHMI—has resisted an increase in the minimum wage for its workers, fought the unionization of its nurses, and lobbied for special legislation to establish its own private police force in and around its campus locations.[101] HopkinsLocal and BLocal cannot be considered initiatives that help to heal a city while workers must continue to fight for the right to earn living wages, the right to unionize, and the right to live in a city where private corporations fully fund public goods.[102] As a private institution, JHMI was a key signatory in a 2016 tax payment agreement in which the institution agreed to pay $3,260,398, or 5.25% of its full tax assessment of $62,094,762.[103] Instead of using its tax savings to lower the cost of patient care and increase worker salaries, JHMI plowed its tax savings into funding its private police force.

The University of Maryland Medical System's (UMMS) actions also undermined the economic well-being of Baltimore residents. Reporter Luke Broadwater found that UMMS board members spent millions of public dollars enriching the pockets of its fellow board members with no-bid contracts.[104] An audit found that UMMS board members never read Mayor Pugh's books and revealed how board members broke the rules regarding board tenure in order to maintain their scheme:

> The audit concluded that certain board members overstayed their five-year terms on the volunteer board, allowing them to "exercise disproportionate influence" over the system. They included former state Sen. Frank Kelly, who was on the board for 33 years; Pugh, who was on the board for 17 years; Pevenstein, who was on the board for 16 years; and John Dillon, who was on the board for 13 years.[105]

Interestingly, 11 UMMS administrators received salaries over $588,000.[106] If those administrators' salaries were cut in half, it would amount to $3.23 million that could have been used to pay its non-administrative workers living in the city a higher salary. The $3.23 million could have been used to build a collective economy in Baltimore in much the same way as Cleveland anchor institutions have supported worker cooperatives with the Evergreen Cooperative Initiative.[107] As a private institution, the UMMS Medical Center was also included in the 2016 tax payment agreement in which the institution agreed to pay $746,576, or 4.66% of its full tax assessment of $16,035,640.[108] Instead of using its tax savings to lower the cost of patient care and support worker cooperatives using the Evergreen model, UMMS enriched board members and administrators alike.

Large corporations, policymakers, and philanthropy are often loath to tackle systemic factors that pilfer wealth from redlined communities and extract resources from Black neighborhoods. When uprisings occur in redlined Black neighborhoods, these same entities vow to "do better" but then proceed to oppose raising the minimum wage and resist the unionization of workers while supporting the creation of private police forces. Making matters worse, large corporations were found to engage in quid pro quo by paying money ostensibly for children's books from Mayor Pugh while expecting and receiving large contracts from the City of Baltimore.[109]

Facilitators for the People's Institute for Survival and Beyond summarize the issues confronting people living in redlined Black neighborhoods in their *Undoing Racism* training when they assert that, "People aren't poor because they lack programs and services. People are poor because they lack power." Black communities are not economically poor because they lack programs and services. Black communities have historically lacked the power to stop the economic destruction, wealth extraction, and resource withdrawals taking place in their communities at the hands of predatory banks, subprime landlords, universities, hospital nonprofits, and city governments. Poverty in Black neighborhoods is not a function of residents' personal attributes, nor their lack of hard work, nor their inability to financially manage money. Poverty is the result of intentional and ill-informed government, corporate, and philanthropic policies and practices that block sustainable public and private allocations of resources to redlined Black neighborhoods, resulting in their severe economic underdevelopment.

White Power and Operative Whiteness in the Chocolate City

Baltimore is one of America's remaining large majority Black cities—or what some call Chocolate Cities. It may be surprising given the city's demographic composition, but the exclusion of Black people in decision making and governance is often found in Chocolate Cities. For instance, a 2017 analysis revealed:

- In 2015, the Baltimore City Department of Transportation selected the Bike Master Plan Steering Committee: 16 members, all White.[110]
- In 2016, key informants contributed to the Sagamore TIF market analysis for Port Covington: 11 informants, all White (and all men).[111]
- In 2017 and 2018, the *Baltimore Business Journal*'s "Future of Baltimore's Waterfront" panels: 5 members, all White.[112]

The dearth of Black perspectives and voices noted previously means that Black futures are discounted and ignored in the economic development and planning of the city. The City of Baltimore is notorious for prosecuting large economic development schemes that result in the uprootings of lower-income Black people (e.g., urban renewal, Hopkins-EBDI, and the Innovation Village). The city also implements economic development devoid of racial equity (e.g., the now defunct Bike Share or Plank's Sagamore Development Corporation in Port Covington). In Baltimore, the executive leaders of wealthy corporations sponsor Black faces in political spaces with campaign donations. Meanwhile, economic development and planning spaces often omit Black people's input.

This campaign funding dynamic highlights the limitations of "diversity" and "inclusion" in city governance and how historical trauma can continue uninterrupted despite Black political leadership. Because of their significant campaign contributions, the concerns of wealthy corporations are prioritized, while the concerns of people living in redlined Black neighborhoods are minimized. The influence of campaign donations—through checks written by wealthy corporate executives—helps explain how Black political leaders end up passing policies that damage Black Lives and decimate Black futures, particularly when Black politicians' election campaigns are funded in large part by White-owned corporate developers and White-led philanthropies.

A clear example of a policy decision that hurt many lower-income Black Baltimoreans can be found with Mayor Pugh's veto of the $15 an hour minimum wage bill in 2017.[113] This was especially damaging because of Baltimore City's drastic racial income gap. With a median annual household income of $38,688, Black households have a median annual income virtually half that of White households', which stands at $76,922 according to 2016 Census Bureau data.[114] Pugh's veto decision was particularly jarring because she promised as a candidate that she would support the bill by responding to a candidate survey: "I am aware of the current initiative to raise the minimum wage in the City Council to $15 per hour and when it reaches my desk I will sign it."[115]

Keeanga-Yamahtta Taylor adroitly explicates the dynamics of Black political leadership:

> The ascendance of Black electoral politics also dramatizes how class differences can lead to different political strategies in the fight for Black liberation. There have always been class differences among African Americans, but this is the first time those class differences have been expressed in the form of a minority of Blacks wielding significant political power and authority over the majority of Black lives. This raises critical questions about the role of the Black elite in the continuing freedom struggle—and about what side are they on.[116]

Although racial representation matters, electing Black political leaders does not automatically mean that the pressing concerns of lower-income Black people will be represented and addressed.[117] This can be the case if Black political elites lack a structural analysis of urban apartheid or if they have internalized toxic perspectives consistent with spatial racism regarding redlined Black neighborhoods. Black political power will not result in racial equity unless Black political leaders directly address and stop ongoing historical trauma, completely dismantle urban apartheid, and advance racial equity in all institutions, policies, practices, systems, and budgets.

Audrey McFarlane has also shed light on this dynamic with her concept of "operative whiteness" or the way in which members of the Black middle class can harm lower-income Black people particularly when it comes to affordable housing and economic inclusion in neighborhood development. McFarlane explains how

> at different decision-making junctures, affluent Blacks sometimes demonstrate that they have similar incentives to Whites—to avoid, run away from, or oppose projects or endeavors that would benefit lower-income Blacks.

> Thus, Blacks with money are privileged in certain limited circumstances to be operatively white. Through their wallets and educational or professional attainments they gain access to some of the privileges, goods, and services formerly reserved exclusively for Whites.[118]

The influence of campaign donations and the concept of operative whiteness both help answer the critical question, *How can racism be an issue in a Chocolate City with Black political leadership?* As Baltimore City has witnessed firsthand, wealthy corporations work to boost their profits and secure their desired outcomes through their executives' campaign donations. When Black political leaders work to secure the interests of wealthy corporations, they deepen the dynamics of urban apartheid and perpetuate historical trauma. As Audrey McFarlane explains in her work, affluent Black people can and do function as operatively White particularly when serving as elected officials or when holding some measure of power. It is not enough to elect Black political leaders who maintain apartheid systems of city government. Black political leaders have the same obligation to engage in a robust racial equity process as everyone else.

The Whiteness and Corruption of Baltimore's Elite Tier Actors

In addition to the public sector and political leaders, the philanthropic and nonprofit sector wields tremendous power in the governance of Baltimore City (and most other large cities as well). A recent national study found that almost 90% of people serving as board members of large philanthropic organizations were White.[119] This racial disproportionality is also found in Baltimore's philanthropic board leadership. Baltimore's top five largest philanthropic organizations by assets are the Annie E. Casey Foundation ($2.6 billion), the Harry & Jeanette Weinberg Foundation ($2.56 billion), the Abell Foundation ($350 million), T. Rowe Price Program for Charitable Giving ($305 million), and the France-Merrick Foundation ($193.6 million).[120] In a 2018 analysis of board member composition for these five philanthropies, 39 board members were counted. Out of 39 such members whose race could be identified, there were 29 White board members, meaning 74.3% of Baltimore's largest five philanthropic board were White.

The disproportionate whiteness of the wealthiest philanthropies' board members has a tremendous influence on the governance of the city especially in the domain of neighborhood redevelopment and revitalization. Baltimore's hierarchy of power and governance corresponds to the level of assets and resources harnessed by the city's philanthropies and large nonprofits. Urban scholar Madeleine Pill divided Baltimore City's governing hierarchy into three major categories:

- *Elite tier actors*: large philanthropies (e.g., Annie E. Casey Foundation, Weinberg Foundation, Abell Foundation);

corporate developers (e.g., H&S Properties Development, Harbor Point Development Group, Beatty Development Group, Sagamore Development Corporation); the Greater Baltimore Committee; major education and medical anchor institutions (e.g., JHMI, UMMS)[121]

- *Middle tier actors*: other education and medical anchor institutions (e.g., Bon Secours, University of Baltimore, Loyola University, Morgan State University, Coppin State University, Notre Dame, and Maryland Institute College of Art); smaller philanthropies (e.g., Goldseker Foundation, Associated Black Charities, Baltimore Community Foundation, and Association of Baltimore Area Grantmakers); Baltimoreans United in Leadership Development (BUILD)
- *Marginal tier actors*: community groups, neighborhood associations, grassroots nonprofits, and activist organizations[122]

As Pill explains, Baltimore's power dynamic can be summarized as this—the city government follows the lead of elite tier actors and thus the city's planning and economic development actions mirror the elite tier actors' prerogatives and imperatives. Elite actor institutions and organizations have historically been able to set the table or determine the agenda for what takes place in Baltimore. The problem is that whoever sets the table is able to determine the city's agenda and thereby constrain which topics are on the agenda while also framing the issue or topic being discussed. This produces a profound and fundamental blindness to the ongoing historical trauma that damages the Black Butterfly and intensifies Baltimore Apartheid. Through this hierarchy of power, elite tier institutions are able to prioritize the White L and neglect the Black Butterfly.[123]

This is especially true when reviewing just how four of the elite and middle tier philanthropic organizations have actually contributed to ongoing historical trauma and Baltimore Apartheid.

- The Abell Foundation is funded with money from Harry Black who ran the A.S. Abell Company that published the *Baltimore Sun* newspaper. As discussed in Track 2, the *Baltimore Sun* pushed and propagated propaganda that ignited the war against the "Negro Invasion," helping to establish racial segregation in Baltimore City.[124]
- The Goldseker Foundation is funded with money obtained by Morris Goldseker's real estate operation which was founded in 1931.[125] Goldseker operated as a predatory contract lender, speculator, and blockbuster in the Black Butterfly—buying homes cheaply from fleeing Whites (at an average of $6,868) and then selling homes at a 85% markup to Black homebuyers (at an average of $12,706).[126]
- In 2016, it was revealed that the Baltimore Community Foundation had accepted a donation from a Texas billionaire to fund secret aerial surveillance of Baltimore residents.[127]
- The Annie E. Casey Foundation partnered with EBDI to displace 732 Black households in the Middle East community. The foundation invested $36.5 million in EBDI.[128]

It is usually accepted as an unquestioned fact that philanthropies help people with less income, access, and opportunity. But how can Baltimore's philanthropies and foundations possibly help or empower the people living in redlined Black neighborhoods when they do not first acknowledge the ongoing historical trauma they have caused? They cannot. There can be no restoration or healing without engaging in deeply restorative actions to help redlined Black communities heal from the damage that they or their institutional predecessors have inflicted.

If $100 million worth of damage was done, it is not fully restorative to dole out $1 million and call things even. All discussions about inclusion, diversity, and even racial equity ring hollow without acknowledgment, apology, and fully restorative actions. Restoration ultimately means returning the wealth that was pilfered from Black communities so that the people and neighborhoods impacted by historical trauma can decide how they want to allocate the funds to rebuild and repair their neighborhoods. This also means that elite and middle tier actors can no longer continue to dominate discussions of development in Baltimore nor set the table for discussions if the work of racial equity is to take place.

In fact, Baltimore's vertically structured hierarchy of power must be altogether flattened if the city is to forge an equitable future. Baltimore's elite actors have aided and abetted the maintenance of Baltimore Apartheid. Recent revelations of rank corruption and conflicts of interest not only underscore the ethical bankruptcy of the elite tier but also reveal the ways racial equity in Baltimore is thwarted. On January 9, 2019, nine executives affiliated with Johns Hopkins University and Johns Hopkins Hospital simultaneously donated to the campaign coffers of then Mayor Catherine Pugh to secure legislative support for the institution's private police force.[129] It was a classic case of quid pro quo. In March 2019, news emerged that nine UMMS board members—including current and former politicians—were receiving millions of dollars in no-bid contracts using public dollars. As Mark Reutter explained:

> Conflicts of interest and lack of accountability suddenly seemed to be rife under [UMMS president and CEO Robert "Bob"] Chrencik's watch, with special friends allegedly receiving special treatment. Perhaps most striking was the case of Francis X. Kelly Jr. As an influential state senator from Baltimore County, Kelly helped Chrencik privatize the University of Maryland Hospital in 1984.

Ever since, Kelly has served on the UMMS board of directors, at times as its chairman. Over the same years, Kelly created one of the country's largest family-owned insurance companies. Among its most loyal clients turn out to be UMMS-controlled hospitals.[130]

In other words, the privatization of UMMS turned out to be a privatize-and-profit scheme where business executives and politicians enriched themselves with public dollars.[131] At the same time, UMMS as an institution was able to ensure that public policies that worked in its favor would be passed even though it was now operating as a private entity.

Baltimore's corporate corruption schemes reveal how elite tier actor institutions are able to use campaign donations and quid pro quo arrangements to distort political outcomes and dictate public policy. These corruption schemes also reveal how elite tier actors—such as UMMS and JHMI—are able to influence Black government officials to push and pass public policies that advance their private interests. As long as elite tier actors' representatives are able to bundle campaign donations and establish quid pro quo arrangements for their benefit, a mockery is made of democracy and the voices of the disenfranchised are muted. The presence of corporate corruption means that racial equity cannot become a reality.

State Takeovers

Another way that local democracy is undermined is through a state takeover or state control of city systems or institutions. The partial state control of the city police department and partial state takeover of the Baltimore public schools have undermined local democratic input and governance in two of the most critical institutions that affect the lives of Black Baltimoreans. The damage that can be done by state takeovers is perhaps most vividly demonstrated by the toxic lead exposure crisis in Flint, Michigan, where the state takeover of a majority Black city gave authority to the city's emergency manager. The emergency manager's decisions concretized saving money over saving lives.

According to education scholar Domingo Morel, state takeovers are most common in cities with larger Black and/or Latino/a populations.[132] Morel found that state takeovers of local education systems in majority Black and Brown cities become a policy option precisely at the point when Black and/or Latino/a political empowerment in cities become a reality.[133] The rationale was clear: to undermine Black and Brown municipal political control.

State takeovers have many of the same deleterious effects as the privatization of public goods—the loss of local political accountability, the removal of democratic decision making, and the disempowerment of people living in redlined neighborhoods. Both privatization and state takeovers block attempts to deepen democracy and empower people living in affected neighborhoods. Only by de-privatizing public goods and finding ways to boost local neighborhood governance can cities foster the participatory engagement and self-determination that will catalyze equitable community economic development, particularly in redlined Black neighborhoods.

Conclusion

After the start of the Great Migration in 1910, the war against the "Negro Invasion" tightened the grip of American Apartheid. As the end of the Great Migration augured the rise of majority Black cities and a wave of Black mayors in 1970, a multiracial array of public and private political and corporate leaders partnered to prosecute a spatial war targeting Black neighborhoods. The spatial war on Black neighborhoods unleashed various components of ongoing historical trauma, including hypersegregation, resource withdrawal, hyperpolicing, economic destruction, and wealth extraction.

To maintain urban apartheid in many cities with large Black populations, these cities are characterized by a hierarchy of power that features what urban scholar John Arena calls a "black public wing" on one side and a "mainly white corporate wing that controls the most important economic institutions" on the other side.[134] Because of the racial wealth and income gaps, the Black public wing is often susceptible to the financial incentives offered by the mainly White corporate wing, whether in campaign donations or quid pro quo arrangements once in office. The combination of ongoing historical trauma and corruption embedded in governing arrangements contributes to Black neighborhoods' exploitation.

During her speech to her fellow Mississippians who were afraid of joining the Civil Rights Movement in September 1964, the great freedom fighter and sharecropper Fannie Lou Hamer prodded the audience and spoke to the reality of American Apartheid:

> It's no need of running and no need of saying,
> "Honey, I'm not going to get in the mess,"
> because if you were born in America with a black face,
> you were born in the mess.

Black people living in Black neighborhoods are in the mess of hypersegregation and hyperpolicing in Baltimore, Chicago, St. Louis, Flint, Detroit, Milwaukee, and beyond. Black neighborhoods are mired in the muck of economic deprivation, corrupted elite tier actors, corrupted politicians, harmful philanthropies, and devastating state takeovers. To get out of this mess, Baltimore City—along with other cities and counties—must engage in a relentless assessment of policies, practices, budgets, and systems to determine what damage has been done to Black Lives and Black neighborhoods. *Municipalities and their elite tier actors—*

philanthropies, nonprofits, and corporations—must work to pass, implement, and enforce policies and practices to swiftly dismantle municipal apartheid, flatten hierarchies of power, root out corruption, and end ongoing historical trauma (Step 2).

This means putting mechanisms in place to prevent corruption and block conflicts of interest so that elite tier actors can no longer disrupt political processes and hijack democracy. This means not only disrupting whiteness in the form of lack of racial representation but also challenging the operative whiteness of middle-class Black political leaders who participate in the project of urban apartheid. This means de-privatizing public goods and undoing state takeovers so that democratic decision making is returned to cities and communities that were disenfranchised based on their racial composition.

Black communities also have a role to play. They must work to disrupt the politics of corruption and ensure that Black leaders work as advocates for racial equity instead of as surrogates for corporate imperatives. In a representative democracy, Black public officials must operate in a way that is ethical and must eschew the quid pro quo arrangements that undermine racial equity. With the advent of open data and computing technology, online information tools can be developed that can facilitate multiple analyses of how corporations are unduly influencing Black elected leaders. This can be used to empower voters to ask serious questions of all elected officials but also to hold all elected officials accountable as advocates for racial equity instead of surrogates for corporate imperatives.

Fostering racial equity is required to build a twenty-first-century America where everyone can thrive and reach their full potential. Racial equity work can and should be done by everyone who lives in Baltimore City and across America. Racial equity involves deep democratic listening and equitable engagement with those who are most affected by apartheid institutions, policies, practices, budgets, and systems. An authentic municipal racial equity process produces spatial equity—with required resources and rich opportunity in all neighborhoods. This can only manifest when people in historically marginalized neighborhoods can participate meaningfully and deeply in economic development discussions and can set the table for what community development should look like in their neighborhood.

But municipalities should be forewarned—the work of racial equity is not a lighthearted affair. Implementing racial equity is not a short term project or quick fix. Fostering racial equity requires a reiterative wrestling with ramifications of American Apartheid. A reckoning is required to accurately assess the costs of American Apartheid as it relates to Black neighborhoods and Black Lives. This reiterative reckoning must account for damages inflicted during America's wars to crush Black Reconstruction, halt the "Negro Invasion," and stymie Black neighborhoods. It might be helpful to think of components of ongoing historical trauma as akin to a cataclysmic meteor shower where massive asteroids rain down on the ground of Black neighborhoods leaving immense craters (i.e., wounds and gashes). The constant orbital bombardment of ongoing historical trauma on Black neighborhoods from the outer space platform of American Apartheid exacts a tremendous toll. What happens to redlined Black neighborhoods when this bombardment does not cease?

Black Neighborhood Destruction

Wacky wizards concocted a spell you see.
It would be the instrument that allowed racial segregation
into housing, education, and financial institutions' policies.
Monique Gardner, "Red Raisin: A Fairytale Story"

Gray skies over Baltimore
Have me craving and wanting more
How can I . . . when I'm equipped
with Hardship and Hood-ish
Governed by Lunatic Politics
-No scholarship or leadership
Just disrespect and neglect/ ed
houses and abandonminiums
And living life at a minimum
Nakisha Gaddy, "Harm City, Murderland"

Black neighborhoods in America have survived two urban wars: the war against the "Negro Invasion" and the war on Black neighborhoods. The challenge for community development and public health in America's redlined Black neighborhoods is understanding how the health and well-being of Black individuals have been undermined by American Apartheid. This means identifying the "spell" that has been cast on Black neighborhoods and addressing the realities of "living life at a minimum." The spell proliferating hardship, hood-ish, and lunatic politics is structural violence, which has undermined Black communities thereby directly diminishing Black health outcomes. Without this context, public health practitioners and researchers fail to successfully combat the diseases and health risks that shorten the life spans of people of African descent in America. Without a reckoning of the damages caused by spatial wars, there can be no healing in the form of spatial equity.

During the mid-twentieth-century push for civil rights, Black neighborhoods were subjected to destruction from successive policies and practices of uprooting: slum clearance, land dispossession, urban renewal, highway construction, the reduction of public goods, gentrification, and mass incarceration. As Black people gained political rights, Black neighborhoods were being torn apart. This weakened their social and cultural integrity and stability. All the while, rural and coastal Black landowners were losing critical farmland and waterfront properties. To borrow a rap music phrasing from Houston, Texas, even as movements for Civil Rights and Black Power were underway, Black neighborhoods were being chopped and screwed.

The Elements of Black Neighborhood Destruction

As a result of spatial racism, there are eight main elements proliferating community health crises and catastrophes in redlined Black neighborhoods: (1) root shock, (2) internal colonization, (3) resource apartheid, (4) toxic lead exposure, (5) housing precarity, (6) racism-based traumatic stress, (7) homicides, and (8) urban uprisings. While these elements do not occur in a neat sequential or linear fashion, they do stack one on top of the other, acting synergistically when mixed together. This is not an exhaustive list of issues, but through this analytical framework, it can be shown how the fabric of redlined Black neighborhoods becomes frayed and how these neighborhoods are pushed to the edge.

Root Shock

Urban scholars and journalists are increasingly knowledgeable about the harms caused by government-enforced racial segregation. Comparatively speaking, the damage caused by serial forced displacement is nearly completely overlooked in national discussions. This is especially true when considering how often Black neighborhoods have been uprooted and destroyed. Nearly 100 Black communities or cities were destroyed by white supremacist urban violence. Two prime examples of such destruction include Black Wall Street in Tulsa, Oklahoma (1921), and Rosewood, Florida (1923). In addition to this urban violence, hundreds of Black neighborhoods were laid waste by the successive rapid fire of federal and local policies and practices such as urban renewal, highway construction, code enforcement, mass incarceration, and land dispossession.

Historically, the federal government has been a primary purveyor of forced displacement in urban areas across the nation. Three pivotal pieces of federal policy helped spark urban upheavals for many Black communities: the Housing Act of 1949, the Housing Act of 1954, and the Federal-Aid Highway Act of 1956.[1] The two housing acts authorized and provided federal funding for urban renewal, while the highway act funded a massive system of freeways that displaced large numbers of Black families. In a televised program in June 1963, writer James Baldwin acidly described urban renewal: "San Francisco is now engaged . . . as most northern cities are now engaged in something called 'urban renewal' which means moving Negroes out. It means Negro Removal—that is what it means."[2]

Making matters worse, urban renewal intensified racial segregation. The Maryland State Conference of the NAACP—led by the activist Lillie Mae Carroll Jackson—argued this exact point in an NAACP 1951 letter to a federal official leading the government's slum clearance and urban redevelopment efforts. The Maryland NAACP warned: "The Baltimore, Maryland slum clearance and redevelopment program deprives colored people of living spaces and places the full strength of the Federal Government behind a policy of rigid racial segregation in that city."[3]

Lillie Mae Carroll Jackson and the Maryland NAACP were proved correct based on empirical research by Jessica Trounstine almost 70 years later. Trounstine found that, as spending on urban renewal in cities across the nation increased, racial segregation increased.[4] Baltimore City was one of the nation's worst offenders. Baltimore City spent a huge amount on urban renewal (i.e., Negro Removal) meaning that Baltimore's urban renewal program not only uprooted tens of thousands of Black residents but also simultaneously boosted Baltimore Apartheid and strengthened the city's spatial racial segregation. Compared to Chicago, which spent more than $200 million on urban renewal, Baltimore spent a whopping $900 million on its urban renewal projects despite having a quarter of Chicago's population.[5]

While urban renewal tore apart Black neighborhoods from the 1950s to the mid-1970s, the Federal-Aid Highway Act of 1956 authorized the construction of over 40,000 miles of new highways across the country. The disruptive construction of many urban highways demolished often solid and stable Black communities in Washington, DC, Atlanta, Memphis, Kansas City, Pittsburgh, Ft. Lauderdale, Birmingham, Seattle, Charlotte, Miami, and Baltimore.[6] Local governments partnered with the federal government to displace millions of Black people in urban areas.[7] Meanwhile, discriminatory policies and practices by officials in the United States Department of Agriculture helped lead to the rapid dispossession and loss of millions of acres of Black-owned farmland in rural areas.

These federal and local forced uprootings and land disposses- sions were carried out amid tremendous global economic and social upheaval. Beginning around 1950, many manufacturing jobs were outsourced to countries outside the United States as manufacturers sought to take advantage of low-wage laborers around the world. This resulted in the cataclysmic reduction of higher-paying jobs for working-class people. In addition, on the heels of the Great Uprising, President Richard Nixon began what became known as the War on Drugs in 1972–1973 by signing Executive Order 11727.[8] The War on Drugs (targeting redlined Black communities) would contribute to the rise of mass incarceration of Black Americans accompanied by the escalation of militarized policing of Black neighborhoods.

This toxic combination of government policies and practices uncorked root shock and triggered a surge of health and social crises in redlined Black neighborhoods by the mid-1980s.[9] Root shock is at the heart of ongoing historical trauma in Black neighborhoods in America. It induces emotional trauma in individuals impacted and ruptures bonds in uprooted communities. The impact of root shock is catastrophic; it disables community cohesion, instigates social chaos, and undermines mental and physical Black health. Repeated forced removals continue to have a destructive impact on the health and wellness of people living in Black neighborhoods.[10]

Writer and playwright Ntozake Shange lamented the effects of uprootings in Black neighborhoods:

> When the freeways came through our communities, the African American ones, my home was disappeared along with thousands of others. We were left with no business districts, no access to each other; what was one neighborhood was now ten, who lived next door was now a threatening six or eight highways away, if there at all. Particularly hurt were the restaurants and theaters where a community shares food and celebrates itself. This we know is already a deathblow to our culture, extraverted, raucous, and spontaneous.[11]

What Shange articulates, and what too few have recognized, is the undoing of the community fabric, the destruction of culture, and the separation of neighbors, family, and friends that took place as a result of forced uprootings. Root shock exacts a toll on people who are uprooted, but it also results in community-wide disruption.[12] The loss of connectedness, "access to each other," and the decimation of places of celebration and sharing were all part of the damage caused by extensive urban renewal and massive highway construction between 1950 and 1975.

In the past 20 or so years, many urban scholars and commentators of urban planning and economic development have often debated the occurrence of gentrification, and its pros and cons, without linking modern occurrences of forced displacement with a long history of America's colonization and the uprooting of existing communities for corporate benefit and demographically whiter residents.[13] Community psychologist Tahira Mahdi clarifies how gentrification is not only about economic impact but also power, control, and self-determination:

> Gentrification means that powerful people, exchanging resources among themselves, can select a disenfranchised location-based community, claim it as their own community, decide what investments are valid and necessary for people to belong to it, and make those investments while pushing out those who cannot make the newly required investments. Do the people who already live there get to declare that the community is their group and that they have the right to belong? Perhaps, but more powerful people and entities can invalidate that right and dismantle the existing community to benefit their own interests.[14]

This is how Black communities can be rebranded and erased with ease in Baltimore City. Gallows Hill becomes Preston Gardens, Middle East becomes Eager Park, and Pigtown becomes Washington Village. Once a wealthier and demographically whiter population moves in, they have the power to change the very name and identity of the community itself. To summarize, America's repeated forced uprootings damage Black health and Black neighborhoods due to root shock.

Internal Colonization

Real estate transactions are an example of internal colonization—the extraction of wealth and resources of a vulnerable community within American borders. Because of American Apartheid, millions of Black people were confined into geographic areas that would become colonized spaces of exploitation. In these redlined neighborhoods, White-owned banks did not offer capital access for home mortgages or for small businesses. In some instances, Black-owned banks could meet the demand for capital access, but Black banks often did not possess the levels of capital needed to provide an equal playing field.

Therefore, third-party financiers called *blockbusters* often filled the gap by deploying extractive homebuying contracts in the absence of more protective traditional mortgages. These homebuying contracts charged Black homebuyers an exorbitant purchase price in order to secure White blockbusters with hefty profits. White blockbusters became wealthy by extracting dollars from Black homebuyers. When those neighborhoods flipped from White to Black, those newly Black neighborhoods were redlined and denied bank lending for homes and small businesses.

In 1966, the Southern Christian Leadership Conference (SCLC)—led by Dr. Martin Luther King Jr.—embarked on a campaign "up South" in Chicago to join the Chicago Freedom Movement to counterattack Chicago Apartheid. In a press statement titled "The Chicago Plan," the SCLC linked the City of Chicago's treatment of Black Chicago neighborhoods with internal colonization.

The Chicago Problem is simply a matter of economic exploitation. Every condition exists simply because someone profits by its existence. This economic exploitation is crystallized in the slum.

A slum is any area which is exploited by the community at large. . . . In a slum, people do not receive comparable care and services for the amount of rent paid on a dwelling. They are forced to purchase property at inflated real estate value. They pay taxes, but their children do not receive an equitable share of those taxes in educational, recreational and civic services. [We] have come to see this as a system of internal colonialism, not unlike the exploitation of the Congo by Belgium.[15]

The SCLC understood the myriad ways that Black people living in redlined Black neighborhoods were subjected to powerful policies and practices that undermine Black Lives. They articulated the relationship of "slums" and the surrounding city as akin to a colonized area exploited by colonizers who extracted resources through predatory rents and taxation while simultaneously receiving inferior municipal resource allocation from cities and counties.

As King's SCLC argued, Chicago's redlined Black neighborhoods were subjected to "a system of internal colonialism." One of the main functions of racial segregation is the facilitation of economic deprivation (i.e., redlining), exploitation (i.e., subprime mortgage lending and predatory rents), and taxation (i.e., receiving an inequitable share of public goods) in urban Black neighborhoods. This is segrenomics in a nutshell. This means that segrenomics and internal colonialism are one and the same.

But a fundamental problem with this arrangement would arise, particularly as many cities became majority Black due to White flight and the Great Migration. How would the purveyors of internal colonialism, or segrenomics, keep such a system in place, especially when Black mayors began to win office in large urban areas? To maintain this system—which produces greater wealth for many White banks and landlords—requires a degree of political control or influence. To achieve this, many corporate interests provide significant campaign funding for Black political candidates who will do little to disturb or disrupt the status quo. By working to serve the corporate interests of banks, developers, and landlords, Black political leaders are often complicit in allowing segrenomics to continue uninterrupted and undisturbed.[16]

As Black mayors began to assume office of large cities in the 1970s, many would serve as surrogates for the interests of the White-dominated corporate and business sector (who still controlled an overwhelming majority of the wealth in a given local area).[17] Internal colonization in many majority Black cities offers the appearance of Black political progress while maintaining the same system of resource extraction based on maintaining spatial racial segregation.

Resource Apartheid

Because of the dynamic of internal colonization, Black neighborhoods are drained of resources and Black residents are overcharged on taxes, mortgages, and rents, thereby fostering economic disadvantages in redlined neighborhoods. This resource extraction subsidizes inequitable growth and prosperity in White neighborhoods and grants structural advantages to greenlined neighborhoods. Segrenomics, however, turns many Black neighborhoods across America into areas characterized by resource apartheid: people lack access to high-quality transit, food, green space, and recreation centers. The implications for health are tremendous.

> Access to more nutritious foods, biking infrastructure, recreation centers, and equitable spending on public parks would help residents in Black Butterfly neighborhoods lower their higher rates of obesity, diabetes, hypertension, and heart disease. Instead, the public policies and practices of city officials proliferate food, transit,

park, and recreation [apartheid]. By greenlining and investing in White L neighborhoods via tax policy and not curbing private bank and public government redlining/subpriming, city officials allow economic despair and high unemployment to cascade into crises we see in terms of crime, violence, and substance abuse in disinvested, redlined Black neighborhoods.[18]

A large part of the reason for resource apartheid is municipal redlining. Municipal redlining means that city governments engage in the redlining of their own communities, especially Black neighborhoods. In her masterpiece *Segregation by Design*, researcher Jessica Trounstine demonstrated empirically that, as the statistical level of racial segregation increases in cities, municipal spending per capita on public goods decreases. This includes municipal spending on roads/streets, police, parks, sewers, General Fund allocations, and a category combining welfare, health, and housing and community development.[19]

In other words, racial segregation itself is a primary negative predictor of city spending per capita on public goods, particularly in Black neighborhoods. City governments help create and maintain resource apartheid through their decreased spending on public goods in Black neighborhoods. Redlining is not just a matter of private investment, but the inequitable under-allocation of public goods.

Public schools in Black neighborhoods are also affected by resource apartheid. Many Black public schools in redlined neighborhoods are deprived of equitable resources thereby denying Black children a quality K–12 education. According to a February 2019 report, school districts that are 75% White in student population receive $23 billion more than school districts that are 75% children of color (despite serving roughly the same number of students).[20]

Resource apartheid is not simply the inequitable underallocation of city budgets or spending disproportionately less in redlined communities. Resource apartheid can take the form of gutting critical public goods, often with a disparate impact on vulnerable populations and neighborhoods. For instance, a national study found that the permanent closures of public schools disproportionately affect Black students.[21] When school boards decide to permanently close public schools, they are also often removing a community hub and polling site from redlined Black neighborhoods.[22] Therefore, resource apartheid deepens poverty and strips wealth in redlined Black neighborhoods due to the inequitable under-allocation of resources and the gutting of public goods.

Toxic Lead Exposure

Compounding the situation, America once allowed the lead paint and gasoline industries to put a known neurotoxin into paint and automobile fuel well after the dangers of lead poisoning were known to the scientific community.[23] This intentional toxic disregard created an environmental crisis in many urban areas across America, particularly in post-industrial cities that were hubs of manufacturing before many jobs began to be outsourced overseas as corporations sought out cheaper labor forces. Because of manufacturing and automobile fuel, toxic lead was often spewed in the air and then it deposed in the soil. The paint industry also was able to keep toxic lead in its paint products for decades even after the devastating damage of lead paint was well known.[24]

The impacts of lead poisoning are destructive for human development and growth. Even at low levels, toxic lead exposure causes damage to the executive reasoning area of the brain. It also causes behavioral difficulties, elevated levels of impulsivity and aggression, and increased odds for depression and panic disorder.[25] Because of these devastating effects, toxic lead exposure is a large contributor to the crime and violence occurring in many urban areas.[26] A 2019 study in Milwaukee found that higher lead blood levels in children age 5 and under was associated with higher levels of firearm violence (both victimization and perpetration).[27] Interestingly, toxic lead exposure also has a differential effect according to biological sex. A study of MRI brain scans of boys and girls exposed to toxic lead revealed that boys' brains are significantly more damaged by lead poisoning compared to girls.[28]

In spite of its long-known neurotoxicity, lead exposure continues to threaten the health of many youth nationwide. A 2016 Reuters investigation identified thousands of census tracts with higher levels of lead poisoning than what was found in Flint, Michigan, after their government-caused lead poisoning crisis became a national story in January 2015.[29] Local governments in nearly all Category 5 hypersegregated cities have perfected the practice of toxic neglect in redlined Black neighborhoods, including those in Flint, Milwaukee, Chicago, St. Louis, Cleveland, Detroit, and Baltimore.[30]

America's lead toxicity crisis is a direct result of toxic government neglect and weaponized indifference regarding Black neighborhoods. American Apartheid intensifies hypersegregation, giving rise to environmentally oppressed neighborhoods where toxic lead exposure festers.[31] Cities with higher levels of racial segregation continue to allocate lower spending levels on public health, often using the money "saved" to subsidize the expansion of private hospitals even as the blood levels of Black babies increase in lead toxicity.[32]

Local public housing authorities also played a role by placing Black children in homes where toxic lead was present and did not conduct the statutorily required pre-rental lead hazard risk assessments.[33] The lead toxicity crisis is compounded by the many Black children who live in areas where their parents are unable to access critical public health and lead testing services, so toxic lead is able to accumulate in the blood of children and eventually reach the bones. At that point, toxic lead can be re-released into the bloodstream later in life, causing further damage.[34]

Given the depth and range of toxic government neglect, drastic action must be taken by public officials. The state of emergency declared to address the lead poisoning crisis in Flint, Michigan, should be declared nationwide—but particularly in lower-income rural and redlined urban communities. With a vigorous national commitment and serious local action, lead poisoning could be nearly eliminated within a five-year period.[35]

Housing Precarity

Research has shown that Black renters pay more rent for their apartments or units (especially in White neighborhoods), while Black homeowners pay more for their mortgages compared to their White counterparts.[36] In rental and mortgage markets, Black people are often subjected to predatory rents by landlords and predatory mortgage loans by banks. This has also been the case historically due to the way government-enforced racial segregation warped the housing market for African Americans. Because Black people were often forced to live in certain restricted areas of cities, many areas became densely populated and overcrowded in the first half of the twentieth century.

Overcrowding was particularly acute in Baltimore.[37] Urban rowhomes and houses were often subdivided into smaller living spaces with Black renters being charged a higher rent than a White renter would be charged.[38] Black homebuyers were often stuck with predatory contracts in order to purchase a home since they were denied access to traditional mortgages due to redlining.

A century later, not much has changed. Because of predatory rents and home loans along with racial inequality in income, many Black renters and homeowners in redlined neighborhoods experience severe housing instability. In many urban areas, large percentages of renters are rent-burdened and homeowners are cost-burdened (i.e., paying more than 30% of their monthly income to cover their rent or mortgage). As a result, millions of Black renters and homeowners constantly worry about rental evictions or mortgage foreclosures.

Federal urban policy has also increased housing instability. President Bill Clinton's HOPE VI policy resulted in the demolition of 250,000 public housing units, while Clinton's Empowerment Zones policy may have also contributed to gentrification and displacement.[39] Large universities have engaged in landbanking and partnering with cities as "anchor institutions" to invoke eminent domain and displace thousands of Black residents in the past 25 or so years.

> Because of their standing as anchor institutions, universities have been endowed with tremendous power to engage in community development in many urban areas. When this occurs, nearby residential communities face demolition and families face forced relocation—particularly when universities have partnered with local, state, and federal governments to invoke the power of eminent domain.[40]

Because of urban policies and practices associated with uprootings, many Black homeowners and renters face instability in housing. Tens of thousands of people have been rendered homeless and have difficulty getting back on their feet. In cities like Baltimore, tax liens were once placed on homes and churches when property owners fell behind on their water bills, owing as little as $750.[41] Several Black homeowners and church congregations lost their homes and cultural institutions based on these tax liens. Collectively, these policies and practices instigate housing instability and create the crisis of homelessness and housing precarity in Black neighborhoods.

Racism-Based Traumatic Stress

America's hyperpolicing of redlined Black neighborhoods arose as an attempt to suppress the Great Uprising of 1963–1971. While many see Nixon's War on Drugs as the pivotal turning point, researcher Elizabeth Hinton has highlighted President Lyndon Johnson's 1965 and 1968 law enforcement legislation as the inception of hyperpolicing Black neighborhoods. Starting with the Great Uprising, hyperpolicing has intensified due to pivotal Supreme Court decisions and the combination of omnibus crime bills and executive orders. As a result, police forces can legally operate differently in different areas. In 1966, during the early stages of the Great Uprising, writer and activist James Baldwin described the nature of policing in cities with large Black populations:

> Now, what I have said about Harlem is true of Chicago, Detroit, Washington, Boston, Philadelphia, Los Angeles and San Francisco—is true of every Northern city with a large Negro population. And the police are simply the hired enemies of this population. They are present to keep the Negro in his place and to protect white business interests, and they have no other function.[42]

For at least a half century, elected leaders in many cities did not direct police to serve and protect people living in Black communities, but to protect and serve White business interests. This core function not only helps explain fatal police shootings of unarmed Black people but helps explicate why America's media outlets tend to automatically trust police accounts, thereby allowing police brutality to remain in the shadows. Only the proliferation of smartphones and social media disrupted this dynamic and helped police brutality emerge as a national political issue beginning around 2014.

The rise in documented police brutality certainly brought more attention to the issue of disproportionate police killings of unarmed African Americans. But the psychological or mental health impacts began to mount as Black people were bombarded with traumatic images and videos on smartphone devices and computer screens. Research showed that when unarmed Black people were killed by police and it was widely reported in the news, a measurable rise in depression and anxiety could be detected among Black Americans overall.[43]

This led to increasing recognition of a phenomenon called *racism-based traumatic stress* for many African Americans. Race-based traumatic stress is "the emotional distress a person may feel after encountering racial harassment or hostility." According to Monnica Williams, "race-based stress reactions can be triggered by events that are experienced vicariously, or externally, through a third party—like social media or national news events."[44] Police brutality and police killings of unarmed Black people are especially potent triggers of racism-based traumatic stress, sparking feelings ranging from anxiety to helplessness or rage to hopelessness.

Perhaps no one expressed these feelings better than Baltimore rapper Young Moose in a song released in the days after the April 2015 Baltimore Uprising entitled "No SunShine":

They wanna throw us in a cage, ain't no letting us out
I want to know why the mayor keep on ducking us out
They labeled us as some killers and some f—ing gorillas
They said the kids criminal, them b——s is tripping . . .

They trying to tie us up—
But we can't get tangled
They trying to treat us like slaves
I'm 'bout to zap out like Django

I'm Young Moose, I'm the future, they wanna do me like Kunta
They said he killed himself, they really spreading a rumor
They said he died in the alley, they said he died in the paddy
Man, them b——s assuming! Them b——s assuming!

No justice, no peace. Man, this s——t really real
They don't want to speak up cause they know it's True Bill
When we gon' wake up and realize it's real?
They did the same thing to Rodney King and Emmett Till[45]

Young Moose's reference to being labeled as "killers" and "gorillas" speaks to the realities of racial stereotyping. His line "they wanna throw us in a cage, ain't no letting us out" speaks precisely to how racism evokes anxiety and feelings of being trapped and locked in a space that cannot be escaped. Whether online by way of social media or offline through experiences living in hypersegregated and hyperpoliced communities, high levels of stress wear down the proper functioning of Black people's bodies over time, accelerating the breakdown of body systems.[46]

The health impacts of hyperpolicing are more clustered and keenly felt in redlined Black communities in cities with higher measures of racial segregation.[47] Although more media attention often goes to Black men who are killed by police, Black women have also faced violence at the hands of police, including murder, rape, and physical and sexual assault.[48] Black people who are gender nonconforming have also been exposed to these and other forms of violence and mistreatment at the hands of police.[49] Research shows police violence increases Black community fragmentation and instigates poor health among Black residents as a result of toxic stress, anxiety, and fear of police harassment.[50] In spite of the epidemic of police killings, public health departments rarely count such deaths or maintain a database of violence inflicted by police.[51] Since many public health departments do not specify and address the dangers of racism-based traumatic stress, the epidemic of police-inflicted trauma goes untreated and unresolved in redlined Black neighborhoods.

Escalating Homicides

For many people, homicides are the most pressing and disturbing issue in urban areas. A city's homicide rate is often touted as the most salient indicator of public safety in media outlets. But for many people living in redlined Black neighborhoods, statistical measures of homicide rates only partially illuminate the issue.

Grieving families are often left with post-traumatic stress and anguish from losing loved ones to what appears to be senseless violence.[52]

But what appears to be senseless begins to make more sense once the downward cycle of Black neighborhood destruction is taken into account. The first six components of Black community destruction are invisible forms of structural and slow violence that wear down the social cohesion and communal bonds of redlined Black neighborhoods.[53] A homicide epidemic erupts when the effects of invisible and slow violence accumulate over time and the cycle of Black community destruction reaches a critical stage.

Ongoing historical trauma is structural violence, and structural violence is slow violence. The damage from slow violence will not be immediately apparent but does manifest over a period of time. The cumulative and synergistic interplay of root shock, internal colonialism, resource apartheid, toxic lead exposure, and housing precarity leads to deadly results. When Black neighborhoods are systemically deprived of resources due to regimes of urban apartheid, crime and violence often escalate. Structural violence slowly becomes manifest through fast and visible street violence. Fast violence is then used as the pretext for hyperpolicing Black neighborhoods as opposed to policymakers addressing the slow violence that structures the toxic environments in which people live.

Empirical research helps elucidate this point. In an innovative study, researchers Dana Goin and colleagues used a sophisticated machine learning methodology to analyze the predictors of firearm violence across urban communities in California. The machine analyzed 242 variables at the outset and came up with 18 final predictors.[54] The top two predictors were Black isolation index and Black segregation index. These machine learning findings help clarify the results of social mobility research by Raj Chetty and Nathaniel Hendren where they found that Baltimore City ranked dead last out of the 100 largest county units in America in terms of income mobility for children who grow up and live in them.[55] Other hypersegregated metropolitan areas were also in the bottom 10 out of the 100 largest county units, including Milwaukee, Wisconsin (93), Wayne County, Michigan (94) (which includes Detroit), and Cook County, Illinois (96) (which includes Chicago).

In other words, redlined Black communities in Category 5 hypersegregated metropolitan areas have both the highest levels of violence and the worst income mobility for Black children. If children are born in lower-income families in hypersegregated metropolitan areas, they are likely to grow up with even lower incomes than their parents. In this spatial and economic context, there is little hope for even *imagining* the American Dream. Recall that Trounstine's findings show that as cities' racial segregation levels increase, spending on public goods per capita decreases. Hence, hypersegregation is a devious form of structural violence that spawns neighborhood conditions that escalate street violence.

The impact of hypersegregation can also be seen when reviewing the cities that led the nation in homicide rates going back to 1990. In 1990, the top five cities in homicide rates were Washington, DC, New Orleans, Richmond, Atlanta, and Birmingham. In 2000, the top five cities were Washington, DC, New Orleans, Detroit, Baltimore, and Richmond. In 2010, the top five cities included New Orleans, St. Louis, Detroit, Baltimore, and Newark.[56] With the sole exception of Newark, all of the aforementioned cities were categorized as Category 4 or 5 hypersegregated areas at some point after 1970.[57] Persistently hypersegregated cities, such as Detroit, Baltimore, and St. Louis, consistently witnessed homicide rates near or above 40 homicides per 100,000 people. In 2017, St. Louis ranked first (66 per 100,000), Baltimore ranked second (56 per 100,000), Detroit ranked third (40 per 100,000), and Chicago ranked fifth (24 per 100,000) in rate of homicides.[58]

Data regarding police killings also reveal the impact of hyper-segregation. Using data from the Mapping Police Violence online tool and examining cities that have a violent crime rate higher than 10 per 100,000 residents reveals that cities at the core of hypersegregated metropolitan areas dominate the list of police killings per million population.[59] In addition, Siegel and colleagues demonstrate that police killings are statistically higher in cities where racial segregation is higher.[60]

Hence, racial segregation—particularly hypersegregation—helps explain why certain cities have higher homicide rates *and* police killing rates compared to others. Redlined Black neighborhoods are often isolated from resources, access, prosperity, and opportunity, which contribute to higher levels of violent crime. Cities at the core of hypersegregated metropolitan areas also have ongoing crises with toxic lead exposures, which also contribute to higher levels of violence. At the same time, redlined Black communities report higher sustained complaints of excessive force from police, which means fewer people will trust police, resulting in unsolved violent criminal cases when people are victimized by violence.

Baltimore lyricist and spoken word artist Martina Lynch captures the sense of residents being doubly trapped by violence both from police and from people in the community.

> We live in poverty—probably seen some things
> That could take you out of your normal state and turn you to a
>   fiend
> Maybe give up your dreams and take you out to the street
> The only place we feel free, but damn we still ain't free
> No, the police don't know me, but they wanna take out my whole
>   team
> But my n——s on the streets they shooting too

No sunshine, it ain't bulletproof

So don't get sunny days, feeling like a slave I wanna run away

But I'm lost in the hood trying to find a way—rest in peace Freddie
Gray[61]

At some point, when all the elements are mixed together, entire neighborhoods are pushed to the edge and things fall apart.

Urban Uprisings

In the 1960s, hundreds of cities began to burn across America. Harlem in 1964. Watts in 1965. Cleveland in 1966. Newark and Detroit in 1967. These large cities—and hundreds of smaller cities—would erupt between 1963 and 1971 in the Great Uprising.[62] After 50-plus years of intense racial segregation bolstered by federal policy that ripped Black neighborhoods apart (urban renewal and highway construction), many Black urban residents became disaffected and disheartened despite the victories won by heroic activists in the Civil Rights and Black Power Movements.

Several explanations have been offered for the Great Uprising. Historians Walter Rucker and James Nathaniel Upton posit that "race riots or urban rebellions began in impoverished black communities typically after incidents of police brutality."[63] In contrast, Peter Levy argues that the Great Uprising as a whole was not a spontaneous outburst, but a reaction to long-standing conditions in Black communities. Levy contends that

> the Great Uprising was a product of the long civil rights movement,
> the Great Migration, and the political economy of the postwar era,
> which raised but left unfulfilled the expectations of black migrants,
> who expected that by changing their geographic place (i.e., moving
> from the rural south to the north), they would change places
> socially and economically. This view contrasts with the classic
> presentation of the urban race revolts of the 1960s as spontaneous
> explosions of anger.[64]

Extending both of these analyses, I argue that the Great Uprising (1963–1971) and the Great Rebellion (2014–2020) are responses to ongoing historical trauma. Urban uprisings are the final stage in the cycle of Black neighborhood destruction. Fatal police shootings of unarmed Black people and the hyperpolicing of Black neighborhoods are perhaps the most visible and visceral triggers, but urban uprisings, riots, and looting are responses to existing exigent conditions in Black neighborhoods. When redlined communities have reached the end of their patience and resilience, especially with respect to police violence, they can and do explode.

When the first seven elements of Black community destruction are in place, excessive police force and brutality are akin to lighting the fuse on a stick of dynamite and throwing it on top of a dynamite pile. Soon thereafter, the city is set on fire.

Health Impacts of Ongoing Historical Trauma and Black Neighborhood Destruction

The constant battering of Black neighborhoods has led to the cascading community health crises and catastrophes that confront the Black Butterfly and other redlined Black communities today. Constantly chopping up Black communities through repeated forced uprootings has contributed to the breakdown of family systems and social bonds. Black businesses, churches, mosques, and cultural institutions (e.g., museums, theaters, jazz and blues clubs) have been demolished by community-destroying policies of urban renewal and highway construction repeatedly across America.

As discussed previously, the onslaught of historical trauma continues to decimate Black neighborhoods in urban areas across the United States. When the first seven elements of Black community destruction are stacked one atop the other, people are pushed to the edge, echoing the immortal words of "The Message" by Grandmaster Flash and the Furious Five. People are trying not to lose their head (i.e., mental health). It makes folks wonder sometimes how they keep from going under.

Elements in the cycle of Black neighborhood destruction are like weather elements—rain, snow, sleet, heat, hail, ice—while Black neighborhoods are like a house exposed to these elements over time. Without maintenance and repair, the exposure to weather elements will eventually wear away at the paint on the house and begin to cause structural damage. When the cycle of Black neighborhood destruction culminates, it can cause the social bonds connecting people living in redlined Black communities together to be torn apart.

In much the same way as the first seven elements wear down many urban Black neighborhoods, ongoing historical trauma wears down Black America as a whole. The structural integrity of Black America is damaged by the seven successive uprootings that displaced Black people and Black neighborhoods throughout American history as listed in appendix A. Black neighborhoods are also undermined by the 29 enumerated policies and practices outlined in appendix B. The cumulative toll of toxic policy after policy is weakened Black community health. Uprisings are the logical result when redlined neighborhoods are pushed to the edge and Black neighborhoods are treated as disposable.

This is what is depicted in figure 5.1. The horizontal bars represent the structural integrity of Black communal bonds. Ongoing historical trauma chops and shortens the length of communal bonds, weakening the capacity of people to work cooperatively to solve problems.[65] The elements of Black neighborhood destruction also damage communal bonds and interconnectedness. Internal colonization and resource apartheid both starve Black neighborhoods from receiving proper allocations of public goods and equitable access to private capital. Toxic lead exposure damages proper cognitive functioning, impairs emotional regulation, and reduces gray matter in the brain responsible for executive functioning.

Housing instability and racism-based traumatic stress combine to induce fear, stress, and anxiety. Community homicides and police brutality steal lives and escalate emotions of rage, anger, trauma, and despair. For many, there is a desire to engage in acts of retaliation spawning sprawling epidemics of homicide.

Ultimately, the public health epidemics produced by the elements of Black neighborhood destruction shorten the length of communal bonds. When people experience root shock, chaos escalates. When people lack resources, conflicts increase. When people are exposed to toxic lead, violence rises. When people are constantly worried about evictions and foreclosures, chronic stress is elevated. When people are being murdered and homicides spike, distrust multiplies. The cooperative work that is needed is unlikely to happen while multiple public health epidemics are raging like wildfire.

Public and private entities often respond to the conditions in redlined Black neighborhoods with urban redevelopment schemes that only work to intensify Black neighborhood destruction. Past government and corporate "solutions" in redlined Black neighborhoods include the permanent closures of Black public schools and recreation centers, the dismantling and demolition of public housing, the privatization of public water and hospitals, the militarization of public safety, and toxic environmental disregard. Little thought is ever given to nurturing Black neighborhoods and residents without displacing people or withdrawing resources.

Often in the field of public health, entire discourses are held and research is discussed about health disparities or health inequities without contextualizing how Black people today are harmed by the weathering effects of Black neighborhood destruction. Community crises and catastrophes diminish the physical and mental health of people living in these geographic areas, resulting in a loss of connectedness and cooperative work.

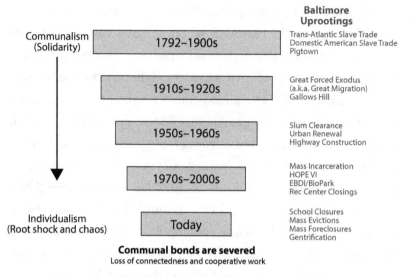

Figure 5.1. Ecosocial Model of Black Neighborhood Destruction
This model was drafted based on various insights and scholarship by the following scholars: Alexander Leighton, Mindy Thompson (Fullilove), Rodrick Wallace, Lawrence Brown, Nyasha Grayman-Simpson, and Jacqueline Mattis.

No discourse of health disparities or health outcomes involving Black people can explain why health disparities or inequities persist without understanding the policies, practices, systems, and budgets that bedevil Black Lives and destroy Black neighborhoods. To make Black health matter, public health must go beyond traditional frameworks of public health and account for what is happening at the individual level and at the neighborhood level. Public health epidemics accelerate Black neighborhood destruction as Black people living in redlined neighborhoods are often abandoned to ward off and recover from a host of diseases and conditions, including tuberculosis, HIV, lead poisoning, environmental oppression, intracommunal violence, police violence, and now the novel coronavirus. Conversely, the loss of connectedness and the ensuing reduction in cooperative work undermines efforts to stop those epidemics and commence community-wide healing.

Only by reversing the cycle of Black neighborhood destruction can cities catalyze the regrowth of communal bonds needed to increase connections and foster cooperative work. Instead of root shock and housing precarity, support neighborhood and housing stability. Instead of internalized colonialism, enforce spatial equity. Instead of resource apartheid, allocate resources and public goods equitably. Instead of ongoing toxic lead exposure, remove lead from the environment. Instead of hyperpolicing violence, engage in peacebuilding. This is how cities can stop Black neighborhood destruction and strengthen communal bonds, connections, and cooperative work. Before moving forward to solutions, it is important to illustrate how Black neighborhood destruction manifests in Black families in order to understand its impact on a human level.

The Gorham Family and Middle East Baltimore

The history of the Gorham family exemplifies how the cycle of Black neighborhood destruction impacts Black families intergenerationally. Lucille Gorham was a child of the Great Migration—born in 1940 in North Carolina and moved with her family to Baltimore in 1943. Later in her adult life, in response to urban renewal and Johns Hopkins–led displacement, Lucille Gorham and other Black residents in East Baltimore formed the Citizens for Fair Housing. She led the organization as Hopkins displaced her community during the 1950s and 1960s in the Broadway Redevelopment Project. She also helped East Baltimore pick up the pieces after the devastating April 1968 Holy Week Uprising, which erupted in the days after the assassination of Dr. Martin Luther King Jr. on April 4.

For decades, she lived at 1931 East Chase Street in East Baltimore, becoming a prominent neighborhood leader in East Baltimore. During urban renewal planning, she named the geographic area in the middle of East Baltimore "Middle East." In the 1980s, many of the homes surrounding the Johns Hopkins medical campus were viewed as blighted, and the institution engaged in landbanking—buying up many of the homes but not fixing them up. The area surrounding Hopkins where Lucille Gorham lived became more distressed and deeply redlined.

During the Clinton administration in 1994, the area was declared an Empowerment Zone, but the pace of improving the neighborhood was deemed too slow by 1999. When Martin O'Malley became mayor of Baltimore City, his administration designated large swaths of the Middle East community for demolition. O'Malley told *Sun* reporters, "I'm not going to force it down anyone's throat" but then proceeded to uproot and displace 732 households in the Black neighborhood using eminent domain.[66]

In 2001, Lucille Gorham predicted how the project would impact the neighborhood informed by her experiences with urban renewal, telling the *Baltimore Sun*: "When you have to move people around, they don't always get where they want to be. You lose part of the neighborhood."[67] In response to their pending uprooting, the Middle East community organized and protested, winning several victories. But by 2008, most of the residents had been forcibly displaced by a newly created proxy entity for Johns Hopkins Medical Institutions called East Baltimore Development Incorporated (EBDI). Gorham succinctly described what had transpired: "They kind of swooped down on the neighborhood and bought property and moved people out without thinking about it."[68]

Although Middle East residents organized to oppose the project through an organization called the Save Middle East Action Coalition, EBDI displaced Lucille Gorham and her family from their home on Chase Street in 2005. EBDI relocated them to a home in Belair Edison in Northeast Baltimore with the assistance of family service coordinators working on behalf of the Annie E.

Casey Foundation and EBDI. She would later explain how she felt the moment she received the relocation letter: "When I got my letter to move, it hurt. It was like sticking a knife in my chest."[69]

Lucille Gorham later suffered a heart attack in the new property and lost much of her mobility. Compounding the problem, the home in Belair Edison was not suited to meet her needs. The house's heating unit was decrepit, aged, and out of order. The house was infested with rodents. Given the list of repairs needed in the home and in desperate need of relief from her mortgage payment, Gorham took out a reverse mortgage, which helped her avoid having to pay the EBDI-secured mortgage ($40,000 mortgage loan, 6.25% interest for 360 months), which had worse terms than her home on East Chase Street ($7,592.58 mortgage loan, 4% interest for 112 months).

EBDI secured Lucille Gorham a wholly predatory mortgage with Harbor Bank that totaled over five times the amount she owed on East Chase Street with an interest rate 50% higher than what she had before. With a relocation assistance package that would pay $151,943.18, all EBDI and the Casey family service coordinators needed to do was place her in a home worth that amount where she would not have owed anything at all. But because of EBDI's and Casey's neglect and disregard, Gorham was placed in a home worth $184,900 in November 2005, thereby necessitating a $40,000 mortgage to cover the gap and pay off the remainder of her East Chase Street home mortgage.[70]

Lucille Gorham's daughter, Sallie Gorham, was a hairdresser during this time. Seeing her mother in need of in-home care (especially after her mother suffered a heart attack), Sallie moved in to help take care of her mother. After Lucille Gorham died in early November 2012, Sallie and her family members still residing in the home were soon threatened by a foreclosure due to the terms of the reverse mortgage (which allowed the bank to take ownership of the home upon the owner's death).[71] Harried and out of money, the family often spent weeks without electric power or water during stretches of 2013.

By 2014, Sallie and her family were without stable housing as foreclosure was finalized, and they were forced to vacate the property. Since then, the family members who lived with Sallie Gorham have bounced around from home to home without a place to call their own. In December 2016, Sallie's son Anthony Lasalle Brown was murdered in West Baltimore, dying of gunshot wounds. Before his death, Anthony had a 1-year-old son. Today, Sallie continues to raise her grandson, even as she and her family continue to battle housing precarity, landlord abuse, depression, and unresolved trauma.

Conclusion

The Gorham family's plight illustrates the tenuous situation confronting many working-class Black families living in redlined neighborhoods in Baltimore City. Four generations of the Gorham family have had to battle repeated forced uprootings:

- from North Carolina to Baltimore during the Great Migration, or Great Forced Exodus
- from one East Baltimore home to another near Johns Hopkins due to urban renewal
- from Middle East to Belair Edison due to EBDI–Hopkins City displacement.
- from Belair Edison to housing precarity in East Baltimore following the reverse mortgage foreclosure

The repeated uprooting of the Gorham family reverberates through subsequent generations and impacts their physical and mental health. Repeated forced uprootings have induced housing instability. These experiences elevated the levels of toxic stress, hypertension, anxiety, and frustration in the family to untold levels and likely contributed to Lucille Gorham's heart attack and Anthony's anxieties before he was killed in 2016.

Lucille Gorham became a powerful and well-respected advocate in East Baltimore at the end of one cycle of Black neighborhood destruction in 1969 (after the 1968 Holy Week Uprising). She would die just three years before the end of another when Freddie Gray was killed by the actions and negligence of the Baltimore Police Department. The experiences of Lucille Gorham and her family are multiplied millions of times in America's hypersegregated cities in deeply redlined Black neighborhoods.

The impacts of ongoing historical trauma are intergenerational. Ongoing historical trauma inflicted in one generation reverberates down through the lives of the youth and the unborn. The question that arises now is, *How do cities create communities where Black families like the Gorhams can thrive in neighborhoods that have historically been and currently remain redlined, subprimed, marginalized, and demonized?*

Make Black Neighborhoods Matter

Black Butterfly Taxonomy
Apartera Segregatus
Working on a Tightrope
With No Safety Net
Toxica Plumbum
Sterling Warren, "Baltimore: A Life"

I got a target on my body,
Somebody—please protect me.
The devil heard I got a message
So he's trying to disconnect me.
The mayor said "do the right thing, doc."
So here I am . . . trying to heal the hood.
Mohamed Tall, "Fire"

In Baltimore's Black Butterfly and in cities across the nation, Black neighborhoods have been neglected and disrespected, gentrified and subdivided, redlined and subprimed. Black neighborhoods have been hypersegregated and hyperpoliced. Many exist in a state of exigency.[1] Once hypersegregation calcified, it was never dismantled under color of law. On top of the spatial platform of hypersegregation, segrenomics was weaponized as a punitive economic system—extracting wealth and health from Black Lives and Black neighborhoods. Over time, the constant battering of weathering elements resulted in Black neighborhood destruction.

To improve health and well-being in redlined Black neighborhoods, the nation must commit to dismantling American Apartheid and reversing Black neighborhood destruction. The mandate for the Baltimore metropolitan area and other hypersegregated areas is to repair the damage inflicted during America's three spatial wars—the war on Black Reconstruction (1865–1909), the war against the "Negro Invasion" (1910–1960), and the war on redlined Black neighborhoods (1961–present). The damage sustained in these three spatial wars is manifested in community health crises and catastrophes America has witnessed recently most especially in Category 5 hypersegregated metropolitan areas.

With this frame and analysis in mind, one thing is crystal clear—to boost Black health and affirm Black Lives, America must make Black neighborhoods matter. The analogy of neighborhoods as gardens can prove useful in this work. When gardeners prep their soil with the right nutrients, the flowers in that garden will flourish and thrive. But if the soil of a garden is nutrient deficient, the flowers in that garden will struggle to grow.

The same is true for neighborhoods in which people live. The "soil" of a neighborhood must be properly prepped to foster optimal human development and health. The soil of a neighborhood is determined by the policies, practices, and systems of the cities and counties where people live. To some extent, neighborhoods are also affected by state and national policies. But local governments usually have the most direct influence on its neighborhoods.

In addition to nutrient-rich soil, a gardener will need ample water to hydrate plants and fuel growth. Similarly, neighborhoods need ample "water" in the form of equitable budgets and public allocations. It is not enough to have the right policies, practices, and systems in place if the proper amounts of funding are not allocated to neighborhoods to implement and enact the changes that must be made to ensure proper human growth and healthy functioning.

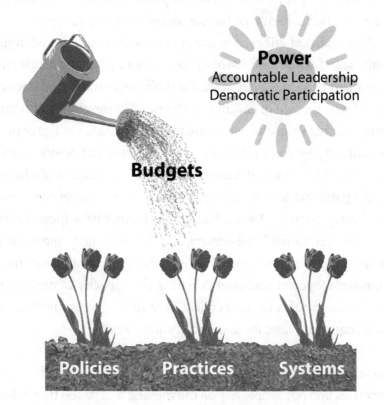

Figure 6.1. The Community Health Garden

To paraphrase a line from "Flashlight," the ebullient funk masterpiece by the music collective Parliament, everybody's got to have a little light under the sun. Flowers in a garden need sunlight for proper growth and development. People living in redlined and neglected neighborhoods need the "sunlight" of accountable leadership from local leaders and deep democratic participation in decision making to reach their highest potential. Corruption, privatization of public goods, and state takeovers of local systems all rob residents in redlined communities of their capacity to hold leaders accountable, to become self-determining, and to contribute to the community economic development process. People must be democratically engaged in the decision-making process.[2]

An important effect of ongoing historical trauma is undercutting the self-determination of a people. That is, denying people the opportunity to make decisions for their community that impact their lives. Instead of continuing the trend of development or urban planning where decisions are made by outside entities or predominantly by corporate developers and elite tier actors, *people in redlined Black neighborhoods need deeply democratic decision-making structures to develop and grow grassroots governance and leadership* (Step 3).[3] Desired outcomes cannot be achieved with top-down, command-and-control, outsider-dominated approaches despite the best intentions of do-gooders. Building democratic community power and strengthening the capacity of marginalized communities to work collectively and collaboratively must be a central aim and focus of racial equity work.

In addition, advocates for community and public health must scrutinize institutions and their budgets, systems, policies, and practices and not simply rely on the rhetoric and jargon that political, nonprofit, and philanthropic leaders often deploy in meetings and the media. Attention must be paid not only to outcomes but also to processes to produce the desired outcomes. How will wealth be generated? Who stands to benefit? Who makes the decisions and calls the shots? Who has ownership of the initiative? These are central questions that residents of redlined Black communities and organizers must demand clear answers on from government, developers, and philanthropy. Wealth generated and benefits derived from development projects must be shared with residents. Community entities should be co-owners of initiatives. *Only by creating meaningful mechanisms of community ownership and wealth-generating stake in all projects can people in redlined neighborhoods have the necessary power, voice, and resources needed to navigate changes that will be taking place in their neighborhoods* (Step 4).

Addressing Ongoing Historical
Trauma with Racial Equity

Once residents and leaders understand the ecological truth that Black Lives cannot matter when Black neighborhoods do not matter, cities and counties can begin to make racial equity a reality. Equity is not the equal allocation of resources. Equity means *doing more* for those who have less due to ongoing historical trauma. Racial equity is *taking corrective action to help communities organize themselves to heal from ongoing historical trauma*. Racial equity is the work required to support Black Lives and foster community health so that entire Black neighborhoods—not just individuals—can begin to thrive.

Take a sick patient in a clinic as an example. A physician or nurse cannot fully foster bodily healing in a sick patient without understanding how the injury occurred. Health professionals' encounters start with the patient history so that health practitioners can understand why a patient might be ill. There is no healing without taking the patient's history. Similarly, there is no healing redlined Black neighborhoods without obtaining a deep understanding of ongoing historical trauma and Black neighborhood destruction. Working to achieve racial equity will only result in more trauma if government officials and nonprofit organizations do not engage in each of the five steps of an authentic and restorative racial equity process.

Across the nation, many organizations and governments claim they are doing racial equity work or using a "racial equity lens" while continuing to inflict harm on deeply redlined Black communities. The Baltimore City Public School System (BCPSS) touts its restorative practices work with students to decrease suspensions while continuing to permanently close public schools, nearly all of them in Black neighborhoods.[4] BCPSS has overseen the mass reduction of Black teachers from 63% in 2005 of the teacher workforce to only 38% in 2015.[5] Since BCPSS continues to inflict disparate impacts on Black schools, teachers, and students, it cannot say it is fully using a racial equity lens, or approach. Doing racial equity means stopping *all* policies and practices that inflict disparate impacts on Black communities.

Racial equity is also misappropriated by organizations and systems that claim to use a racial equity approach, or lens, but continue to allocate budgets and funding in an inequitable manner. One approach to sidestepping racial equity would be if a Baltimore City mayor decided to allocate funds equally to all communities even though the White L has received decades of inequitable and favorable treatment. *Equity does not mean equal* when corrective action is the goal. Racial equity means allocating more resources to redlined communities than are allocated to greenlined communities for as long as it takes to create more equal outcomes.

Authentic racial equity also means ensuring Black communities have an ownership and a wealth-generating stake in projects, programs, developments, and interventions that affect their lives. This includes decision making, but also includes financial projects that will create profit. If there is profit to be made on projects, particularly when outside developers come into redlined Black neighborhoods, the profit should be shared by the developer with the entire community so that the community can be enhanced, enriched, and empowered. This also means that members of redlined neighborhoods and developers both can be "winners" in community economic development. An intentional focus on development without displacement can produce a win-win scenario for everyone involved.

America must be rigorously serious about fostering and implementing racial equity in public and in private budgets, systems, policies, and practices. The phrase *racial equity* has become a popular nonprofit and government catchphrase that people discuss with aplomb but do not implement nor enforce. This is counterfeit racial equity. In the wake of the Great Rebellion in the spring of 2020, many White-run organizations and corporations issued ringing statements of support for Black Lives Matter. These statements are utterly meaningless unless and until they are backed up and accompanied by deep changes in policies, practices, systems, and budgets. Funding must flow to redlined Black communities for restoration. The still existing exclusionary White labor spaces must be desegregated. American Apartheid must be dismantled with the same intense energy and effort that went into creating and maintaining it for over 150 years.

To ensure authentic racial equity strategies, members of redlined Black communities must become adept at analyzing budgets, systems, policies, and practices to see whether corrective actions are undertaken commensurate to the scale of the traumas inflicted on their neighborhoods and to ensure that community ownership is embedded in the implementation of change efforts. To make Black neighborhoods matter, all people and policymakers must demand racial equity in city budgets, systems, policies, and practices.

How can city systems implement a robust racial equity process? I use several systems and policy domains in Baltimore to provide concrete examples of what racial equity entails to foster healing, transformation, and growth for redlined communities in the Black Butterfly. Although these examples center on Baltimore City, the same type of system analysis can be applied in cities and counties across the nation.

Racial Equity in Public Education

BCPSS currently receives funding from the City of Baltimore (roughly 25%) and the State of Maryland (roughly 75%). Both the city and state drastically underfund the school system. The state's Kirwan Commission has convened the past several years to determine the formula for allocating the per pupil amount for districts statewide. On May 7, 2020, the Maryland General Assembly passed legislation entitled the Blueprint for Maryland's Future to implement the Kirwan Commission's recommendations. However, Governor Larry Hogan vetoed the legislation, leaving Baltimore City public schools deeply underfunded.

It is imperative to unpack how the state and city both perpetuate education apartheid in Baltimore City. As the student population has fallen in BCPSS, state funding has fallen because state funding for public schools is allocated on a per pupil basis. In other words, more students equal more funding. This arrangement financially punishes public schools in Baltimore City based on something beyond their control.

Baltimore City's tax policy also plays a role in deepening education apartheid. Between 2014 and 2017, Maryland's funding for BCPSS declined as land assessments for Baltimore increased due to tax incremental financing (TIFs), payments in lieu of taxes (PILOTs), and tax breaks. These mechanisms raised the wealth of the city on paper but delay the receipt of corporate taxes for 20 to 40 years in the future.[6] Without tax diversion mechanisms, corporate tax dollars would be placed in the city's General Fund where they could help pay for better schools. Baltimore's tax policies unfairly enrich and benefit White-run corporate developers and businesses while damaging and defunding the city's more than 80% Black public schools. Baltimore City's elected officials have made tax policy decisions that divert and delay the receipts of tax revenue desperately needed now to pay for public education.

Like all of Maryland's jurisdictions, Baltimore City relies on the State of Maryland for funding a large amount of its education budget. But because of the state's relationship to the city—which included partial state control of the BCPSS school board for nearly 23 years—the state dictated unfavorable terms to the city. This was reflected in the 21st Century Schools initiative where the State of Maryland agreed to allocate $1 billion to BCPSS to build new or to refurbish older schools as a part of the Baltimore City Public

Schools Construction and Revitalization Act of 2013. But the agreement was contingent on BCPSS permanently closing roughly the same number of public schools, nearly all of them in redlined Black communities. With partial control of the BCPSS board, the state could help ensure that any community pushback to this stipulation would be ignored.

While $1 billion may seem to be a sufficient amount of funding, another $3 billion or more is still needed to address the critical issues found as it relates to deferred maintenance in many BCPSS buildings—roofs, windows, plumbing, electrical heating systems, ventilation, and air-conditioning. The State of Maryland did not fund these critical maintenance issues as a part of the 2013 legislation, so buildings that could have been refurbished were instead left in disrepair. The state lottery system was set up to provide funding for public schools but no additional dollars were allocated to schools due to a loophole in the law legalizing casinos in the state.[7] Hence, the State of Maryland intentionally authorized budgets that deeply underfunded Baltimore City public schools and contributed to the closing of public schools in redlined Black communities.

The consequences of decades of funding neglect were laid bare during the winter of January 2018. With temperatures well below freezing, BCPSS administrators allowed Baltimore's children to attend schools in buildings without functioning heating systems. Many students were forced to wear coats, gloves, and blankets. As pictures and videos circulated on social media, many were outraged at the conditions Black youth were forced to endure. But the conditions reflected in the pictures were produced by over a century's worth of Baltimore Apartheid and funding neglect impacting Black public schools. A January 4, 2018, *Baltimore Sun* editorial entitled "City Schools' Deep Freeze" revealed the depth of the need for capital spending to improve school facilities: "Ultimately, officials expect the 21st Century Schools funding will allow the district to rebuild, renovate or replace between 23 and 28 schools. [But] that's in a district with 183 permanent buildings on 163 campuses, 49 of which the consultants concluded needed to be replaced or scrapped. The condition of another 75 was rated as 'very poor.'"[8]

Issues with repairs on older campuses are not new.[9] Indeed, problems in BCPSS are multifaceted: restrictive state rules, insufficient repair funding, slow repairs, nondemocratic school board governance, and old infrastructure. However, many of these problems are rooted in the apartheid education system that Baltimore City operated for 87 years until the eve of *Brown v. Board of Education*. While desegregation did occur in terms of Black children attending formerly White public schools, White resistance to desegregation prompted massive White flight from the city followed by the deep underfunding of increasingly Black public schools in the city. This spatial chain reaction undermined the true aim of desegregation—to provide Black children with access to resources hoarded in White public schools.

Desegregation did not secure racially equitable funding for school buildings in redlined Black neighborhoods. As BCPSS became primarily attended by Black students, neither the state nor the city took steps to address the issue of racially inequitable funding in a system increasingly funded through segrenomics. In BCPSS, segrenomics has resulted in mass closures of Black public schools, an increased emphasis on school choice and charter schools, and running the district on a portfolio model (treating schools like they are on the stock market).[10]

Baltimore City's policy agenda of desegregation did not account for the damage inflicted by White desegregation resistance nor the devastating impacts of hypersegregation and segrenomics. No funds were ever allocated to address the harms inflicted by Baltimore Apartheid. No attempt at compensatory spending was ever allocated to Black public schools by BCPSS or the State of Maryland for maintaining a racially segregated system for 86 years or for an exclusionary system during enslavement for nearly 40 years before that.

As the needs of the children attending Baltimore City's public schools changed and the city population declined due to White desegregation resistance and flight after the 1950s, funding for the newly majority Black education system lagged. By 1983, officials from Baltimore City and the Eastern Shore filed lawsuits alleging the State of Maryland was not funding their schools equitably. Although the suit would fail, the ACLU filed another suit in 1994 on behalf of Keith and Stephanie Bradford. Baltimore City would also file another lawsuit arguing the state underfunded city schools. The suits were combined in the Bradford suit, and the day before going to trial, the city and the ACLU settled with the State of Maryland on November 25, 1996, leading to a funding agreement for an additional $230 million over five years.

But the settlement also authorized a partial state takeover of Baltimore City's public schools as Maryland's governor could now select some of the members of the Board of Commissioners. The threat of still more lawsuits against the state due to inequitable funding inspired the state legislature in 1999 to establish the Thornton Commission on Education Finance, Equity, and Excellence to revamp Maryland's funding formula.[11] Although the Thornton Commission required the state to fund the city with an additional $1.3 billion over six years after 2002, by fiscal year 2008 Baltimore City had received only $258 million.[12]

To make matters worse, during the Great Recession under the leadership of the Democratic governor Martin O'Malley, the inflation factor in the education funding formula was nixed, which contributed to a shortfall of over $290 million in state funding for city schools annually.[13] As a result of this systemic underfunding, BCPSS is currently forced to operate with a yearly structural deficit—lacking sufficient funds to provide health services for

Baltimore's youth (many of whom are often coping with toxic lead exposure and post-traumatic stress disorder from exposure to violence) and refurbish school buildings in severe disrepair.

Compounding the state's underinvestment, a 2017 internal study by the Baltimore City Planning Department found that the city's capital budget spending in wealthy majority White communities was nearly double the amount allocated to majority communities of color.[14] Baltimore City's capital budget spending could have been allocated toward addressing the maintenance needs of BCPSS buildings, but the city itself redlines Black neighborhoods and schools. Hence, both the City of Baltimore and the State of Maryland have underfunded BCPSS as a district and intensified the disinvestment in Black public schools by not adequately funding repairs and fixing the massive maintenance issues in many Black public schools.

Given such structural disinvestment in BCPSS rooted in Maryland's deep underfunding and Baltimore's municipal segrenomics, merely working to obtain "adequate funding" is insufficient to make Black schools, teachers, and students truly matter. A color-blind adequate funding approach does not address the long legacy of Jim Crow in Baltimore's public schools and neighborhoods. As Sonya Douglass Horsford argues in her book *Learning in a Burning House*: "Racial liberalism's focus on the ideals of color-blindness (color or race doesn't matter), meritocracy (access and achievement are based on individual worthiness), and neutrality of the law (all persons are treated equally under the law) was based on a definition of equality as 'the absence of formal, legal barriers that separated the races' rather than 'a fair and just distribution of resources.'"[15]

In other words, desegregation based on equality was only one of several means to an end. What desegregation has never included is racial equity in school funding or "a fair and just distribution of resources." Merely removing "legal barriers that separated the races" does not address the deeper and more fundamental issue of "a fair and just distribution of resources" in BCPSS. In Maryland, public schools within districts are disbursed a roughly equal amount of money per pupil (although, in Baltimore, charter schools are disbursed a slightly higher amount of funding per pupil). But neither the current funding formula for the State of Maryland established by the Thornton Commission nor the BCPSS Fair Student Funding formula are consistent with racial equity. Roughly equal per pupil funding is neither fair nor just for Black children living in redlined Black neighborhoods attending dilapidated school facilities where Black children are confronted with health issues such as toxic lead exposure, traumatic stress, and the ensuing root shock that follows the permanent closure of Black public schools.

Relying on a per pupil approach to funding also means that individual public schools with declining student populations receive less funding for dynamics beyond their control, including when Black residents are forced to leave their homes (e.g., rental evictions, mortgage foreclosures, public housing demolition, eminent domain) or when housing mobility programs give families a chance to go to the suburbs (a good thing for those families). Per pupil funding punishes Black public schools with declining student enrollment and forces them to have to cut staff and services for children. To make matters worse, the decline in funding, staff, and student enrollment is often stated as part of the basis for BCPSS (or other school districts such as Chicago Public Schools) to permanently close Black public schools.

While a step forward from the past, both the Blueprint for Maryland's Future and BCPSS's Fair Student Funding formula still fall short of the imperative for racial equity—even with their emphasis on concentrated poverty and "high poverty schools." Concentrated poverty is a misleading phrase that fails to highlight *who* concentrated the poverty, *how* it became concentrated, and *what* damage was caused. Only city and state funding formulas that explicitly center on racial equity can address the ongoing historical trauma affecting redlined Black communities and the various policies and practices that negatively affect Black public schools.

Because of this history of deep underfunding of Black public schools, the State of Maryland and the City of Baltimore must make racial equity central in their funding of Baltimore City public schools and Black schools located in redlined Black communities. One approach to achieving this would be to adopt a "per school" funding formula instead of a per pupil funding formula (or perhaps as a complement to it). A per school funding formula could be developed that takes into account the types of neighborhoods in which schools are located and how neighborhoods and schools may have been structurally advantaged or disadvantaged according to inequitable policies based on race, class, industrial pollution, and toxic exposures that damage brain functioning (i.e., lead poison, air pollution, violence, and extreme poverty).

With a per school funding formula approach, the city and state could then allocate Racial Equity Block Grants (REBG) directly to Black public schools and schools in redlined Black communities.[16] This amount could be as much as $10 million per school annually, depending on thresholds determined in the per school funding formula. A democratically elected REBG Parent and Community Council should be put in place to help allocate and administer the funds—with the advisement of school administrators and teachers. REBG funds would be designated to help people living in redlined Black neighborhoods address the needs of students in Black schools, especially lead poisoning, toxic stress, trauma, housing instability, and exposure to other pollutants in the physical and social environment. REBG funds should also be used to hire more mental health professionals, community health workers, social workers, public health professionals, and others to address the health needs of students.

Along with a per school funding formula, REBG funds, and REBG Parent and Community Councils, racial equity in public education can also be advanced by doing the following:

- Allocating $290 million more annually to Baltimore City Public Schools in operational spending according to the Thornton Commission funding formula (after the state no longer accounted for inflation).
- Allocating the needed $3 billion in capital spending needed to rebuild and repair all of Baltimore City's aging schools in redlined Black neighborhoods.[17]
- Ensuring TIFs and school declines in population do not result in reduced funding.
- Suspending all public school closures in Black neighborhoods.
- Funding a community-driven process that creates a culturally relevant and abolitionist curriculum instead of a Common Core curriculum that responds to high stakes testing.[18]

BCPSS is also a nondemocratic institution in terms of governance. Commissioners on the school board have been political appointees since the partial state takeover after 1996.[19] The school board must be fully turned back over to city residents and converted into a democratically driven education system. The democratization of BCPSS should also extend to all individual schools. If the State of Maryland and city schools deploy these approaches—centering racial equity in funding, democratizing school governance, and implementing a broader version of its newly passed equity policy—then Black schools, Black teachers, and Black students will matter.[20]

Thankfully, some changes are on the way. The BCPSS Board of Commissioners adopted a new equity policy in June 2019. The BCPSS equity policy states that the school district will focus on unequal academic and education outcomes along with disproportionality in disciplinary action.[21] The policy acknowledges the district's complicity in creating an apartheid system of public education, but it remains to be seen whether other issues such as disproportionate and disruptive school closures and inequitable funding within the school district will be addressed. BCPSS and the State of Maryland must take concrete measures to repair the damage to both Black students and Black neighborhoods that has been caused by the tremendous number of permanent school closures since 2000. This means halting permanent school closures in the Black Butterfly and then allocating more resources to schools with higher percentages of students and teachers who have been uprooted from their neighborhood school.

Racial Equity in Community Economic Development

Given the long history of redlining, subpriming, and uprooting Black neighborhoods in Baltimore City, it is incumbent upon the city's Department of Housing and Community Development (DHCD) to develop strategies for community economic development in the Black Butterfly. Baltimore cannot continue boosting wealthy White L neighborhoods while economically starving Black Butterfly neighborhoods. Like many urban areas in America, Baltimore has not implemented a spatially equitable community economic development plan. Instead, the city's strategies have amounted to Black depopulation and Black community uprooting.

DHCD would seem to be the best city agency to implement equitable strategies for community economic development. But it is vital to understand the department's history. DHCD was once the Baltimore Redevelopment Commission in the early 1950s and subsequently became the Baltimore Urban Renewal and Housing Agency (BURHA). Mayor Thomas D'Alesandro II created BURHA in 1956 by combining multiple housing and development agencies into one massive municipal agency.[22] Baltimore's urban renewal program cost a staggering $900 million over 20 years with $300 million paid for by the city and $600 million paid for by the federal government. In other words, DHCD is the same agency that carried out the destructive policy of urban renewal and highway displacement, uprooting a total of 16,505 households and upending multiple Black neighborhoods between 1951 and 1971.[23] Hence, DHCD must acknowledge the damage it has caused to redlined Black neighborhoods and the way it has disproportionately uprooted Black households throughout its history.

In 2018, Mayor Catherine Pugh created the Neighborhood Impact Investment Fund (NIIF). While the fund seems to answer the call for racial equity, the strategy behind NIIF highlights the need to both call for more spending in Black neighborhoods and to pay close attention to *how* the money will be spent. NIIF is predicated on giving away approximately $250 million in future revenues for the next 40 years (from city parking garages) in exchange for $55 million now—a net loss of $195 million to the city. In addition, Pugh's plan called for a private nonprofit structure where meetings can be closed to the public.[24] As the University of Maryland Medical System's (UMMS) corporate privatize-and-profit scheme revealed in March 2019, the private NIIF structure sets the stage for corruption to flourish and for outside investors to benefit.[25]

But NIIF was simply part of the Baltimore way. Long before the NIIF proposal, city officials had also structured the Baltimore Development Corporation (BDC) and East Baltimore Development Incorporated (EBDI) to operate as quasi-governmental organizations that funneled public dollars to the pockets of private corporate developers. The privatization of publicly funded entities—such as UMMS, NIIF, BDC, and EBDI—allows private corporate entities to siphon off public dollars designated for the development of the city's redlined Black neighborhoods. The prerogatives of private corporate developers are satisfied while the community economic development needs of the Black Butterfly remain neglected or go unaddressed. Hence, racial equity in community economic development must involve a process of de-privatization and re-claiming public dollars for the public good. It is imperative that public dollars are used to the fullest extent possible by public agencies or community enterprises so that the racial equity in community economic development can become a reality.[26]

The State of Maryland also plays a role in community economic development. But its approach also reifies existing racial inequities. State economic development policies, such as Project CORE (Creating Opportunities for Renewal and Enterprise) and Enterprise Zone tax credits, help maintain Baltimore Apartheid. Project CORE is a $694 million initiative that was designed to allocate $94 million to the demolition of vacant housing and allocate $600 million to subsidies and tax breaks for developers to build in redlined areas of Baltimore City. The $600 million is slated for outside developers to come in and develop their vision without existing Black residents having a decision-making say in what happens or obtaining a co-ownership stake in the development projects. Project CORE is an example of how a seemingly large amount of money can be purportedly directed to redlined Black neighborhoods but not for the benefit of people living in those neighborhoods.[27]

Another example of corporate largesse can be found in Maryland's Enterprise Zone policy. Enterprise Zones were created to give businesses tax credits if they located in blighted communities and hired people from designated communities. In Baltimore, the legislation establishing the $117 million Harbor Point TIF (obtained by developer Michael Beatty) and $660 million Sagamore TIF (obtained by Under Armour CEO and developer Kevin Plank) both included Enterprise Zone tax credits, totaling $88,383,724 and $313,298,890, respectively.[28] Given the large amounts of money gained by the Enterprise Zones legislation, city residents should expect tremendous employment opportunities for people living in redlined neighborhoods.

However, the drafters of the Harbor Point TIF cunningly used the demographics of the Perkins Homes public housing community without providing any sort of employment guarantee for its residents. Similarly, the drafters of the Sagamore TIF only mandated that 33% of the construction employees would have to be Baltimore City residents, and no mention was made of targeted hiring from redlined Black communities.[29] These corporate actions make sense in light of a report by the State of Maryland's Department of Legislative Services, which found that the state's Enterprise Zones fail to produce a significant number of jobs for residents who live in the zones.[30] Thus, Enterprise Zones are just another way to claim Black neighborhoods will be helped while corporations reap the tax avoidance rewards. While a meager amount of Black workers are hired, corporations pocket hundreds of millions in tax payments that could have otherwise gone to funding public goods, such as schools and recreation centers.

Making matters worse, federal economic development policies also increase benefits for large real estate developers when such policies are purportedly designed to combat poverty. The latest example of this is the Trump administration's Opportunity Zones— i.e., Trump Zones—that bundle benefits for private corporate developers and real estate profiteers.[31] In Baltimore City, wealthier White L neighborhoods—Downtown and Port Covington—received Trump Zone designations although both areas are flush with private capital and do not need more government assistance.

However, ProPublica reporters discovered an email showing that Sagamore Development Corporation met with Governor Hogan's administrative officials in order to lobby for Port Covington to be designated as a Trump Zone. Based on a "random" mapping error by the Treasury Department, Kevin Plank's Sagamore was able to obtain a Trump Zone designation for an area that did not qualify as low income.[32] But Plank was not alone in receiving a Trump Zone. *New York Times* reporters found wealthy and well-connected Trump associates were positioned to profit from Opportunity Zones and that capital investments were not going to low-income communities in urban areas as intended.[33]

Corporate developers exploit local, state, and federal economic development policies to enrich themselves under the guise of helping redlined Black neighborhoods. Meanwhile, redlined Black neighborhoods remain in the same desperate economic condition or worse after receiving such "help." This corporate enrichment undermines community economic development. The subversive implementation of past economic development policies should teach advocates for racial equity a valuable lesson: policies that initially look good on paper can fail due to inattention to the intricacies of implementation or an absence of enforcement to ensure spatial equity is achieved.

Undoing redlining requires that the right policies are implemented with a strong racial equity process at the center and in every phase. Diversions from an equitable process must be identified and corrected by vigorous government enforcement so that private interests and corporate developers do not end up being the primary or only beneficiaries. Prepping Black communities for corporate gentrification and handing them over to outside developers subverts racial equity. Diversions from and subversions of racial equity continue the long history of uprootings and forced displacement in redlined Black neighborhoods.

Racial equity, as a robust process, is not simply "investing in disadvantaged areas." In fact, *investing* is a term that carries corporate overtones and implies that there will be a financial return—that is, profit—on money spent. A better frame and term is *public allocation*. A robust racial equity process engages people living in redlined Black neighborhoods in a democratic process to publicly allocate resources. This process is intentionally undertaken in order to help first identify and then heal the damage caused by ongoing historical trauma. Black communities must be strengthened in their capacity to facilitate community economic development as long-term residents work to envision and transform their communities in ways that will uplift their lives.

The path to racial equity must center collective economics so that people living in redlined communities can work together to address their economic needs while building community wealth for all.[34] While it is fine to develop strategies for individual entrepreneurs and traditional small businesses, such strategies ultimately lift up the financial fortunes for a few. *A racial equity strategy requires collective economics and community wealth-building approaches that will lift up the financial fortunes for entire communities.*[35] Collective economic approaches help build Black community political power and knit the social fabric of Black communities closer together. Collective economics and community wealth building must be foremost among strategies for fostering community economic development in redlined Black neighborhoods.

Another issue to address in community economic development is the drastic racial income gap. Much of this gap is due to racial disparities in the labor market. The Baltimore Black Worker Center identified the labor needs of Black workers in Baltimore City and outlined solutions rooted in an equitable community development strategy.[36] In sync with their solutions, here are four approaches to catalyze community economic development in the Black Butterfly.

1. *Center racial equity in community economic development.* To center racial equity in Baltimore City, DHCD must adopt the recommendations of the Fair Development Roundtable (FDR) with respect to the Affordable Housing Trust Fund (AHTF). In their 2019 report, FDR proposes a racial equity scoring criteria for the city. Two recommendations are "threshold criteria," and one is

points-based. A threshold criteria means that the proposed building project must meet the stated threshold before receiving funding, while the points-based criteria results in a score. The three racial equity criteria are geographic area (threshold criteria), permanent affordability (threshold criteria), and building financial equity (points-based criteria).

The FDR scoring criteria should not only be adopted by the DHCD for the AHTF but also other development-oriented tools and strategies.[37] The brilliance of the FDR scoring criteria is that it addresses the ongoing redlining of Black Butterfly neighborhoods through the geographic area criteria, the racial income gap through the permanent affordability criteria, and the racial wealth gap through building financial equity criteria. Once approved by DHCD, the racial equity scoring criteria would allow for the passage of a Black Butterfly TIF that funds and supports the work of Black social entrepreneurs and community enterprises in rebuilding redlined Black neighborhoods.

One such collective of Black developers, architects, and designers is currently positioned for a TIF in West Baltimore—Veronica Owens's Monarch Butterfly Enterprises, Sarsfield Williams's Aspire Homes, LaQuida Chancey's Smalltimore Homes, and Bree Jones's Parity Homes. With the proper amounts of funding for property acquisition combined with seed and gap funding for construction and rehabilitating vacant units, central West Baltimore can begin a process of equitable redevelopment without displacing existing residents. In South Baltimore, this TIF could be used to fund and expand community gardens, place them in community land trusts, and provide funding for expanding distribution of healthy foods to residents in South Baltimore communities.[38] In Northeast Baltimore, residents have advocated for a community land trust as a part of the North East Housing Initiative. In East Baltimore, residents and churches formed the Charm

City Land Trust. These grassroots efforts, in addition to many others, often are neglected by DHCD and BDC. A Black Butterfly TIF would foster equitable community development in the Black Butterfly and in environmentally oppressed neighborhoods.

2. *Community Reinvestment Act lending/granting.* Current redlining and subpriming are evident when examining maps and data presented by the National Community Reinvestment Coalition.[39] This means Black small businesses, community enterprises, and cooperatives are not able to receive financing to boost Black communities' economic well-being or hire Black workers to boost employment. Baltimore's Community Reinvestment Act (CRA) advocacy groups should focus on ensuring that CRA funds go directly to Black neighborhoods and Black social enterprises, especially cooperatives and community enterprises. In addition to these advocacy efforts, the Baltimore Office of Equity and Civil Rights and the City Solicitor should focus on the real-time enforcement of the 1977 CRA in order to monitor and eliminate the redlining and subpriming currently taking place in Black neighborhoods.

3. *Black-owned resource cooperatives.* Baltimore must create and fund worker, housing, energy, food, and transit cooperatives to provide services and encourage collective wealth-building activity and growth. The city's wealthy anchor institutions—universities and hospitals in particular—can and should be sponsoring the creation and sustainability of Black-owned cooperatives through consistent contracting to Black cooperative enterprises. The Cleveland Model, with Evergreen cooperatives, provides an example of how this could be done in Baltimore.[40] The Cleveland Model involves anchor institutions—hospitals and universities—contracting with local cooperatives and community enterprises. In Cleveland, worker-owned cooperatives help provide anchor institutions with solar power, fruits and vegetables, and laundry services.[41] Worker-owned cooperatives foster the democratization

of wealth where many more people are able to share in the profits and secure a living wage while anchor institutions help to support local community economic development.

4. *Community investment trusts.* Community investment trusts are a form of real estate investment trusts (REITs). In southeast Portland, Oregon, Mercy Corps Northwest used a community investment trust to help lower-income Portland residents gain ownership in a small commercial mall.[42] This is another community economic development strategy that can be used so people with lower incomes can take ownership of property in their neighborhood and ensure that the enterprises in the REIT serve essential community needs.

Racial Equity in Housing and Ending Homelessness

Housing is a human right. Yet most Americans are so accustomed to think of housing as a commodity that the notion of housing for all sounds like a utopian fantasy to implement. With its vast supply of vacant properties, Baltimore City possesses a potential resource to actually provide housing for all if the political will existed. To become a great city, Baltimore must center racial equity in housing and in the fight to end homelessness. Here are three strategies that should be employed.

1. *Keep people in their homes.* Given the myriad ways Baltimore's laws, landlords, and financial institutions kick people out of their homes—including rental evictions, mortgage foreclosures, tax sale foreclosures, reverse mortgages, and eminent domain—many Baltimore residents are undergoing a massive housing crisis. Predatory mortgage lending by big banks, exorbitant rents charged by landlords, and forced relocation by universities are threats to housing stability for many Baltimoreans. Housing instability is a threat against Black Lives and undermines entire communities, especially in Black Butterfly neighborhoods. Approximately 10,000 Black families in Baltimore are uprooted and kicked

out of their homes every single year through foreclosures and rental evictions.[43] This housing churn has devastating health effects on children and adults alike.[44]

Hence, keeping people in their homes is desperately needed for community and family stability. Keeping people in their homes entails rethinking the way that evictions and foreclosures feed the very homelessness cities should work to prevent. A great deal of charity is aimed at helping people after they are homeless as opposed to helping prevent people from losing their homes in the first place. A few nonprofits work with people to help them prevent foreclosure, but this usually relies on people in the foreclosure process having sufficient liquid cash assets on hand, which many do not have.

Baltimore City could set up a foreclosure and eviction prevention fund that bridges homeowners and renters for a period of six months—helping them to gain employment and boost income during the time period (perhaps with a growing cooperative or community enterprise if they are unemployed). Then, instead of having people pay back the amount to the fund, the imperiled homeowner or renter could provide services to their community. In effect, this strategy involves community service in exchange for foreclosure or eviction assistance. Part of this community service could be to allow recipients to join efforts like Baltimore Ceasefire or Safe Streets to learn conflict mediation and help boost violence reduction throughout the city. Or they could help conduct community cleanups or perform health checkups on the elderly and shut-in. Cities could also pay people for this work so that they can boost their incomes in the process of saving their homes. In this way, foreclosure and eviction prevention could serve as a way to bring stability to housing and address community needs.

2. *Reinvigorate public housing.* Since 1992 and the rise of President Bill Clinton's HOPE VI policy—which resulted in 250,000 public housing units nationwide—public housing has been

dramatically reduced in Baltimore City. The number of public housing units in Baltimore dropped from over 15,000 to just around 9,000 units as large public housing communities were demolished by the Housing Authority of Baltimore City (HABC). Plans are currently underway to demolish the Perkins Homes public housing community although HABC promises to bring current eligible residents back (a legal requirement under Obama's Choice Neighborhood policy). However, the Trump administration may at some point drastically cut the Department of Housing and Urban Development's budget which would threaten the funding for Housing Choice Vouchers (more commonly known as Section 8).

The drastic reductions in public housing contribute to the housing instability crisis. To reverse the drastic reduction of public housing units, the city must find ways to reinvigorate public housing. Given the existence of 31,000 vacant homes in Baltimore, a tremendous opportunity exists for the city to create a "New Deal" type of initiative that would renovate homes, abate toxic lead in vacant housing units, and provide locally owned and deeply affordable public housing for people earning less than $30,000. Community land trusts could be expanded to allow people in redlined neighborhoods to take ownership of vacant houses and use public funds to turn vacant properties into homes for their neighbors as United Workers and Free Your Voice have pushed for in Curtis Bay.

The FDR has also advocated for a 20/20 plan to boost affordable housing in the city through the use of community land trusts. FDR's 20/20 plan would allocate $20 million for community-driven redevelopment and housing made deeply affordable with community land trusts. Another $20 million would be deployed to "deconstruct vacants into parks, urban farms, and other green space."[45] Their plan articulates a solid vision for reinvigorating public housing using community land trusts. Baltimore City can issue general obligation, or GO, bonds and use the recently created Affordable Housing Trust Fund to pay for deeply affordable public housing.

Another way to reinvigorate public housing is to strengthen Baltimore's current inclusionary housing ordinance by eliminating waivers for corporate developers. The city must pass a mandatory inclusionary housing ordinance for new housing developments in White L neighborhoods. Baltimore City can look at the way that Montgomery County, Maryland, implements their inclusionary housing policy and learn from their Maryland neighbor. A mandatory inclusionary housing ordinance can do more than simply expand housing for lower-income folks in wealthier communities—it can also help with desegregating neighborhoods. Such an ordinance must include a strong component to "affirmatively furthering fair housing"—as stated in the Fair Housing Act of 1968— to ensure that racial desegregation is effectuated in the city's housing and development policy.

3. *Build autonomous transitional housing communities and implement Housing First.* Many of the principles of an autonomous community were inspired by the members of the Coalition of Friends/Tubman House collective in Sandtown-Winchester at Gilmor Homes.[46] The collective—led by former political prisoner and Black Panther Eddie Conway—occupied a vacant house owned by the city, started multiple community gardens, and provided services to neighborhood children. They did not wait for the city to give them permission to use vacant homes and empty lots. Instead, they exercised their autonomy to make decisions to begin building a thriving community. Black autonomous communities build on the legacy of Black maroons—forming communities amid apartheid conditions that create life-enhancing and sustainable spaces for Black people to thrive and determine the course for their lives.[47]

Tiny houses can be a central part of autonomous transitional housing communities (ATHC). The tiny house design by Davin

Hong offers the type of innovative green housing that can help residents build an ATHC.[48] The nonprofit Civic Works estimates the cost would run $50,000 to $60,000 for each unit. Another tiny home and micro shelter designer and builder LaQuida Chancey runs Smalltimore Homes. Chancey's firm estimates that fully outfitted tiny homes can cost between $28,000 and $60,000 each.[49] If the materials for construction were bought at bulk for a citywide program, the cost could be driven down further. Fifteen tiny houses could possibly be built for anywhere between $420,000 and $900,000 or perhaps lower. The City of Baltimore can establish multiple ATHC locales throughout the city that would allow clusters of 20 to 30 tiny houses on lots of unused land. Perhaps abandoned school lots in redlined neighborhoods could serve as the hub facility for such locales and be transformed into ATHCs.

However, fighting homelessness and building ATHCs is also tied up with the quest for dismantling Baltimore Apartheid and implementing racial equity. Therefore, it is vitally important that ATHCs are also located in White L communities so that residents without homes can live and thrive in communities that have secured structural advantages. The white supremacist legacy of Baltimore's racial zoning and exclusionary zoning must be confronted. The city council and mayor must amend the zoning code to allow for ATHCs in White L communities that fought to exclude Black people for decades—especially communities such as Roland Park, Guilford, Homeland, Hampden, Mount Washington, Lauraville, and Bolton Hill. Baltimore's historically greenlined and bluelined White neighborhoods must now do their part and host ATHCs so that people without homes can share the wealth unfairly bestowed on White L neighborhoods through racist urban policies and practices.

Funding for ATHCs could be obtained from a variety of sources: HUD, HABC, the city, CDFIs, CRA funds, and philanthropies through donations or social impact bonds. This funding should be directed toward financing autonomous versions of the following: (1) housing cooperatives that would put residents in control of constructing and managing tiny houses in ATHCs, (2) solar cooperatives that would put residents in control of energy production, (3) food cooperatives so that residents can grow their food and achieve food security, and (4) worker cooperatives that would allow residents to control their own labor.

These cooperative mechanisms allow residents to build their collective power and chart their own destiny and develop cooperative communities. But alongside autonomous transitional housing communities, Baltimore City must also begin to more rapidly and effectively implement Housing First to provide permanent housing for people without homes in the city. Given the large levels of vacant properties and the potential of tiny homes, the city could expand the amount of funds allocated toward permanent housing for people without homes in addition to using some of the same funding sources for ATHCs already mentioned.

4. *Account for the racial income gap in housing.* Even so-called affordable housing is often unaffordable for lower-income Black households. This is due to an unrecognized racial income gap. Baltimore City's median annual household income (MAHI) is $62,820 a year. But White Baltimoreans' MAHI is $76,992 while Black Baltimore's MAHI is $38,688 according to 2016 Census Bureau data.[50] Therefore, racial equity in calculations for affordable housing should use the $38,688 figure as a reference point so that the MAHI used for affordable housing considers that the Black MAHI is nearly half that of the White MAHI.

The racial income gap means many Black renters in Baltimore are confronted with unaffordable rents. It is no surprise then that Baltimore leads the nation in rental evictions per capita.[51] Even among those who are not evicted, a high number of Black Baltimoreans are cost-burdened when it comes to paying their rent. The lack of housing affordability is rooted in the aforementioned racial income gap, which in turn, is exacerbated by inequities in wealth by race. While one way to address this would be for the City of Baltimore and the State of Maryland to pass legislation raising the minimum wage to $20 an hour for the workers of all larger employers in the city (corporations with 50-plus workers), it is also necessary to ensure that families and households are not paying more than they can afford to secure housing. Hence, the city council should pass and the mayor should sign rent control legislation for renters in Black Butterfly neighborhoods. This could be done by capping tenants' rents at 30% of their annual income and perhaps providing some sort of subsidy to landlords to make up the difference.

Another way to ensure the racial income gap is incorporated in affordable housing is to ensure a broad range of incomes are included in the mandatory 20% requirement for inclusionary housing in publicly sponsored residential development projects. A diverse range of incomes might look like the following: 30% of the inclusionary units go to households making between $60,000 and $80,000, 30% will go to households making between $38,688 and $59,999, and 40% will go to households making less than $38,688. With this approach, deeply affordable and inclusionary housing is achieved for lower- and middle-income families in Baltimore City and the MAHI calculation is properly calibrated to produce racial equity in inclusionary housing.

5. *Stay Where You Are Housing Voucher.* Employees for large corporate employers are able to use a public/private grant program called Live Near Your Work to move within a certain proximity to their employer in Baltimore City. This grant subsidizes wealthier incoming residents and provides them with an economic advantage over existing lower-income residents. While wealthier White residents are given subsidies to move in, many Black residents are given housing mobility vouchers to move out of the city (to communities of opportunity).[52]

The problem with this subsidy-mobility dynamic is lower-income Black residents are rarely afforded the chance to stay in communities on the upswing. Black neighborhoods should also be afforded the chance to become "opportunity neighborhoods" without longtime Black residents being uprooted by publicly subsidized gentrification. When development dollars begin knocking on the door of redlined Black neighborhoods, Black residents should receive the same type of incentives to stay where they are and benefit from improved conditions. A Stay Where You Are Housing Voucher could accomplish this by providing a subsidy to cover the cost of any increases in rents and taxes for longtime Black residents. A Stay Where You Are Housing Voucher would help prevent gentrification and give existing residents the ability to fix up their properties so they will not be displaced.

Racial Equity in Public Health

The Baltimore City Health Department (BCHD) has long played a primary role in the erection and maintenance of Baltimore Apartheid. In addition to operating a segregated public health system, Baltimore's public health officials helped justify racial segregation during the James Preston administration (1911–1919). In May 1916, BCHD Health Commissioner John Blake told a joke mocking Black people at a health conference and joined a chorus of other White health professionals in blaming White exposure to tuberculosis on Black domestic workers and their supposed lack of individual hygiene practices (as opposed to the slum housing conditions in unpaved alleys with a lack of a sewer system where many lower-income Black people were forced to live at the time).[53] In February 1917, Acting Commissioner of Health William Howard presented health data at Mayor Preston's conference to consider the partial relocation of Black Baltimoreans and formation of a Negro colony in Baltimore County.[54] In July 1918, Blake along with William Howard (now as assistant health commissioner) presented data to bolster Preston's plan for a suburban Negro colony using tuberculosis disparities by race as a rationale.[55] BCHD officials were accomplices in Preston's racial segregation and forced uprooting schemes.

In 1921, the Hospital Commission under Mayor William Broening advocated for a racially segregated hospital. The plan was detailed by BCHD Commissioner Jones who wrote to the mayor stating that the city needed "a hospital of sufficient capacity for the segregation and care of persons, both white and colored, suffering from diseases such as scarlet fever, diphtheria, etc."[56] The chairman of the commission (Dr. John M. T. Finney) and the Johns Hopkins Hospital superintendent (Dr. Winford H. Smith) cooperated and agreed with the health commissioner's plan.

Two decades later, the City of Baltimore passed a health ordinance on March 6, 1941, that gave BCHD's new Division of Housing the authority to engage in slum clearance, resulting in the displacement of Baltimore's Black residents.[57] Although the health department was given wide-ranging code enforcement authority, BCHD never moved systematically to halt the lead poisoning crisis by abating homes of toxic lead, even though much of the research discovering the various dangers of lead poisoning was conducted in Baltimore. The director of health and safety for the Lead Industries Association, Manfred Bowditch, was able to warmly joke with BCHD's Charles E. Couchman in a December 28, 1955, letter about "Baltimore's human rodents," derisively referring to Black children who were eating lead paint chips off of walls.[58]

In the 1963 annual health report, Baltimore City Health Commissioner Dr. Robert Farber wrote callously regarding the health issues in lower-income communities in Baltimore:

> Some of the health problems which face the community exist because adult individuals fail to take the initiative or exert the

discipline which can gain for themselves and their children a better state of health or a longer lifetime. . . . Logical efforts at control can only be based on efforts to encourage a change in moral climate among residents of the city living in socially distressed conditions.[59]

Farber's discussion regarding a "change in moral climate" and the lack of initiative or discipline among community members is telling. His report omits the responsibility of Baltimore City to improve the social determinants of health and is silent on BCHD's responsibility to dismantle racial segregation in hospitals and public health facilities. The tendency to blame the behaviors of lower-income Black people for their poor health while doing little to change social determinants of health is a Baltimore pastime. Indeed, it is a hallmark of traditional public health thinking and approaches.

But in addition to racist attitudes by BCHD leaders historically, public health operates in a racially exclusionary manner. For over a century, BCHD has leaned heavily on collaborations with predominantly White and historically segregating institutions, particularly Johns Hopkins Medical Institutions (JHMI) and the University of Maryland (UM). JHMI and UM have functioned often as the brains and arms of BCHD. As such, much of the framing of public health in Baltimore has centered on a research and intervention orientation as opposed to dismantling Baltimore Apartheid and addressing social determinants of health, attributable to the fact that BCHD receives 70% of its funding from state and federal sources often in the form of competitive grant applications. Much like the education system, Baltimore's public health system has been chronically underfunded by the city.

One of the first things needed to foster racial equity in public health in the city is to allocate at least $50 million more from the Baltimore City General Fund to BCHD so that the health department can focus on the community health crises in the city instead of chasing grant dollars from external sources. With more stable yearly funding, BCHD can better focus on the five following strategies:

1. *Declare racism a public health emergency.* Given the levels of hyperpolicing in Baltimore City that spawn police brutality, rough rides, and the lack of medical intake for injured detainees, BCHD has failed to articulate clearly that police-inflicted trauma and racism-based traumatic stress are threats to public health. The city's health department should track health outcomes related to hyper-policing and racism-based traumatic stress. BCHD should follow the examples of two Wisconsin cities—Madison and Milwaukee—and declare racism a public health emergency. This would make tracking and reporting police-inflicted trauma, racism-based traumatic stress, and other forms of harms from racism an imperative.

2. *Declare a state of emergency on toxic lead exposure.* One of the most damaging failures of BCHD has been allowing lead poisoning to continue instead of declaring a state of emergency so that resources can be marshaled to abate and remediate toxic lead from homes, soil, and water. Since 1993, over 65,000 children in Baltimore, nearly all of them African American, have been poisoned by lead at over 10 milligrams per deciliter blood lead level.[60] Even more Baltimore youth have been exposed to lower levels of toxic lead, although there is no safe level of toxic lead for human beings. Most children have never received treatments or interventions to ameliorate the toxic impacts of lead exposure.[61]

Therefore, a state of emergency would bring a renewed urgency to the fight to stop toxic lead exposure from robbing Black children of their full cognitive capacity and future potential. Yet despite this bleak situation, there are guiding lights for solutions. At Morgan State University, faculty and students created a lead awareness and solution-driven campaign entitled #BmoreLEADfree. Morgan State is partnering with Coppin State University faculty and students to create a science-based approach to testing for lead poison in redlined neighborhoods, remediating lead in contaminated soils, abating lead in housing structures, and developing citizen scientists who can engage in this vital work in partnership with these historically black colleges and universities (HBCUs). The Baltimore City Health Department should help fund and amplify this burgeoning effort to identify lead hotspots and eliminate, by any scientific means, the toxic amounts of lead (and other heavy metals) found in the city's air, water, soils, and homes.

3. *Boost health in the Black Butterfly.* In many ways, BCHD bears responsibility for being a negative social determinant of health for Black people, especially those living in redlined neighborhoods. Part of the work of racial equity for BCHD is to acknowledge its own history and then work to remedy the social determinants of health it has neglected and ignored. Racial equity for BCHD means apologizing to Black residents for helping to diminish Black health in Baltimore City and declaring explicitly that Black health matters.

BCHD has a plan entitled *Healthy Baltimore 2020* that addresses four core areas: behavioral health, violence, chronic disease, and life course and core services. But between *Healthy Baltimore 2020* and the *White Paper: State of Health in Baltimore*, health issues such as hypersegregation, forced displacement, root shock, racism-based traumatic stress, police brutality, toxic lead exposure, and the harms of Baltimore's economic development strategy are either barely mentioned or completely absent from BCHD's guiding vision.

The Baltimore City Health Department cannot improve the health of people living in the Black Butterfly with tepid colorblind approaches and race neutral language and policies. BCHD must become a radiant and active force in the fight to dismantle Baltimore Apartheid. It must amplify racial equity in all of its work to make Black health truly matter and heal the damage it has inflicted.

4. *Conduct health impact assessments of new public policy and large tax spending proposals.* A common catchphrase public health researchers and practitioners say is, "Health is in all policy." But to ensure health is truly in all policy, BCHD must conduct health impact assessments for all local policies, especially for new economic community development, public transit, public housing, public education, tax policy, school closures, public capital spending, public recreation centers, and public water. BCHD should be a leading agency in the city—along with the Baltimore Office of Equity and Civil Rights—examining the health impacts of new city policy *before* it becomes law. The results of the health impact assessment should be released to the city council and mayor before legislation and projects come up for a vote, so that their votes can be informed by the BCHD's work.

5. *Practice public health from the grassroots.* BCHD must begin to practice public health from the grassroots by training and employing a sizable cadre of community health workers to address community health needs in every redlined neighborhood. BCHD historically has done this most effectively with Safe Streets—a program of violence interrupters. But Safe Streets should be placed in 30 communities as opposed to 5. To make this a reality, the City of Baltimore must fund community health workers with a stable line-item allocation from the city's budget at the amount of at least $25 million every year so that community health workers are not dependent on fickle grant funding. BCHD must deploy community health workers widely throughout the Black Butterfly. These critical city workers should be well compensated (at least $80,000 a year) and live in the communities they serve so that they are constantly fostering relationships and helping connect residents to resources they need.

Scholars and practitioners in Morgan State University's School of Community Health and Policy have built a track record of community engagement and work in partnership with a variety of grassroots health-serving organizations. Coppin State University health professionals and scholars are also conducting research on environmental health threats to develop health information systems. BCHD has a long history of partnering with Johns Hopkins Schools of Public Health and Medicine and the University of Maryland's School of Medicine but has not worked with HBCUs in any sustained and impactful way. The only way to effectively boost the health of residents in the Black Butterfly and environmentally oppressed communities is to bolster the work and efforts of scholars, practitioners, and students in the city's illustrious HBCUs.

Racial Equity in Public Transit

Baltimore City's extensive streetcar system once provided racial equity in public transit. However, the streetcar system was dismantled by the automobile and tire lobby at precisely the point that many Southern Black migrants arrived in Baltimore during the Great Migration after 1948.[62] Today, Baltimore is devoid of racial equity in public transit. A rapid rail system runs along the north-south corridor of the White L. But no east-west rapid rail system connects the two separate sides of the Black Butterfly (i.e., East Baltimore and West Baltimore). The free Charm City Circulator—a subsidized bus system that operates largely for the benefit of downtown and the waterfront areas—avoids redlined Black communities altogether, except for stops near the University of Maryland and the Johns Hopkins medical campus.

To make matters worse, in 2017, the new Baltimore Bike Share system was launched to much fanfare. However, it became clear that 41 out of the first 50 stations would be located in the White L.[63] In addition, protected bike lanes were built along Maryland Avenue and in the Inner Harbor, two of the main corridors in the White L. Other maps revealed that bike infrastructure such as bike racks were nearly exclusively clustered in majority White neighborhoods throughout the city. Zipcar—which receives city permits for its parking spaces—did not have any stations for its cars in the Black Butterfly until the fall of 2017 when Zipcars were placed at Morgan State University. Much more needs to be done by the Baltimore City Department of Transportation (BCDOT), Zipcar, and biking advocates to ensure transit equity for all.

Elected officials had previously lined up funding for the east-west Red Line, which would have provided rapid rail services along an east-west axis in the city—especially through West Baltimore. But Governor Larry Hogan rejected federal funding for the rapid rail system and soon thereafter spent tens of millions of dollars in highway funds in White suburban and rural areas in the state. In 2017, Hogan announced a massive $9 billion highway expansion project—an amount that could have paid for the Red Line two times over.[64]

Racial equity in public transit means the State of Maryland must build an east-west rapid rail line—to reduce travel times to work for many Black Baltimoreans. Without this critical transit, people living in redlined Black neighborhoods suffer from what the Baltimore Transit Equity Coalition (BTEC) calls "transit detention." BTEC's Samuel Jordan defines *transit detention* as being stuck on transit for over 45 minutes in order to get to work or school. Many of the regional jobs in the Baltimore region are located either in the White L or in surrounding counties. Therefore, the lack of transit equity means many Black commuters must travel more than 45 minutes to get to work. Given that BCPSS does not maintain a large scale public school bus system and many of Baltimore's schoolchildren rely on public transportation to get to school, both Black youth and Black adults alike suffer from transit detention in Baltimore City.

BCDOT must therefore center racial equity in its work. Black mobility matters. Racial equity in public transit means expanding free bus systems such as the Charm City Circulator. BCDOT can set up a Butterfly Circulator that runs east-west through the city and give people living in the Black Butterfly the same free transit opportunity as people who have access to the Charm City Circulator in the White L. Perhaps one innovative way to do this is for BCDOT to fund an electric road train with virtual tracks.[65] With a relatively low cost of $2 million per kilometer, such a Butterfly Circulator could be set up for less than $15 million (compared to the Red Line's cost of over $2 billion).

Racial equity in public transit also means communicating and building a consensus so that protected bike lanes (or transit lanes) can be built in East Baltimore and West Baltimore. Protected transit lanes can promote physical exercise and boost community health while connecting the city's fragmented and segregated neighborhoods.

These mobility solutions should be paired with the construction of deeply inclusionary and affordable units near transit stops to decrease transit detention for Black residents in the city. Since greater transit access (via the Butterfly Circulator and transit lanes) will invite new homebuyers, the city must provide Stay Where You Are Vouchers to guard against gentrification.

Racial Equity in Public Works

A 2017 analysis of the public capital budget by the Baltimore City Department of Planning (BCDP) revealed that predominantly White communities received nearly twice the allocations of capital spending compared to predominantly Black neighborhoods over a five-year span.[66] Reporter Ian Duncan explained the significance of Baltimore's capital budget and how it is allocated for infrastructure: "Money in the capital budget shapes the city's public spaces—helping to renovate schools, libraries and museums, upgrade community centers, pave streets and overhaul sewer lines. [In 2017], the city is budgeted to spend $1.1 billion on such projects."[67]

According to data from the BCDP study, led by Stephanie Smith, Baltimore allocated an average of $15 million in community statistical areas (CSAs) that are 75% White in population, but only $8.3 million in 75% non-White CSAs (very likely Black neighborhoods). The study would likely have revealed even starker capital budget allocation disparities if BCDP employees had examined CSAs that were less than 10% Black compared to CSAs over 90% Black in population. Their analysis covers only a recent five-year span, so one can imagine how much the city has inequitably funded Black areas going back to the early 1900s, especially after 1910 when Baltimore passed the racial zoning law.[68]

The Department of Public Works (DPW) is the agency in charge of the capital budget of the city and has perpetuated apartheid in city infrastructure and operations, including water systems, sewer systems, and trash pickup. DPW apartheid is found not only in inequitable public capital budget spending but also in water billing, trash pickup, and alley cleanup. WBAL-TV investigators uncovered that residents of nearly 200 Ritz Carlton condominiums in Fells Point had not paid water bills in twelve years due to not receiving a bill from DPW.[69] *Baltimore Brew* reporters found that a wealthy neighborhood—The Village of Cross Keys—continued receiving an extra day of DPW trash pickup every week for 10 years, at the same time when many redlined Black neighborhoods suffer from illegal dumping and would benefit from a second day of trash pickup.[70] *Baltimore Sun* reporters found that the wealthier and whiter southeastern part of the city had quicker response and a higher completion rate of cleaning dirty alleys compared to the less wealthy southwestern part of the city.[71]

Given these racial and spatial inequities, Baltimore City desperately needs racial equity in public works.[72] Racial equity in public capital spending means reversing CSA spending so that historically redlined Black CSAs receive significantly more dollars than CSAs in the White L. It is incumbent for DPW to do this given infrastructure in redlined Black neighborhoods. Many public facilities in Black neighborhoods have fallen into disrepair because of the city's redlining of its own neighborhoods with respect to trash pickup, alley cleanup, and capital budget spending. It is likely that a sizable number of public schools and recreation centers would not have been condemned or permanently closed had DPW funded facilities in redlined Black neighborhoods equitably.

Racial Equity in Tax Policy

Baltimore City's TIFs and PILOTs have been used to structurally benefit and boost wealthy White developers. Historically segregating and/or private White institutions have also garnered tremendous benefits from TIFs, PILOTs, and tax breaks. Since 2000, Baltimore City mayors and city councils have catered to the whims of private corporations with inequitable TIFs and PILOTs.[73] In the process, city leaders deepened Baltimore Apartheid and intensified inequitable economic development. While Baltimore's TIFs and PILOTs may not seem as impactful as police and schools, they are vitally important. It is critical for city residents to understand how they work in order to see how city leaders confer structural advantages to large corporations while spawning structural disadvantages in redlined Black neighborhoods.

When the city council approves a TIF and the mayor signs it into law, the city proceeds to issue bonds to pay for approved costs— usually public infrastructure such as streets, sewers, and utilities— so a private developer can build on property they have purchased. Whatever taxes are collected before the TIF is approved continue to go to the General Fund, but once tax revenue increases above that amount, the new taxes (i.e., increments) are diverted to pay off the bondholders. TIFs were designed to be public tools to spur private development in so-called blighted areas such that "but for" the TIF funds, a project would not be built by private developers. But in practice, TIFs often function as a tax diversion—as new tax revenues go to pay off the bonds instead of going to the city's General Fund. TIFs can last anywhere from 20 to 40 years, meaning that new tax revenues are not going into the General Fund for two decades or more. PILOTs are payment agreements between the city and private corporations that replace taxes. PILOTs often function as tools of tax evasion—as they help developers and corporations pay much lower amounts to cities compared to the taxes they would normally be assessed.

Therefore, TIFs and PILOTs are, respectively, forms of tax diversions and tax evasions. They are sought after by wealthy corporations to delay, divert, and decrease full tax assessments. This results in diminished city budgets to pay for public goods and shortchanges the funds needed to build and maintain public schools, recreation centers, mass transit, and more. These tax policies constitute the crux of corporate corruption and help explain why a hypersegregated city keeps moving in a downward spiral instead of soaring to higher ground.

Baltimore's TIFs are rife with racial inequity. In 2002, JHMI and the City of Baltimore joined forces to create EBDI in order to facilitate the use of eminent domain to force 732 Black families to relocate to make room for the expansion of JHMI and their planned biotechnology park. EBDI secured $81.6 million in TIF dollars issued by the city and has spent $212.6 million in public dollars overall to subsidize forced displacement. In 2013, Baltimore City approved $107 million in TIF bonds for Michael Beatty in Harbor East. The Beatty Development Group was also able to procure Enterprise Zone tax credits after adding in the demographic information of people living in the Perkins Homes public housing development. Perkins Homes, like nearly all public housing in Baltimore City, has nearly 100% Black residents with lower incomes. While Beatty Development Group obtained Enterprise Zone tax credits by using the demographics of Perkins Homes residents, it did not sign a community benefits agreement so that

Perkins Homes residents could also benefit from the TIF deal the way that Michael Beatty's development group would.[74]

In 2016, Kevin Plank's Sagamore Development Company pushed for a $660 million TIF deal in Port Covington. Baltimore City's TIF legislation allows TIF funds to be used for affordable housing, but Sagamore representatives fought housing advocates—particularly People Organized for Responsible TIFs, Tax Breaks, and Transformation (PORT³)—to keep the amount of on-site affordable housing at a minimum. The Sagamore TIF allocated $139.8 million to be spent on parks in Port Covington, which the alliance of PORT³ and Build Up Baltimore argued could be better spent on providing affordable and inclusionary housing.[75] During the planning commission approval meetings, large summer hearings, and final negotiations for the Sagamore TIF, affordable and fair housing advocates testified regarding the need to include public housing residents and inclusionary housing in Port Covington for lower-income residents of the city and to desegregate the city. This push, however, was rejected by the Baltimore City Council, and the Sagamore TIF was signed without deep and significant inclusionary and fair housing provisions.[76]

Private nonprofit corporations have been among the chief beneficiaries of city PILOTs. Baltimore's wealthy private hospitals and universities signed PILOT agreements in 2010 and 2016 to pay a low amount of taxes to the city.[77] In 2010, Mayor Stephanie Rawlings-Blake and private universities and hospitals negotiated a six-year deal to avoid a bed tax that was being discussed by the city—paying only $20.4 million over the time span.[78] In 2016, a group of 15 private universities and hospitals signed a $60 million PILOT to avoid paying a higher share of taxes over a 10-year period.[79] With flat annual payments of $6 million, each private institution paid a measly average of $545,454 annually over the 10-year period.[80]

By signing the 2016 PILOT agreement, Mayor Stephanie Rawlings-Blake allowed 15 private universities and hospitals to avoid paying the $1.16 billion they would have paid if they were fully assessed and taxed. Instead of obtaining 100% on the $1.16 billion, Baltimore City now only received 5.15% of their full tax assessment. The corporate sweetheart PILOT resulted in a staggering loss of $1.1 billion in tax revenues from 2016 to 2026. Since past mayors have signed such deeply inequitable tax diversion and evasion deals, Baltimore City collects far less tax revenues than it should given its needs. To further illustrate this point, a 2012 study of the nation's 20 most populous cities found that Baltimore has the fourth highest percentage of tax-exempt properties (30.9%), meaning that Baltimore only collects property taxes on 69.1% of its properties.[81]

To make up for the lost corporate tax revenues, the city charges residents a higher tax rate. According to a 2019 report,

> Baltimore's homeowners and renters bear the burden that is shifted onto them as not-for-profit institutions are exempted from property taxes. Baltimore's property tax rate of $2.248 per $100 in assessed value is by far the highest in the state of Maryland, at 222% of the state average. While home-owners suffer directly from the increased burden of taxation, renters suffer indirectly as high property taxes are passed on to them in the form of higher rent.[82]

This means people living in the Black Butterfly are disproportionately property tax punished while people living in White L neighborhoods are disproportionately property tax privileged.[83] Lower-income Black Baltimoreans often pay a higher property tax rate than their higher-income White counterparts. Because of Baltimore's racially regressive property tax rates, a Black family living in redlined Sandtown-Winchester may end up paying more total taxes than retailers in The Shops at Canton Crossing in the White L.

Baltimore's tax credit policies also bolster racial inequality. The most glaring example of tax credit inequity was the 2019 property tax bill sponsored by Councilmember Eric Costello. Council Bill 19-0414 offered a tax credit for owners of "high-performance newly constructed dwellings." The bill was submitted after the passage of then Councilmember Brandon Scott's 2018 equity assessment bill (18-0223), so the Finance Department assessed Costello's property tax bill according to the new policy. In the Finance Department's equity assessment, the department wrote incisively:

> Recipients of this tax credit are likely to be higher income compared to the average resident purchasing from the City's existing housing stock. This suggests that the Credit has a regressive effect whereby marginal home purchasers are subsidizing benefits which accrue to relatively prosperous residents in neighborhoods where adequate market incentives already exist. . . . Only 10% of City neighborhoods received 90% of the benefits from Fiscal 2015 through Fiscal 2019. In order, the top ten recipient neighborhoods include Greektown, Uplands, Canton, Locust Point, Downtown, Inner Harbor, Brewers Hill, Middle East, Pigtown, and Hampden.[84]

In other words, the Finance Department made it exceedingly clear that Council Bill 19-0414 would perpetuate racial and spatial inequity if passed. Seven out of the top 10 neighborhoods receiving disproportionate benefits from the bill are in the White L. Of the remaining three, one would receive the tax credit due to HUD and HABC subsidized housing (Uplands) while the remaining two are close to historically White and segregating universities (Middle East near the Johns Hopkins medical campus and Pigtown near the University of Maryland). All but one city councilmember voted for the bill: Councilmember Ryan Dorsey. Even after the passage of the equity assessment bill and a superbly written equity assessment, the Baltimore City Council failed to block a discriminatory tax credit bill and ensure racial and spatial equity would be implemented in the city's tax policy.

Solutions here are clear. Baltimore's elected leaders must dismantle and revamp the city's deeply inequitable system of taxation to center racial equity in the tax code. Racial equity should become institutionalized in city-sponsored TIFs, PILOTs, and tax breaks. Baltimore's tax rate should be made racially and spatially progressive to ensure that large businesses, corporate developers, and nonprofits are paying their equitable share of taxes commensurate with their wealth and assets.

Racial equity in Baltimore's tax policy also means a mandatory 20% requirement for inclusionary housing units for all developments that include new housing in Baltimore City when the developers receive TIFs, PILOTs, or tax credits. Corporate developers have a responsibility to help desegregate Baltimore City and foster racial equity as they have long profited from the city's segrenomics. Therefore, large redevelopment projects must be accompanied by a robust and legally binding community equity agreement, to ensure that existing city residents and redlined Black communities are able to share in the benefits and profits. A community equity agreement would be an agreement between the developer(s) and the community affected by the development. The agreement should be drawn up with the assistance of community lawyers and incorporate the five-step racial equity process outlined at the beginning of this book.

Conclusion

Racial equity is not a vision of a fantasy or a utopia. It is a concrete process for creating and manifesting bright futures. The process acknowledges ongoing historical trauma has inflicted damage that must be healed and addressed. But acknowledgment must be followed by sustained and transformative action. Institutionalizing racial equity in all relevant institutions, budgets, systems, policies, and practices is necessary for making Black Butterfly neighborhoods healthy and whole. *Implementing racial equity in city systems means undoing the processes and legacies of disempowerment (e.g., privatization) with participatory democracy and equitable public allocations to ensure that Black communities have an ownership stake in new development* (Steps 3 and 4).

Although Baltimore City is discussed here to show how racial equity should be institutionalized, this department-by-department analytical approach can be applied to cities and counties across America. Racial equity must be intentionally implemented in all relevant institutions, budgets, systems, policies, and practices to heal the damage caused by the war against Black Reconstruction, the protracted war against the "Negro Invasion," and the ongoing spatial war against Black communities waged by governments across the nation. By rigorously examining each city's and county's institutions, systems, budgets, policies, and practices—in philanthropy, nonprofits, and government—racial equity processes can be put in place and implemented to stop ongoing historical trauma and address the damage inflicted over the course of decades and centuries.[85]

Baltimore's Black Butterfly has been gravely wounded because of urban apartheid. As Morgan State University student Sterling Warren highlighted, many people in the Black Butterfly are "walking on a tightrope, with no safety net." Across the nation, millions of Black families and thousands of Black communities have been deeply wounded by American Apartheid. The process of Black neighborhood destruction has weathered and worn down many redlined Black neighborhoods to the point of hopelessness and despair. Spoken word champion Mohamed Tall argues the nation's task now is to "heal the hood." Racial equity is the work of healing Black neighborhoods and making Black neighborhoods matter so that Black people living in redlined neighborhoods can be made whole.

Healing the Black Butterfly

> . . . healing for the oppressed
> is not going to come
> through neoliberal peacebuilding
> where privileged and pulverised
> hug and cry for the cameras
> and world peace;
> then go back to their structurally unequal lives
> off camera, with not a hint of irony.
> Sarah Malotane, "Invisible Violence, Invisible Wounding"

The Case for Radical Change

When the *New York Times Magazine* covered the passage of Mayor Mahool's groundbreaking racial zoning ordinance in 1910, it described the ordinance as "radical and far-reaching." When the *Baltimore Municipal Journal* discussed the Preston administration's uprooting of the Black Gallows Hill community in 1917, the uprooting was described as a "radical measure." Since the burgeoning efforts of apartheid policies and practices were described as both "radical and far-reaching" and a "radical measure," it only makes sense that radical measures and far-reaching government policies and practices will be needed to dismantle Baltimore Apartheid and by extension, American Apartheid.

The radical imposition of racial segregation and uprootings cannot be equitably addressed with incremental changes.[1] It is not sufficient to simply tinker on the edges with piecemeal solutions that sprinkle a few million dollars here and there for a few nice projects and programs. Entire systems must be rethought. Entirely new approaches must be created. A new vision for building and developing cities and neglected spaces must come forth.

Rejuvenating the Black Butterfly and other redlined Black communities across America will require expansive and substantial structural, social, and economic interventions. Healing the damage inflicted by ongoing historical trauma will require billions of dollars and tectonic shifts in resource allocation. While the concrete strategies for racial equity discussed in Track 6 will move Baltimore City in the right direction, comprehensively healing the Black Butterfly means thinking imaginatively beyond the status quo.

Baltimore Apartheid was erected and maintained by intentional public and private policies, practices, systems, and budgets. Therefore, it can be undone and dismantled by those very same means. To do so will require that Baltimore residents develop a politics of public service and means of accountability that stops corrosive corruption. Public officials can no longer cater to corporate imperatives based on campaign finance sponsorship and quid pro quo arrangements. Corruption ultimately disrupts democracy and mutes the voices of people living in redlined Black neighborhoods.[2] Corporate corruption upholds urban apartheid and must be upended if redlined Black neighborhoods are to survive and then thrive. The voices of powerful corporate interests and people living in structurally advantaged neighborhoods should carry less weight when future decisions are made.

Healing redlined and environmentally oppressed communities begins with a robust reckoning—an accounting of the effects of ongoing historical trauma in many Black neighborhoods. The descendants of Africans enslaved in the United States have been subjected to government-enforced racial segregation, seven successive uprootings, violent hyperpolicing, destructive segrenomics, and cultural dispossession. They have experienced land dispossession in rural areas and recurring uprootings in urban areas. Ongoing historical trauma has directly damaged Black neighborhoods and blocked Black neighborhoods from reaching their potential across America. In Baltimore, this is the case for the Black Butterfly.

How to Heal the Black Butterfly

The following eight strategies are designed to jump-start the healing process for Baltimore's Black Butterfly. These ideas can be adapted, scaled, tweaked, and tailored to help heal redlined Black communities in cities and counties across the nation. These following are each big ideas because big problems require big solutions to fix what is fundamentally broken. *Making restorative and equitable funding allocations to help heal and restore redlined Black communities is a necessity* (Step 5).

To be clear, money alone will not foster healing for redlined Black communities. But it is also true that healing Black neighborhoods cannot take place without significant and equitable funding. Step 5 should take place after the first step and as Steps 2, 3, and 4 are underway—while ongoing historical trauma is halted and community members are learning and working to co-manage and co-own the resources that will be allocated and located in their neighborhoods. Through this process, people living in redlined Black neighborhoods will be increasingly comfortable and prepared to participate in and lead the healing and redevelopment of their communities.

A $3 Billion Racial Equity Social Impact Bond

The $3 billion Racial Equity Social Impact Bond is designed to jump-start the Black Butterfly's renewal by channeling philanthropic and public dollars toward pressing issues that need addressing now.[3] I propose a $3 billion social impact bond to begin to bolster racial equity in Baltimore. The proposed social impact bonds would be allocated as follows:

- $1.245 billion to abate toxic lead in homes, remediate toxic lead in the soil, replace lead pipes, and halt toxic lead air emissions
- $200 million to train, to hire, and to pay local residents to perform lead abatement/remediation, home weatherization, solar panel installation, community gardening and clean up, climate change mitigation, and so forth
- $255 million for infrastructure to eliminate transit, biking, and food apartheid in the Black Butterfly
- $100 million for expanding violence prevention (Safe Streets) to 30 neighborhoods
- $100 million for substance abuse treatment, social work, and counseling
- $500 million for the top 20 redlined Community Statistical Areas for community-driven redevelopment
- $500 million for a Black Butterfly Community Economic Development TIF to augment and amplify the Department of Housing and Community Development's work to boost affordable housing, community land trusts, and various cooperatives (e.g., housing, food, solar, internet)
- $100 million for the Baltimore Office of Equity and Civil Rights to coordinate the fund and to hire more personnel to build a more robust office

The use of social impact bonds to address pressing social issues is not a new idea. The City of Denver has used a social impact bond to help house people without homes.[4] Baltimore can follow Denver's example but on a much larger scale. The $3 billion raised from private and public sources can be directed toward solving and preventing many of Baltimore's most pressing issues—toxic lead exposure, violence, resource apartheid, substance abuse, homelessness, and inequitable community economic development. The Racial Equity Social Impact Bond could be broken into several smaller bonds so that once certain amounts are raised, work can commence without waiting for the entire $3 billion to be raised.

In terms of financing the Racial Equity Social Impact Bond, funding could come from Baltimore City developing an aggressive strategy to negotiate with big banks pursuant to the Community Reinvestment Act (CRA) of 1977. Large financial institutions have redlined Baltimore's Black communities over the years; therefore, their CRA dollars should be used to undo redlining. Another way the Racial Equity Social Impact Bond could be financed is through philanthropic and corporate donations. Philanthropies such as the Harry and Jeanette Weinberg Foundation, Plank Enterprises, Abell Foundation, Annie E. Casey Foundation, Goldseker Foundation, Baltimore Community Foundation, and others could foster racial equity in Baltimore by funding the social impact bond. The top 25 philanthropic institutions operating in Baltimore possess over $7 billion in assets.[5] If each of these 25 philanthropies donated half of their respective assets, the Racial Equity Social Impact Bond could be quickly and fully funded. Religious organizations in the city's faith communities can also contribute toward the fund along with social groups and clubs.

The emerging literature on the future direction of philanthropy focuses on systems change and collective impact.[6] The prevalence of ongoing historical trauma and the nature of Black community destruction demands more than philanthropies simply funding programs and services. Entire systems must be changed and collective impact must be maximized. The Racial Equity Social Impact Bond is designed to catalyze systems change—to remove toxic lead, to kick-start Black neighborhood development, to expand violence prevention, and to catalyze a more green, sustainable, and climate-resilient Baltimore. The challenge for philanthropy in Baltimore and beyond is to step forward and fully fund the movement of cities and counties away from American Apartheid and toward racial equity. Just as philanthropic organizations had a hand in creating many problems, they can and must have a hand in funding and supporting the healing of the Black Butterfly.

However, cities and counties should be judicious with this approach. Municipalities should not depend on private dollars to finance the provision of basic public goods. That would result in local governments privatizing the very services that public dollars should fund and support. The Racial Equity Social Impact Bond is proposed mainly to address seemingly intractable and urgent problems, such as the toxic lead crisis, the deadly opioid epidemic, and homicide epidemic—or in cases where a city or county government cannot rapidly muster the large infusion of funds needed to tackle issues decisively. In this instance, a large-scale Racial Equity Social Impact Bond is needed to move swiftly to address the urgent state of affairs and is more of a onetime proposal to kick-start the healing of redlined Black neighborhoods.

Fund Freedom Budgets and Black Neighborhood Reparations

The second major strategy for healing the Black Butterfly in Baltimore City is to dismantle the city's apartheid budget. This can be done by diverting money from policing or social control and allocating money toward expenditures that support the health and growth of redlined Black neighborhoods. Baltimore maintains an apartheid budget where police spending has tripled since the 1990s while spending in other areas has remained flat or not kept pace.[7] The following list includes the fiscal year 2018 expenditures for each of the aforementioned budget categories according to Open Budget Baltimore—the city's budget website. The amount allocated for each municipal system or funding area is followed by the percentage of each line item paid by city dollars through the General Fund.[8]

- Baltimore Police Department—$493.74 million (95.59%)
- Baltimore City Health Department—$141.90 million (28.75%)
- Housing and Community Development—$62.02 million (56.38%)
- Recreation and Parks—$47.13 million (80.51%)
- Mayor's Office of Employment Development—$27.98 million (28.78%)
- Permanent Housing for the Homeless—$27.13 million (2.71%)
- Office of Equity and Civil Rights—$2.1 million (100%)
- Arts and Culture—$8.41 million (99.55%)[9]

In other words, Baltimore City allocated $493.74 million toward policing and social control, but only $316.67 million on supporting life (i.e., health, housing, parks, workforce development, permanent housing for the homeless, and arts and culture) *combined*. When federal, state, and other outside funding are removed, the City of Baltimore's allocation to each of these seven budget areas is even more striking:

- Baltimore Police Department—$471.97 million
- Baltimore City Health Department—$40.8 million
- Housing and Community Development—$34.97 million
- Recreation and Parks—$37.94 million
- Mayor's Office of Employment Development—$8.05 million
- Permanent Housing for the Homeless—$736,260
- Office of Civil Rights and Wage Enforcement—$2.1 million
- Arts and Culture—$8.37 million[10]

For FY2018, Baltimore City spent a massive $471.97 million on policing, but only $132.97 million on health, housing, parks, workforce development, permanent housing for the homeless, and arts and culture. The total amount Baltimore City spent on schools in FY2018—a total of $280.9 million—can be added to the aforementioned $132.97 million and Baltimore City still spent more of its own dollars on policing ($471.96 million) than it spent from the General Fund on public schools, health, housing, parks, employment development, permanent housing for the homeless, civil rights, and arts and culture collectively ($413.86 million).

Baltimore City maintains an apartheid budget. A recent report has found that Baltimore spends more per capita on police than other large cities in the nation. In *Freedom to Thrive: Reimagining Safety and Security in Our Communities*, the Center for Public Democracy, Law for Black Lives, and Black Youth Project 100 found that Baltimore City spends more per capita on police compared to nine other cities it profiled—Atlanta, Chicago, Detroit, Houston, Los Angeles, Minneapolis, New York City, Oakland, and Orlando.[11] Baltimore's current budget approach upholds urban apartheid and social control instead of allocating deep funding for the systems that support life.

Many Baltimore City residents envision another way of allocating public dollars. In 2019, OSI Baltimore sponsored a survey, which was filled out by over 5,000 people.[12] When asking Black Baltimoreans what the mayor should prioritize when spending $1 billion in discretionary funds, 39% of Black respondents prioritized youth programs as their top choice, followed by affordable housing and community-based safety programs (both at 15%), small businesses and neighborhood development (13%), policing (8%), and public health (6%). OSI Baltimore also found that respondents living in the six wealthiest Community Statistical Areas (CSAs) were less likely to support community-based safety programs and more likely to support policing even though less wealthy CSAs are more impacted by violence and crime. These data reveal that Black Baltimoreans envision a more equitable distribution of public dollars compared to White Baltimoreans. This must change if Baltimore City is to seize an equitable future for all. As organizer Tre Murphy said, "This is a chance for our elected officials to lead by example and fund Black futures."[13]

Funding Black futures is not a new strategy. In the 1960s, civil rights activists such as Asa Philip Randolph, Martin Luther King Jr., Bayard Rustin, Ruby Dee, and Oscar Davis proposed a Freedom Budget for the federal government that would drastically increase social spending in areas such as housing and education to address racial injustice impacting Black people. The Baltimore Freedom Budget constitutes a similar approach. A Baltimore Freedom Budget would mean significantly decreasing spending on police and significantly increasing spending for public schools, public health, housing and community development, recreation, libraries, and workforce development. The goal should be to decrease police spending by $200 million in eight years with resulting amounts allocated toward spending that supports human growth and thriving.

As a part of the Baltimore Freedom Budget, Baltimore City should allocate 10% of its annual budget—currently $290 million—to support the establishment of a Baltimore Neighborhood Reparations Fund. Given that mayors will come and go, the BNRF should be enshrined in the city charter via ballot initiative. The money from the BNRF would be allocated to redlined Black neighborhoods to help undo the damage caused by Baltimore City actively adopting, enforcing, and condoning racial zoning ordinances, racially restrictive covenants, code enforcement, discriminatory tax breaks, and repeated uprootings. Baltimore City segregated its own neighborhoods and allows modern segrenomics to flourish. During the 1910s through the 1950s, White government officials, civic leaders, religious organizations, and neighborhood associations waged a devastating war against the "Negro Invasion" from which the Black Butterfly has never recovered. In addition, Baltimore City contributed to redlining Black neighborhoods, assisting the federal government with creating the 1937 Residential Security Map and disproportionately funneling dollars from the capital budget to greenlined White L communities instead of redlined Black neighborhoods.

Hence, Baltimore City should allocate 10% of its budget for at least the next 50 years to undo the redline surrounding Black communities that were intentionally segregated from opportunity and restricted from access to public and private capital for over 80 years. To implement neighborhood reparations as a strategy, the top 20 most redlined neighborhoods should be identified and funds would be divided according to the severity of redlining in those communities. A democratically elected BNRF neighborhood council of 15 people living in each community would convene to decide how the money should be spent with the assistance of neighborhood residents and with technical capacity provided by the city. This participatory budgeting approach would empower neighborhood residents to make critical decisions about how they would like to see their communities developed and rebuilt.

Create the Baltimore Peacebuilding Authority

The third major strategy for healing the Black Butterfly is dismantling the Baltimore Police Department and disbanding the Baltimore Fraternal Order of Police that have proved to be engaged in hyperpolicing redlined Black neighborhoods. In its place, the Baltimore Peacebuilding Authority (BPA) should be organized to address crime and violence in Baltimore City. This does not mean that BPA officers would not carry guns or would not be authorized to use deadly force in certain situations. But the BPA would be organized on the premise that the authority's officers' first jobs are to build peace in communities, de-escalate tense situations, promote public safety, and protect and serve all neighborhoods as community guardians.

Sarah Malotane, a transdisciplinary scholar of restorative justice in South Africa, maintains that peacebuilding must incorporate a deep understanding of historical trauma.[14] Peacebuilding must be more than simply targeting individuals who commit violence. Peacebuilding works to reduce visible violence by addressing the three forms of invisible violence—structural, cultural, and psychological—that are deeply enmeshed in societies with histories of imperialism, enslavement, colonization, genocide, apartheid, and caste systems.[15] Invisible structural violence eventually becomes visible as shootings, stabbings, robberies, and homicides. Malotane's analysis makes it clear that invisible violence *precedes* visible violence and municipalities cannot build peace in societies based on imperialism, enslavement, colonialism, genocide, apartheid, and caste without first addressing the invisible violence and ongoing historical trauma festering in the structures, cultures, and neighborhoods where people live.[16]

Timothy Akers, a Morgan State University epidemiological criminologist, also had an intriguing idea—blending the police and health departments and "have the commissioners of each agency plan budgets together."[17] This approach could be taken with the Baltimore Peacebuilding Authority (BPA) so that public safety—established through peacebuilding and violence reduction—would have a public health orientation instead of a war orientation. Operating public safety from a public health perspective would mean that BPA officers would work with communities to build peace and reduce violence. Peacebuilding officers would work with public health officials to reduce lead poisoning and connect residents to mental health services, workforce development programs, and substance abuse treatment. Peacebuilding officers would be partners with the violence interrupters of Safe Streets instead of the antagonists that Baltimore police officers have often been.

This dramatic change would be difficult given the different cultures and orientation of public health workers and police officers. It might be wise to start with a pilot peacebuilding program that could begin to enact principles and approaches. Over time, the two departments could become a cohesive force for peacebuilding, violence prevention, and health equity throughout the city. A transformational change like this cannot function on its own. It must be paired with the push for racial equity in all multiple systems as discussed in Track 6 and with other strategies for healing the Black Butterfly discussed in this track.

What would a peacebuilding officer do? Peacebuilding officers would learn the history of the communities and cities where they patrol. They would understand that American Apartheid imposes structural violence in redlined Black neighborhoods. After swearing in, a peacebuilding officer would always work to first de-escalate violence and would be trained in mental health to better interact with people who may be suffering from mental illnesses. A peacebuilding officer would maintain regular appointments with mental health professionals to process and deal with their own traumatic experiences. A peacebuilding officer would work with neighborhoods' community economic development efforts to connect youth offenders to burgeoning efforts to build up their community.

Dismantling an entire police force and moving toward a peacebuilding strategy has been done before. The City of Camden, New Jersey, disbanded their entire police force in 2013. Since then, crime and violence have dropped to new lows as the new police department focused on being guardians instead of warriors. According to Chief of Police J. Scott Thompson, "It's more of a protect-and-serve approach to dealing with the residents, rather than kicking down doors and locking our way out of the problem."[18]

Desegregate the City and Suburbs

A fourth major strategy for healing the Black Butterfly is to deseg-regate the city and the suburbs. Ultimately, many of the issues faced in deeply racially segregated areas are rooted in the ways greenlined White communities hoard resources and opportunity, while starving redlined Black communities from equitable access to the same level of resources and opportunity.

To desegregate the city and suburbs, equitable resource alloca-tion must be a priority. Desegregation cannot solely be a matter of moving Black people next door to White people or vice versa. The true damage of racial segregation has been and continues to be segrenomics—the economic weaponization of racial segrega-tion achieved through public and private redlining, subpriming (i.e., predatory lending and renting), repeated uprootings, and other exploitative practices. Desegregation therefore must also mean desegregating public and private budgets and capital flows into Black neighborhoods without displacing existing residents. This is particularly the case for public budgets as research has shown that municipalities decrease spending on public goods as measures of racial segregation and ethnic fractionalization increase.[19]

Another way to achieve desegregation is to boost housing mo-bility within the city. Certainly, consent decrees such as the one spelled out in *Thompson v. HUD* are helpful as over 3,300 families have been given special court-mandated Housing Choice Vouch-ers to move to neighborhoods or suburbs with structured advan-tages outside of Baltimore City. However, roughly only 400–500 families have been given the same special vouchers to move to greenlined wealthy White communities in Baltimore City. More can and should be done to create housing mobility to neighbor-hoods with structured advantages within the city. Baltimore City and the State of Maryland should expand the usage of "desegregation vouchers" so that more Black families are able to move to White L communities within the city if they so choose. Desegregation can be more effectively implemented if the State of Maryland passes and enforces the HOME Act that has been proposed by Delegate Stephen Lafferty.[20] Baltimore City and Baltimore County must also vigorously enforce their newly passed HOME Acts (both passed in 2019) making discrimination against voucher holders illegal.

However, many fair housing advocates overemphasize housing mobility as the spatial strategy for racial equity while ignoring the need to repair and rejuvenate redlined Black neighborhoods without displacing existing residents. Housing mobility must be balanced with making Black neighborhoods matter. The balance can come from ensuring Black residents have a real choice: to live in an "opportunity neighborhood" whether they decide to move to neighborhoods with structured advantages or stay where they are.[21] This is why previously mentioned solutions such as Racial Equity Social Impact Bond, Stay Where You Are Vouchers, and Black Neighborhood Reparations are so vital. These strategies aim to turn Black neighborhoods into opportunity neighborhoods. Without equitable resource allocation to repair the damage inflicted on Black neighborhoods, housing mobility can contribute to the depopulation and destabilization of existing Black communities.

If Baltimore City and the State of Maryland equitably allocate resources to redlined Black neighborhoods with funding strategies such as the Racial Equity Social Impact Bond, the Baltimore Freedom Budget, and Black Neighborhood Reparations, then Black Butterfly neighborhoods would become more attractive to all residents. More people would want to live in previously redlined Black neighborhoods experiencing gains in resources and opportunity. But extreme care must be taken so that before this happens and during capital influx, legal and economic protections are in place (i.e., Stay Where You Are Vouchers), so that as

Black neighborhoods become more livable and attractive, existing Black residents are not displaced.

Another crucial desegregation strategy involves White L neighborhoods playing their role in funding and hosting autonomous transitional housing communities (ATHCs) along with eliminating exclusionary zoning restrictions to allow inclusionary housing. White L neighborhoods that have engaged in practices of racial exclusion—Roland Park, Guilford, Homeland, Bolton Hill, Mount Washington, Locust Point, Hampden, and Remington to name a few—must dismantle their de facto restrictive covenants and zoning laws to accommodate ATHCs and housing units with higher densities to make recompense for decades of racial segregation.

Many of the same neighborhood associations, religious organizations, and institutions that helped promote and enforce racial segregation in the 1910s to 1950s still exist. These entities were actively weaponized in the war against the "Negro Invasion." Given their central role, it is not enough to simply apologize and "have a conversation." As Malotane sharply argues: "healing for the oppressed is not going to come through neoliberal peacebuilding where privileged and pulverised hug and cry for the cameras and world peace; then go back to their structurally unequal lives."[22]

Entities that helped erect the walls of Baltimore Apartheid have a special obligation to help tear them down. Concretely, this means people who are a part of such entities should be organizing to implement the five steps for racial equity and lobbying city government for the desegregation of resources and the end of White L structural advantages. Tearing down Baltimore Apartheid means actively supporting inclusionary policies in White L neighborhoods and shifting the massive resources needed to boost the Black Butterfly. It means revoking the tax-privileged status that many White L entities and homeowners enjoy and ending the tax-punished status of many entities and homeowners in the Black Butterfly.

With billions of dollars in damages over the course of centuries, a $12 million Youth Fund or a $55 million Neighborhood Investment Impact Fund, operated as a privatized nonprofit, is simply not enough. It took over a hundred years to institutionalize apartheid, hence the process for healing will take decades. Entities must remain deeply committed and engaged from beginning to end.

Strengthen the Baltimore Office of Equity and Civil Rights

A fifth strategy for healing the Black Butterfly is to strengthen the newly renamed Baltimore Office of Equity and Civil Rights (OECR). In 2018, Baltimore City councilmember Brandon Scott introduced parallel bills to kick-start the push for racial equity in Baltimore City. The racial equity assessment legislation has already led to vital city agency and departmental reflections and staff training. However, the OECR should have full monitoring authority and subpoena power to enforce the legislation. With investigatory power to subpoena city agencies and compel enforcement, the OECR can work to mandate and monitor the practice of racial equity in city agencies and departments. Given past conflicts over the civilian review of police, OECR should be completely independent from the city solicitor to avoid a conflict of interest (as the city solicitor represents other city agencies, such as the police).

None of this can be achieved without adequate funding. The OECR budget should be at least $20 million. Currently, the office is anemically funded at a paltry $2.1 million. Baltimore's agency to enforce equity and civil rights must be a powerful agent of reckoning.

To make the OECR more effective, community members, historians, and lawyers should be hired as full-time workers to serve on the Community Relations Commission (CRC). According to Ordinance 103 (passed in 1964), the CRC was given the authority to effect systemic remedies for structural inequities. Ordinance

103 was a good start but is lacking in enforcement power and limited by its members being unpaid volunteers. Fostering racial equity requires enforcement and focused attention. Therefore, Ordinance 103 must be strengthened to broaden the scope of the work of the CRC so that the commission can conduct independent and robust equity audits of departments and agencies that operate in the city. Following this, the CRC can propose binding remedies consistent with existing civil rights laws and the racial equity assessment legislation.

Racial equity department/agency assessment committees should work with OECR staff to produce a racial equity plan complete with the amount of funding each agency needs to allocate to stop hurting Black communities and to take meaningful corrective actions where damage was done in the past. This work can be done according to the 10 steps identified by Race Forward in its Racial Equity Impact Assessment.[23] The 10th step in the Racial Equity Impact Assessment is to identify success indicators. OECR can use Community Equity Metrics to determine progress toward citywide spatial equity, although these metrics should continue to be refined and improved.

OECR should also fight to ensure banks are living up to the mandate to undo redlining as outlined in the 1977 CRA. The office should work to attract additional CRA funds to be placed into credit unions and Black banks so that CRA dollars are used to fund community wealth building approaches. Or perhaps the office can create a public banking entity to finance the work that needs to be done.

Bolster Community Wealth Building and Cooperative Enterprises

While addressing historical trauma and implementing racial equity within city government should be the work of the OECR, a separate office should focus on boosting community wealth in the

Black Butterfly. The Baltimore Office of Community Wealth Building (BOCWB) would engage in lending, funding, allocating, and investing dollars in redlined Black neighborhoods so that existing residents can establish cooperatives where they co-own community enterprises, share in equitable decision making, and benefit collectively from the wealth generated by their efforts. Cooperatives are businesses that are collectively owned and democratically governed by people, and they exist to satisfy a need or to address a problem in the community.[24] One of the most pernicious impacts of ongoing historical trauma is that it prevents people from owning the means of the production of their labor and diminishes their decision-making capacity. Therefore, BOCWB should work to empower people living in redlined neighborhoods to build economic power and become more self-sufficient and self-determining.

Richmond, Virginia, has taken an innovative step in this area by starting an Office of Community Wealth Building. For hypersegregated core cities such as Baltimore, such an office must focus on funding redlined and environmentally oppressed neighborhoods—through community land trusts, community investment trusts, utility and solar cooperatives, food composting, community gardens or urban farms, and ATHCs—to help expand economic prosperity and to undo the damage caused by segrenomics. This BOCWB can also duplicate and expand projects like the one created by Agatha So, a Baltimore fellow at the Open Society Institute. Working with a Philadelphia-based community development financial institution (CDFI), So created an alternative credit mortgage initiative that allowed prospective Latino/a homebuyers to show creditworthiness without the traditional credit score. This allowed 200 families to purchase homes in Southeast Baltimore after they saved and were able to put a fairly significant down payment on a home without subprime penalties.[25] This approach could be used by the BOCWB and affiliated

CDFIs so that Black homebuyers can also use a similar approach. However, this homebuying approach should be used in concert with other collective ownership models such as the housing cooperative put into practice by members of the Potomac Association of Housing Cooperatives.[26]

Another way to boost community wealth would be to provide funding for Baltimore's burgeoning community garden movement. Community gardens should be viewed as cooperative community enterprises by the BOCWB. Community garden efforts are underway in redlined and environmentally oppressed communities, such as Cherry Hill (Black Yield Institute), Sandtown-Winchester (Tubman House), and Curtis Bay (Filbert Street Community Garden). These efforts represent resident-led empowerment projects and beacons of hope. With significant funding and support, community gardens can boost food security and nutrition, increase residents' employment, and provide green space that improves mental health for residents.

Other solutions can be paired with cooperative community gardens. Open Society Institute fellow Marvin Hayes is leading an effort to compost food scraps to create what he calls "black gold," or fertile soil, in partnership with Filbert Street Community Garden director Rodette Jones. Cooperative community gardens combined with citywide composting sites could form the basis of a sustainable solidarity economy. According to Hayes, such a robust citywide effort could provide viable employment for youth who clean windshields and help them earn a living wage while providing a tremendous service to the city. Further, by reducing trash sent to the waste incinerators in Curtis Bay, air pollution would be reduced and public health would be improved. The generative potential of this strategy—as envisioned by Marvin Hayes—is tremendous for the Black Butterfly and the environmentally oppressed communities in South Baltimore.

Across the nation, Black banks play a central role in the project of boosting community wealth in Black neighborhoods. But Black banks are no silver bullet or panacea for what ails Black neighborhoods.[27] They certainly cannot eliminate the racial wealth gap on their own.[28] But Black banks can support community wealth building and alternative credit mortgage initiatives. Black banks can and should financially support more cooperatives in Black communities, underwrite projects in community land trusts, and set up community investment trusts to allow people to co-own commercial property in their neighborhood.

Another effort called BankBlack, led by architect and scholar Justin Garrett Moore, aims to track the lending portfolios of Black banks and their funding of Black cooperatives. This effort can help encourage Black banks to underwrite the rise of collective economics in redlined Black communities. Black banks that are federally qualified CDFIs, in particular, should make these collective economic mechanisms at least 15–20% of their portfolio by 2025 and 30% by 2030. At least one Black bank has already made strides in this direction. OneUnited, the largest Black-owned bank in the country, has financed affordable housing in South Central Los Angeles, Compton, Liberty City (Miami), and Roxbury (Boston).[29] In addition, OneUnited offers an official Community Land Trust Home Loan and provided such loans to Dudley Street Neighborhood Initiative and the South Florida Community Land Trust.[30] Working together with cities' Offices of Community Wealth Building, Black banks (and other banks) can play a pivotal role in promoting community wealth building in redlined Black neighborhoods.

The Evergreen Cooperative model in Cleveland is also a model for Baltimore's universities and hospitals often referred to as *anchor institutions*. In Cleveland, anchor institutions have partnered with Evergreen Cooperatives to provide support for laundry, greenhouse, and solar energy cooperatives.[31] Baltimore universities and hospitals can replicate the Evergreen Cooperative model and boost community wealth building by contracting with Black Butterfly collective economic enterprises such as worker, food, energy, utility, solar, and housing cooperatives. Although the HopkinsLocal initiative has helped hire 1,017 people and to distribute $58 million in contracts to minority-owned firms, this activity only helps individual employees and small-business owners.[32] It does not boost wealth for redlined Black communities as a whole.

Cooperative enterprises, however, fuel the engine of community wealth building and democratize the ownership of work. Worker-owners are able to have a strong decision-making say in how their community enterprise operates and enhance their voice in governance. Building community wealth has to be about more than generating money; it is also about building power and meeting the needs of redlined Black communities. Anchor institutions must do much more than hire people into low-wage positions. The goal for anchor institutions is to underwrite the development and growth of community enterprises in redlined Black neighborhoods. In the final analysis, the existing residents who live in redlined Black communities must be seen and regarded as anchor institutions, too.

Finance Racial Equity Efforts with Funds from the 1977 Community Reinvestment Act

The Community Reinvestment Act was passed in 1977 to combat redlining in Black neighborhoods. It is the only federal tool designed to address the legacy of bank redlining in Black communities. While billions of dollars have been awarded based on violations of the 1977 CRA, the CRA has not been used to specifically help heal and restore redlined Black neighborhoods. One major problem is that the act has focused primarily on lending to Black and lower-income homebuyers instead of being set up to address the broader damage caused by private bank redlining in Black neighborhoods specifically. Redlining not only damaged home-buying and small-business expansion for Black neighborhoods, it contributed to increased levels of crime and violence, vacant homes, substance abuse, and toxic lead exposure.

A second major problem is that the CRA, like other federal urban policies, has not addressed the root issue of urban apartheid. Previous federal urban policy efforts (including the CRA) are implemented in cities and counties that still practice apartheid. Federal funds obtained via the CRA and other federal urban policies are not distributed to redlined Black neighborhoods in a manner consistent with the five steps to foster racial equity. Like the CRA, federal urban policies such as Model Cities (President Johnson), Enterprise Zones (President Reagan), Empowerment Zones (President Clinton), and Promise Zones (President Obama) have failed to produce the desired results.[33] President Trump's Opportunity Zones will also fail.

History is clear—it is not enough to purportedly allocate dollars to Black communities, when large corporations and developers are the actual beneficiaries. The CRA and other federal urban policies have not materially improved the lives of Black residents because American Apartheid has been left unaddressed. Without dismantling urban apartheid and carrying out a robust racial equity approach—including setting up democratic structures of local community decision making, increasing resident participation in community economic development, and cooperatively sharing the wealth produced by particular initiatives with Black communities—the dollars spent will not and cannot produce the desired outcomes.

With this in mind, the CRA (and all federal urban economic policies) should be revamped to foster the economic empowerment of Black neighborhoods and fund racial equity work. Since redlined Black neighborhoods were damaged historically and are still damaged specifically due to the denial of capital access in specific communities, CRA dollars should be allocated directly toward the communities that were most affected and deeply redlined. Existing data and analysis from national research now allows researchers and communities to specify the damage done by banks and financial institutions engaging in redlining and subpriming.[34] With this empirical research, many of the financial harms of redlining and subprime lending have already been quantified and calculated.

It makes sense then to use this data to create a redlining/subpriming index for each Baltimore neighborhood so that the allocation of CRA dollars can be disbursed to Black neighborhoods according to how severely they were impacted by banking segrenomics. In other words, more CRA dollars should be allocated to the Black neighborhoods most damaged by banking segrenomics and fewer CRA dollars should be allocated to communities that have not been damaged as much.[35] This is what a racially equitable approach entails not only for CRA dollars but also for all capital spending and allocations of resources.

In addition to indexing CRA allocation amounts to the intensity of banking segrenomics, CRA dollars should be allocated directly to a democratically elected council of 15 people in redlined Black communities. This could be the same council that would administer the dollars allocated as a part of the Baltimore Neighborhood Reparations Fund (see the section "Fund Freedom Budgets and Black Neighborhood Reparations"), or it could be a separate second neighborhood council. A CRA neighborhood council would foster the governance capacity of people in redlined communities and give them a decision-making voice on how they would like to see their community developed. CRA dollars should be used to fund a neighborhood development leadership program to train CRA neighborhood councilmembers on the ins and outs of community economic development from a holistic perspective. Leadership programs could be housed at HBCUs such as Coppin State and Morgan State Universities in Baltimore to inform and bolster the work of building healthy communities in the Black Butterfly.

Funds from the CRA can also be used to subsidize wealth-enhancing strategies such as "baby bonds" for lower-income residents living in redlined Black neighborhoods. Senator Cory Booker's American Opportunities Account Act can serve as the model for funding baby bonds for Black residents with lower incomes throughout the city.[36] Another approach is to use CRA dollars to fund a universal basic income program. Universal basic income can be distributed to lower-income residents in households earning less than $50,000. The lower a household's income, the higher the level of their disbursement from the CRA neighborhood council.

Several efforts are underway to pilot universal basic income approaches in cities across the nation. In Jackson, Mississippi, Magnolia Mother's Trust started providing 16 Black mothers with lower incomes $1,000 a month in income support.[37] Stockton, California, is piloting a guaranteed income starting in February 2019 with $1 million donated by a private entity.[38] Other cities are also rolling out similar programs.[39] Baltimore can create a larger guaranteed income program to help eliminate the racial income gap. Another strategy is to follow the lead of New York City, which is starting a municipal health care program.[40] Baltimore can fund expansive universal basic income or universal municipal health care programs if it secures billions in CRA dollars through vigorous CRA advocacy and determines how to structure social impact bonds using CRA dollars. If Baltimore City works seriously to enforce the CRA, the necessary funding can be secured to make Black neighborhoods matter.

Center Black Planning Principles
in Redlined Black Neighborhoods

In 1960, the League of Women Voters of Baltimore City published a report detailing how urban renewal was being carried out in the city. The League asked a powerful question, *Who then is doing the planning?* They listed three organizations: City Planning Commission, BURHA (the Baltimore Urban Renewal and Housing Agency), and the Greater Baltimore Committee. After this list, they wrote the word "cooperatively." In other words, residents of the city were not among those planning the city and certainly not Black residents.

The question posed by the League of Women Voters 60 years ago is a compelling question for people living in redlined Black neighborhoods today. Who is doing the planning now? Who is planning Black futures in hypersegregated cities? Who is planning for thriving Black neighborhoods to emerge out of the constrictions of urban apartheid? Who is planning for healthy and whole Black Lives today in America today?

It is vitally important to ask and answer these questions in order to ensure inclusionary Black planning approaches are centered when developing Black neighborhoods. Black planning and development are not a new phenomenon in America. Black Reconstruction—the period immediately following the Civil War—can serve as a planning inspiration for healing and redeveloping redlined Black neighborhoods in hypersegregated cities. After winning and securing emancipation, formerly enslaved Black people made tremendous strides in the 50 years post-enslavement. Black educators helped start HBCUs and Black congregations built churches. Black communities helped democratize the allocation of public goods. Black economic practitioners collectively built economic districts, such as Black Wall Street in Tulsa, Sweet Auburn Avenue in Atlanta, Hayti in Durham, and Springfield in Illinois.

Black people engaged in collective economics, secured ownership of land, and managed entire cities and towns (such as Rosewood in Florida or Freedom Colonies in Texas).

Today, there is an abundance of wisdom and visionary insight worth considering when it comes to making Black neighborhoods matter in planning. Mindy Fullilove and colleagues have expanded the insights of her work on root shock while laying out a compelling urban redevelopment framework in her book *Urban Alchemy.*[41] A variety of Black planners and urbanists recently articulated approaches to developing Black neighborhoods in the journal *Planning Theory and Practice.*[42]

Alongside these Black planning visions, the simplicity and beauty of the BlackSpace Manifesto developed by BlackSpace NYC—a group of Black professionals in New York City trained in architecture, urban planning, design, and art—stands out. They succinctly articulate planning principles that should guide the work of building and developing Black neighborhoods.[43] BlackSpace Manifesto principles and the accompanying explanations exemplify the ways that planners, architects, designers, developers, and government officials should operate while planning and developing redlined Black neighborhoods. Without trust, deep listening, planning with, designing with, cultivating wealth, and centering lived experience, economic development efforts in Black neighborhoods result in repeated uprootings and economic destruction while deepening cultural dispossession.

The BlackSpace Manifesto principle "manifest the future" is especially important given the exigent conditions found in many redlined Black neighborhoods. BlackSpace NYC encourages planners to remember that "Black people, Black culture, and Black spaces exist in the future! Imagine and design the future into existence now working inside and outside social and political systems." Manifesting the future is linked to Afrofuturism. As Ingrid LaFleur argues: "Afrofuturism [is] a way to encourage experimentation, reimagine identities, and activate liberation." Manifesting the future of Black neighborhoods is supremely important in a society that cannot even imagine thriving Black neighborhoods. Experimentation—the grace to try and fail and try again—should be encouraged and nurtured.

Afrofuturistic ecological thinking is needed to imagine and envision thriving Black neighborhoods (figure 7.1). Afrofuturistic ecological thinking generates a scientifically seasoned faith, which allows practitioners to know that planting the seeds today will bring forth beautiful flowers (i.e., healthy people) in due season if nutrient-rich soil (i.e., systems, policies, and practices), abundant water (i.e., budgets and funding), and ample sunlight (i.e., accountability and participatory democracy) are put in place.

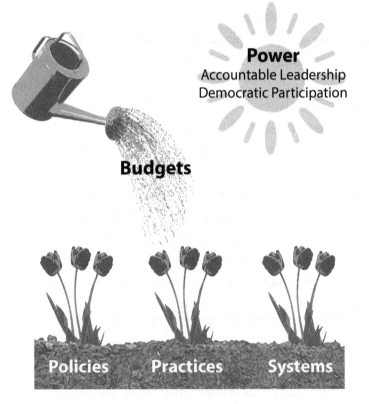

Figure 7.1. The Community Health Garden

Black neighborhoods can flourish if cities and counties engage in a robust racial equity process. Black Lives will blossom if cities and residents work diligently to build healthy Black neighborhoods and nurture them to reach their fullest potential. When cities and counties engage in the work to grow the flowers in the *community health garden*, Black neighborhoods and Black Lives will finally matter.

Financing Healing for the Black Butterfly

Each of the eight solutions outlined to heal the Black Butterfly addresses at least one of the four major components of historical trauma. Desegregating the city and suburbs addresses the harm of racial hypersegregation. The Racial Equity Social Impact Bond addresses the damage wrought by economic destruction. The Baltimore Peacebuilding Authority and Baltimore Office of Equity and Civil Rights would help attend to the damage inflicted by physical, psychological, and structural violence. The proposed Freedom Budget, Baltimore Neighborhood Reparations, Office of Community Wealth Building, and CRA advocacy are all designed to heal the Black Butterfly from the damage of economic destruction. Finally, centering Black planning principles is designed to help prevent future cultural dispossession. With these types of strategies, hypersegregated cities can stop ongoing historical trauma and catalyze the healing needed using a robust racial equity approach.

Although wealthy and powerful corporations should no longer be privileged in city planning, they still have a pivotal role to play. Corporations and people with wealth and power may be asked to provide resources, capacity-building assistance, or technical expertise in certain areas, and they should do so with humility and a mindset of service instead of profit. Going forward, corporate interests should no longer be privileged to the detriment of people living in redlined Black neighborhoods.

Table 7.1.   Financial solutions for Black Butterfly neighborhoods

Name of Initiative	Time Frame	Annual Allotment	Source of Financing	Cost
Racial Equity Social Impact Bond	5 years	Onetime allotment	Banks, philanthropy, donations, CRA dollars	$3,000,000,000
Baltimore Neighborhood Reparations	40 years	~$350 million in the top 20 most redlined neighborhoods	10% Baltimore city budget, TIF districts after bond repayment	$14,000,000,000
BCPSS capital budget	Onetime allotment	Onetime allotment	Maryland state bonds	$5,000,000,000
BCPSS Thornton payment	Onetime allotment	Onetime allotment	Maryland state General Fund	$2,000,000,000+
Racial Equity Block Grants for schools	20 years	$250 million at 50 schools— $5 million each	City and state General Fund; CRA dollars	$5,000,000,000
Universal Basic Income & Assets	20 years	Average $20,000 for 150,000 households	CRA Social Impact Bonds from banks	$60,000,000,000
CRA Neighborhood Reparations	20 years	$500 million in redlined neighborhoods	CRA Social Impact Bonds from banks	$10,000,000,000
Total Cost				$99,000,000,000

The solutions to make Black Butterfly neighborhoods matter must be fully financed. A rough estimate of how much money major proposals would cost, how money would be allotted over time, and possible sources of financing are presented in table 7.1. Since institutions that are both public (city, state, and federal governments) and private (banks, philanthropy, and nonprofits) played a role in damaging Black communities, they all have a role to play in financing the mechanisms needed for healing the Black Butterfly. Over the course of 20 years, a total cost of nearly $99 billion will be needed—with $12 billion allocated to public schools, $60 billion to close the racial income gap, and $27 billion to heal and repair Black neighborhoods.

If cities and counties implement similarly tailored solutions in the course of applying a racial equity approach to all relevant policies, practices, systems, and budgets, then environmentally oppressed and redlined Black neighborhoods will receive the needed resources to thrive.[44] From a community health standpoint, these solutions are vital to improving the health of environmentally oppressed and redlined Black neighborhoods that have been subjected to sustained segrenomics, repeated uprootings, toxic lead exposures, polluted environments, post-traumatic stress disorder due to intracommunal violence, and racism-based traumatic stress due to hyperpolicing. Chronic diseases would be improved by creating healthier environments that encourage physical activity (e.g., building recreation centers, planting trees and gardens, protected bike/transit lanes with community input) and by boosting nutrient-rich food access to combat food apartheid. Other health conditions such as opioid overdoses, sexually transmitted infections, and homicides would decrease as economic security increases and community health workers connect people to services and resources.

Conclusion

While these eight strategies would be the responsibility of Baltimore City, various entities in city neighborhoods should not wait on the city to start making racial and spatial equity real. Implementing racial equity strategies in Baltimore will require White L neighborhoods to play a supportive role in dismantling Baltimore Apartheid, especially those neighborhoods that practiced racial exclusion or enforced racially restrictive covenants. Neighborhood associations in the White L must also stand in solidarity with and economically support the people living in environmentally oppressed and historically redlined Black neighborhoods. This is an ethical mandate particularly since many historic neighborhood associations vigorously lobbied Baltimore's mayors to "build that wall"—the same apartheid wall that now separates Black Butterfly neighborhoods from the wealth hoarded in the White L.

Now is the time to lift up the neighborhoods that have been systematically put down. Developing an equitable city for all people—especially for Black residents in redlined neighborhoods—requires a concrete sharing of power and resources by structurally advantaged White L communities and wealthy corporate interests. However, the notion of healing Black neighborhoods should never devolve into a warm and fuzzy rhetoric devoid of addressing dynamics of power. As Sarah Malotane argues:

> I do NOT position myself as a victim because I refuse to hand my power over to oppressors and some beneficiaries who seek to individualise and pathologise my response. I position myself as someone who was victimised in the domestic, intra-group, inter-group and political spheres; and who must of necessity acknowledge and tend to my wounds as an act of power, not defeat.[45]

Healing the Black Butterfly means empowering everyday residents in the Butterfly to assume governing roles and collectively confront the impacts of ongoing historical trauma. This will allow environmentally oppressed and redlined Black communities to "tend to their wounds" as an action of empowerment. As Malotane argues in her book *Disrupting Denial*, people impacted by ongoing historical trauma need symbolic, psychological, structural, and physical healing.[46] Concrete healing must take place at every level where damage has been done. This includes stopping structural violence and providing the necessary resources for redlined Black communities to reach their full potential.

Baltimoreans in redlined Black communities deserve structural healing, deep resources, and shared power. Only by intentionally taking each of the five steps of an authentic racial equity process, highlighted throughout this work, can Baltimore City and other cities at the core of hypersegregated metropolitan areas across America first openly acknowledge, then halt, and finally structurally heal from ongoing historical trauma. America can only make Black neighborhoods matter once policymakers—in places ranging from hypersegregated cities to small towns—concretely address the damage caused by ongoing historical trauma and employ large-scale strategies to secure spatial equity.

Outro:
Organize!

Like liberation is any. other. place.
than under our sternums
Like we ain't been surviving
Like we ain't been needin freedom
Like the time ain't now
Tariq Touré, "Like This Road Been Crystal"

America is now over 150 years removed from the end of the Civil War and the ratifications of the Thirteenth and Fourteenth Reconstruction Amendments, which ended chattel slavery and extended citizenship to people of African descent. In many ways, the questions posed by the Civil War have yet to be resolved. Whether Black people are considered full citizens in America remains a question to be fully and affirmatively answered. Despite tangible political and legal progress, America's repeated whitelashes result in a retrenchment and retreat from fulfilling the nation's promises.

America is now over 50 years removed from the passage of the Fair Housing Act. For millions of Black homebuyers and renters, the ability to live in prosperous neighborhoods has remained an illusory dream. For Black people living in redlined neighborhoods, racial equity is but a fairy tale as spatial equity has been neglected. In its fullness, fair housing means not just housing mobility but also spatial equity to remedy spatial racism. Black people should have fair access to public dollars and private capital, whether they live in demographically whiter suburbs or urban

Black neighborhoods. Instead of basking in the sunlight of spatial equity, Black neighborhoods continue to be redlined, subprimed, and targeted for wealth extraction.[1]

Across the nation, 21 large metropolitan areas remain hyper-segregated—a number that could very well increase during the Trump presidency once the numbers are crunched from the 2020 Census. Evidence already indicates that racial segregation is increasing. When faced with increasing racial diversity in their communities, many White families hunker down and move into less diverse neighborhoods.[2] Wealthy White breakaway school districts are on the rise—indicating a retreat from a shared commitment to education as a common good.[3] Meanwhile, the nation's K–12 public school systems continue to resegregate.[4] With America playing the Trump card in the 2016 presidential election, America is racing backward in terms of progress on dismantling the white supremacist policies, practices, systems, and budgets that extract both health and wealth from Black neighborhoods.

Only blood and fire seem to motivate America to pass strong policies to confront the racism deeply embedded in the legal and social DNA of the nation. Blood and fire rained down on America during the brutal Civil War and Wars of Reconstruction. The blood of Dr. King and fires of urban rioting shook America to its core during the Great Uprising. Since 2014, the blood of victims of police violence sparked the fires of uprisings and militant protests in Ferguson, Baltimore, Cleveland, Baton Rouge, Milwaukee, Kenosha, Charlotte, Minneapolis, St. Louis, and Chicago.

America's history reveals ongoing racial turmoil and the repeated emergence of whitelash. After making progress on eliminating racism, America reverts to patterns and practices of racial dominance and reconstitutes its systems of oppression. The whitelash of White Redemption and the war on the "Negro Invasion" undercut many advances made during Black Reconstruction. The whitelash of the war on Black neighborhoods undermined advances made during the Civil Rights and Black Power Movements. The whitelash of the 2010 Tea Party and the 2016 election of Trump blocked and rolled back advances gained during the Obama presidency. With such a cyclical history, the question becomes whether America will ever be a nation with liberty and justice for all or whether racism is a permanent feature of American social and political life (as posited by critical race theorist, legal scholar, and writer Derrick Bell).

Confronting Urban Democrats

The GOP–Tea Party has not been alone in damaging Black neighborhoods and Black people with lower incomes. Democrats in large urban areas have repeatedly harmed Black neighborhoods by rejecting a minimum wage increase (Baltimore), repealing a corporate head tax (Seattle), and uprooting Black neighborhoods (Austin, Washington, DC, Denver, Atlanta, San Francisco, Oakland, Chicago, etc.). Although damage caused by state and federal policies is severe, urban Democrats are in a position to inflict severe damage as local governments are more proximate to redlined Black neighborhoods. Local governments have tremendous power to shape how state and federal policies are implemented and enforced.

It may be politically expedient to direct all attention to the GOP–Tea Party given the alarming policies currently passed and enforced at the national level, but from an organizing and outcomes perspective, doing so represents a huge tactical error. It is akin to being pummeled by two people—one on the left and the other on the right—but ignoring the person on the left and directing all energy to the attacker on the right. Black neighborhoods and Black Lives are being attacked on both sides—by a resurgent whitelash party on the right and by a pro-corporate apartheid party on the left. Therefore, organizing strategies are needed to challenge the policies, practices, systems, and budgets enacted and implemented by the two dominant parties in America.

Organizing Strategy

Education and commemoration should constitute the foundation of organizing for positive political change. Before rushing straight to solutions, Americans must spend the time to reflect and study the nation's history. Reflecting and studying requires reinvigorating public education and historical commemoration, particularly as it relates to the history throughout this work. Americans will never pass radical progressive legislation if they do not come to terms with the radically oppressive legislation that created and now upholds American Apartheid.

The National Peace and Justice Museum located in Montgomery, Alabama—often called the National Lynching Museum—is a sobering yet powerful example of public education and historical commemoration that lifts up a prominent aspect of American history many Americans would like to forget or ignore. The museum should serve as inspiration for cities like Baltimore, which does not lift up its own sordid history in a forthright and compelling way. The history of the extensive Baltimore Slave Trade centered at the Inner Harbor, the Underground Railroad stations in Black churches such as Orchard Street Church in Seton Hill, and the slave pens and jails that were located on Pratt Street have been relegated to books and archives. Baltimore City must make this history come *alive*. Without this critical context, most residents will not understand why Baltimore continues to wrestle with the demons of its past and why the city is doomed unless it makes amends for inflicting ongoing historical trauma and for giving birth to urban American Apartheid. It is this education and commemoration that can catalyze the redeeming of Baltimore's soul and making Black neighborhoods whole.

This education and commemoration should inform the organizing work in the city. Recent Baltimore organizers have repeatedly called attention to Baltimore's apartheid policies, practices, systems, and budgets.[5] In the wake of the April 2015 Uprising, important victories have been won by local activists, including establishing and funding the Affordable Housing Trust Fund and Youth Fund, calling for Housing First policies for people experiencing homelessness, passing important ballot initiatives, and ensuring the water system remains a publicly owned entity. Advocates have also won the passage of the Baltimore Clean Air Act, the Water Taxpayer Protection Act, and a statewide $15 per hour minimum wage bill. Other organizers are pushing for increased wages for nurses at Johns Hopkins Hospital and renegotiating the 2016 payments in lieu of taxes agreement so that private universities and hospitals will pay their proportionate share of taxes.

The city council's passage and voters' approval of the Equity Assessment Program legislation in 2018 also constituted advancement in the push for racial equity.[6] The bill requires city agencies and departments to "assess existing and proposed policies and practices for disparate outcomes based on race, gender, sexual orientation, or income and to proactively develop policies, practices, and investments to prevent and redress those disparate outcomes."[7] The same assessment should be applied to the Baltimore City Council itself as the council continued to pass inequitable legislation in 2019. Hence, there is much more work to be done to make racial equity a reality. The next step is to go to the heart of Baltimore Apartheid and dismantle its infrastructure root and branch.

Across the nation, powerful local organizing is taking place. The National Black Worker Center is building power in local communities by supporting worker centers in multiple cities. In Washington, DC, groups such as ONE DC and BlackLivesMatter DC have been organizing for racial equity and social justice. In Los Angeles, BlackLivesMatter LA has been engaged in a consistent critical demand against police brutality. In Seattle, the Seattle People's Party has emerged as a potentially viable third party. In Jackson, Mississippi, an effort named Cooperation Jackson continues the legacy and work of Chokwe Lumumba and the push for cooperative development. In Chicago, Black Youth Project 100 and other advocates have pushed for radical change in the city. In North Carolina, the Moral Mondays movement continues to call for social justice. In 2018, the national Poor People's Campaign organized demonstrations around the country reviving the 1968 organizing push by Dr. Martin Luther King Jr. and the Southern Christian Leadership Conference. In the voting sphere, gubernatorial candidates Stacey Abrams and Andrew Gillum electrified electorates in Georgia and Florida. Only massive voting violations and voter disenfranchisement by their respective states stopped them from assuming office.

These efforts highlight hope for a brighter future. To dismantle American Apartheid in urban areas, local movements must coalesce to make Black neighborhoods matter. In his West Indian Emancipation speech, Frederick Douglass observed: "Power concedes nothing without a demand. It never has and it never will." Student Nonviolent Coordinating Committee (SNCC) organizer and chairman Stokely Carmichael later echoed Douglass: "When improvements within the system have been made, they resulted from pressure—pressure from below. Nothing has been given away; governments don't hand out justice because it's a nice thing to do."[8] Black neighborhoods will not matter without a demand or without pressure. Black neighborhoods will not thrive without securing voting rights and polling sites. Given this, organizers and residents must increasingly focus on dismantling urban apartheid policies, practices, systems, and budgets enacted and enforced by mayors and city councils in order to make racial equity a reality.

Importantly, organizing to make Black neighborhoods matter should be a both-and proposition instead of an either-or dichotomy.

That is, confrontational strategies should be deployed when needed, but it is equally important to employ Afrofuturistic ecological thinking to build and foster healthy Black neighborhoods. Strengthening Black neighborhoods is essential even though it may not receive the press or accolades as radical protests against power. Organizers should also maintain flexibility in the type of strategies they employ and consider the lay of the land in different urban areas. In some urban areas, it may make more sense to organize within the Democratic Party (Jackson, Mississippi) while in other areas it may make more sense to organize outside of the Democratic Party (Seattle People's Party).

The organizing challenge is to identify and stop segrenomics, apartheid budgeting, hyperpolicing, and resource withdrawal that both Democrats and Republicans have advanced and enacted. During his speech at the University of California Berkeley on October 29, 1966, SNCC chairman Stokely Carmichael—who would later be known as Kwame Ture—indicated how both major political parties do not protect Black Lives nor uplift Black neighborhoods:

> The political parties in this country do not meet the needs of people on a day-to-day basis. The question is: how can we build new political institutions that will become the political expressions of people on a day-to-day basis? The question is: how can you build political institutions that will begin to meet the needs of Oakland, California? And the needs of Oakland, California, is not 1,000 policemen with submachine guns. They don't need that. They need that least of all. The question is: how can we build institutions where those people can begin to function on a day-to-day basis, where they can get decent jobs, where they can get decent houses, and where they can begin to participate in the policy and major decisions that affect their lives?[9]

SNCC's work was rooted in understanding local conditions and empowering local people to organize to dismantle Jim and Jane

Crow. Carmichael himself was mentored by the great Ella Baker. In the 1940s and 1950s, Ella Baker served as an assistant field secretary, national director of branches, and director of the New York branch of the NAACP. In the 1960s, she helped co-found three pivotal organizations that advanced the struggle for Black freedom—the Southern Christian Leadership Conference, the Student Nonviolent Coordinating Committee, and the Mississippi Freedom Democratic Party.

While there were multiple factors and many people involved, it was Baker's organizing principles that proved vital to mobilizing rural Southern Black people so that they could confront and overthrow Jim and Jane Crow in the Deep South. In "Developing Community Leadership," Baker articulated:

> Black people who were living in the South were constantly living with violence. Part of the job was to help them to understand what that violence was and how they in an organized fashion could help to stem it. The major job was getting people to understand that they had something within their power that they could use, and it could only be used if they understood what was happening and how group action could counter violence even when it was perpetrated by the police or, in some instances, the state. My basic sense of it has always been to get people to understand that in the long run they themselves are the only protection they have against violence or injustice.[10]

In spite of violence and whitelash, people have succeeded in dismantling previous forms of racial dominance. The challenge for today's organizers is to use the Ella Baker model of organizing to build community power in redlined Black neighborhoods and hypersegregated cities. The same organizing model used to defeat Jim and Jane Crow in yesteryear—group-centered leadership, building local leaders, eschewing the charismatic model of leadership, political education, and direct action—will also be effective in dismantling American Apartheid.[11] By employing Baker's model of organizing, people can build power at local levels that can then be brought together to carry out a national struggle to make Black neighborhoods matter.

Along these lines, organizers should consider forming local political action committees that can link together and form a Movement for Black Lives (M4BL) or #BlackLivesMatter (BLM) SuperPAC. A BLM/M4BL SuperPAC can support electoral candidates who will work to make Black Lives and Black neighborhoods matter. A nationwide BLM/M4BL SuperPAC can support candidates in the Democratic Party or in third parties who best reflect the values of the movement, giving organizers electoral flexibility and preventing BLM/M4BL from being co-opted by the Democratic Party.

Ultimately, the push for racial equity and social justice is a marathon, not a sprint. However, an organized community can often spur rapid changes. As Baker revealed in a short but powerful speech:

> It takes organization. It takes dedication. It takes the willingness to stand and do what has to be done, when it has to be done . . . until we can get people to recognize that they themselves have to make the struggle and have to make the fight for freedom everyday, in the year, every year, until they win it.[12]

Let a new America rise. Let a new America be born. Let every city and county engage in deep reflection and then implement the five steps of an authentic racial equity process. Let the activists, organizers, and everyday people heal, build, organize, and "make the fight for freedom"—each and every generation—until Black Lives and Black neighborhoods truly matter.

Album Credits

Many times we picture a scholar and their work as arising from them individually sui generis. Given that this work is about Black neighborhoods, it is important to note that I am a product of Black communities, and this work emerges from that spatial and cultural context. My work is a product of the training, opportunities, and support bestowed upon me by Black women—Sharon Parker, Aressa Parker, Sharon Brown, Shelley White-Means, Kim Dobson Sydnor, LeConte Dill, Beverly Inman, Mamie Simpson, Anita Hawkins, Marisela Gomez, Tahira Mahdi, Nicolette Louissaint, Sheryl Gaston-Garcia, Corrine Harley, Rubye Johnson, and Adama Afrika. This work could not exist without their fierce brilliance and support. I am also the product of Black men who helped hone my scholarly potential, particularly at Morehouse College—Marcellus Barksdale, Aaron Parker, Mwalimu Buruti, and Kurt Young. In addition, I am grateful for the Black men who have modeled to me what it means to be a Black man in America—Rev. S. J. Parker, Joseph L. Taylor, Ronald McCullough, and Shabaka Afrika.

There are also Baltimore scholars I drew inspiration and knowledge from—Lorece Edwards, Marisela Gomez, Lester Spence, Karsonya "Kaye" Whitehead, Michael Scott, Nadine Finigan-Carr, Roland Thorpe, Nyasha Grayman-Simpson, Ailish Hooper, Tahira Mahdi, Nicole Fabricant, Audrey McFarlane, Khalilah Harris, Jessica Schiller, Garrett Power, Corey Henderson, Angel King Wilson, Sabriya Linton, Myra Margolin, Camika Royal, and

Ashanté Reese. I thank Renee Hatcher and Joseph Fioramontti for the Equity Baltimore project work. I also extend my gratitude to Nadine Finigan-Carr, Edward J. Blum, Tracy Rone, George Lipsitz, Nicole King, Nicolette Louissaint, Lorece Edwards, and Audrey McFarlane for providing me with publishing opportunities that helped propel my career as an academic scholar. I also thank my teachers from Ross Elementary to Clear Creek High School and my professors at Morehouse College, the University of Houston, and the University of Tennessee Health Science Center—especially Dr. Marcellus Barksdale at Morehouse College who started the African American Studies program there and encouraged us to achieve academic excellence.

I am thankful for Fatima Wilkerson, Shannon Freeland, Union Baptist Head Start (Gayle Headen, Sherise Yow, Sonya Hawkins, Amil Saboor), and Leon Purnell at the Men's and Family Center for welcoming me to Baltimore in 2010. You all gave me my education about what it means to render service in redlined Black neighborhoods. Thank you especially to my brother Dwayne Johnson at Union Baptist Head Start for your steady friendship and for showing me what is real in Baltimore. I give thanks to my activists-colleagues in Baltimore—Donald Gresham, Lucille Gorham, Sallie Gorham, Lisa Francis, Reginald Fitzgerald, Marc Steiner, Richie Armstrong, Sylvia Chappelle, Destiny Watford, Michael Rogers, Doug Armstrong, Joan Floyd, Kenneth Gwee, Robert Moore, Kim Trueheart, Charly Carter, Carol Ott, Barbara Samuels, Dorcas Gilmore, Betty Garman, Nicole Fabricant, Marceline White, Lydia Waither-Rodriguez, and more. I give a special thanks to Nikkia Rowe for helping me understand the issue of the permanent closures of public schools in Baltimore and Keisha Leverette for helping me understand the nuances of philanthropy. Kimberlyn Peal and Sharlimar Douglass, I appreciate you both for your advocacy work and for greatly contributing to my knowledge of Baltimore's public education system. I also thank Jehan Reaves for providing support with citations and for helping to inspire the Black Butterfly Project.

I am grateful for the work of my colleagues in Baltimore Bloc—both present and past. I want to also thank my colleagues in PORT³. I would also like to thank local journalists, especially Melody Simmons, Lisa Snowden-McCray, Baynard Woods, Luke Broadwater, Stephen Roblin, Talia Richman, Fern Shen, Brandon Soderberg, Caitlin Goldblatt, Jaisal Noor, Dharna Noor, Joan Jacobson, and many more who helped explain systems, budgets, policies, and practices in Baltimore City. National journalists I'd like to thank include Brentin Mock, Nikole Hannah-Jones, Tanvi Masri, Emily Badger, Wesley Lowery, Erica Green, and many others.

Thanks to the Maryland Historical Society, Baltimore City Archives, the Enoch Pratt Central Library's Maryland Department, the University of Baltimore Langsdale Library's Special Collections, and my sister, Sharon Brown, for the writing spaces and/or research assistance provided during the course of writing this book. I am particularly thankful for the funding and support provided to me during the summer of 2017 by the Archival Research Fellowship on Structural Inequality at the University of Baltimore. The work on Baltimore's forced displacement between 1940 and 2010 is a direct result of research conducted in the Langsdale Library Special Collections section at the University of Baltimore. Many thanks to Aiden, Angela, and the rest of the archivists on staff. Thanks to Saul at the Baltimore City Archives for locating files of mayors and Paul at the George Peabody Library for locating the *Baltimore Municipal Journal*.

If the streets of the city are akin to blood veins and arteries, then the city's libraries must be considered the brain and the accumulation of memories of the metaphorical body. From the archives and libraries, we can recall "memories" of the city as it has lived for over 200 years. From the archives and libraries, we can understand where the city has fallen short and perhaps create new brain cells—scholarship and research—that will inform the city to act differently and become truly equitable for all.

I would also like to lift up the Kellogg Health Scholars program and Open Society Institute (OSI) Baltimore for fellowships that supported my work and scholarship early in my career. I remain inspired by the work of Kellogg Health Scholars who were at Morgan State while I served as a postdoctoral fellow—Caree Jackson, Taqi Tirmazi, Ndidi Amutah, and Shalon Irving. I am uplifted when I think of the work of OSI Baltimore fellows such as Agatha So, on building alternative credit for Latina/o homebuyers, and Marvin Hayes, leading a crusade to compost and create that "black gold." Thank you also to Pam King and Evan Serpick for your support through the years. I appreciate you both. Thank you to everyone at Baltimore Corps (particularly Fagan Harris and Karon McFarlane) and the Bunting Neighborhood Leadership Program (Rebkha Atnafou) for the opportunity to facilitate learning with your fellows and staff members.

Thank you also to the mighty Morgan State University! I am thankful for colleagues across the university that I had the pleasure of working with—folks such as Natasha Pratt-Harris, Raymond Terry, Maija Anderson, Celeste Chavis, Alexander Wooten, Ray Winbush, Jared Ball, Randy Rowel, E. R. Shipp, Yvonne Bronner, Lenwood Hayman, Anne Marie O'Keefe, Keisha Baptiste-Roberts, Kimberly Coleman, Ian Lindong, Mamie Simpson, Beverly Inman, Mian Hossain, Payam Sheikhattari, and all the staff and faculty of the School of Community Health and Policy. Many of the world's greatest students, scholars, and thinkers teach at Morgan State University. I am especially thankful for Kamaria Massey who served as a critical research associate in the last stages of the book. Thank you for giving me your impressions, offering critical suggestions, and reading drafts to help strengthen the text.

I owe a tremendous debt of gratitude to the students I had the pleasure of teaching at Morgan State University, especially students who took my Community Needs and Solutions and my Public Health and Health Disparities courses. I am grateful for students who have helped me to publish in the past (Alicia Sherrell and Imani Bryan) and those whose creative and poetic genius appears in this book (Aja Cross, Nakisha Gaddy, Monique Gardner, Sterling Warren, and Mohamed Tall). I have learned a great deal from you all. You allowed me to share my work and listened to my stories. I pray you have been inspired by me as I have been inspired you.

Finally, I thank my editor, Robin W. Coleman, who had the vision to see that a book like this needed to be written and for affording me the opportunity to write it. I also appreciate the work of everyone at Johns Hopkins University Press—Andre Barnett, Juliana McCarthy, Kathryn Marguy, Hilary Jacqmin, and Jane Medrano—for all that each of you have already done to support this manuscript and increase my excitement about bringing this book to the world. If I have forgotten anyone, please accept my sincerest apologies.

> May the words of my mouth
> and the meditation of my heart
> be acceptable in Thy sight,
> O Lord, my rock and my redeemer.
> Psalm 19:4

Appendixes

A: The Seven Great Displacements in African American History

Uprooting	Time Frame	Name of Displacement	Details and Description of Black Community Displacement
1	1619–1820s	Trans-Atlantic Slave Trade	Roughly 389,000 Africans were transported as cargo by European and American slave ships for the purpose of forced labor
2	1820s–1861	American Domestic Slave Trade	White slavers bred African Americans and White slave traders transported Black people from the Chesapeake region to the Deep South to pick cotton on Southern plantations
3	1866–1909	Black Exodus during the War of Reconstruction	After Whites engaged in barbaric violence against individuals (lynchings) or communities (mob violence, pogroms, coup d'états), Black people would often flee by the thousands
4	1910–1980	Black Land Dispossession	Whites stole and confiscated millions of acres of farmland and waterfront property owned by Black farmers and landowners
5	1910–1970	The Great Migrations	The movement of 6.5 million Black people from the Deep South to states in the North, West, and Midwest regions of the United States
6	1940–1974	The Great Urban Displacements	Destruction of Black neighborhood villages, which includes massive policies of displacement and disruption of Black neighborhoods through slum clearance, urban renewal (Housing Act of 1949), university-led displacement (Housing Act of 1954), and highway construction through Black neighborhoods (Federal Highway Act of 1956); introduction of the war on Black communities
7	1975–present	Resource Withdrawal and Neighborhood Destabilization	Includes the demolition of a quarter of a million public housing units (HOPE VI); the rise of mass incarceration; mass foreclosures due to subprime lending to Black homeowners and mass rental eviction of Black renters; gentrification due to local incentives and public housing demolition; New Orleans evacuees displaced by Hurricane Katrina and levee destruction; national mass Black school closures, mass reduction of Black teachers, and school pushout

B: Racist Wealth-Extracting Systems, Policies, and Practices in American History

1. International slave trading—allowed by British, then American colonial and federal governments: 1619–1820
2. Domestic slave trading and human breeding—after number 1 was outlawed and cotton became king: 1820–1865
3. Enslavement, forced labor, torture, rape—allowed by multiple states and the federal government: 1619–1865
4. President Andrew Johnson rescinded General William T. Sherman's Special Field Order 15—40 acres redistribution: 1865
5. Convict leasing and peonage: 1865–1960
6. Sharecropping: 1865–1970
7. Destruction of independent Black cities and economic districts by white mob violence and lynchings: 1825–1930
8. Racial zoning, racial steering, local government real estate conspiracy: 1910–present
9. Racially restrictive covenants—legally enforceable barring of Black homeownership in White areas: 1912–1948
10. Federal Housing Administration White suburban subsidization using racially restrictive covenants: 1937–1968
11. Discriminatory Federal Housing Administration and Veterans' Administration mortgage lending: 1937–1968
12. Blockbusting and contract buying homeownership schemes due to number 11: 1940–1980
13. Home Owners' Loan Corporation/Federal Housing Administration Residential Security Maps—the federal government sponsors redlining: 1937–present
14. Black farmland dispossession—millions of acres lost due to US Department of Agriculture white supremacist actions: 1940–present
15. Urban renewal a.k.a. "Negro Removal"—downtown revitalization and university/hospital expansion: 1949–1975
16. Beachfront and waterfront property dispossession: 1940–present
17. Federal Highway Administration's construction of highways through Black communities: 1956–1975
18. Predatory finance in Black communities—check cashing, payday loans, pawn shops, rent-to-own, predatory rental payments, subprime mortgage lending: 1950–present
19. Mass incarceration—legal financial obligations, high bail bonds, criminal disenfranchisement: 1980–present
20. Urban land dispossession through gentrification—boosted by assistance for incoming homebuyers: 1990–present
21. US Housing and Urban Development's HOPE VI public housing land disposition for private developers: 1994–2007
22. Big banks' reverse redlining—a.k.a. subprime mortgage lending: 2000–present
23. HUD's CHOICE Neighborhoods and Rental Assistance Demonstration—more land disposition, privatizing public housing: 2008–present
24. Mass school closures and private charter conversions in Black neighborhoods: 2000–present
25. The Neo-Confederate Nullification of the Affordable Care Act by Supreme Court Medicaid Opt-Out and GOP: 2012–present

26. Discriminatory consumer debt collection lawsuits by banks, utilities, hospitals, debt buyers: 2000–present
27. Predatory tax sales by hedge funds and big banks—over small tax liens such as a water bill: 2000–present
28. Contemporary redlining in hypersegregated metropolitan areas such as Milwaukee, St. Louis, Baltimore: 2007–present
29. Discriminatory urban tax policy via tax increment financing (TIF), payment in lieu of taxes (PILOTs), tax breaks, and so forth, for White developers and neighborhoods: 1980–present

C: Tools and Tactics of Racial Segregation in Baltimore

Wave	Time Frame	Description	Details and Description of White Baltimore's Racial Segregation Tactics and Tools
1	1820s–1867	White-only public school system	During this time, free Black Baltimoreans operated their own private school system
2	1867–1954	Segregated public schools	The Baltimore City Public School System operated an apartheid school system
3	1880s–1950s	Segregated public transportation	Steamboats, trolleys, and railroads often segregated passengers by race
4	1910–1917	Racial zoning city ordinances	Initially passed by Mayor John Berry Mahool and then pushed by Mayor James Preston
5	1912–1948	Anti-Black restrictive covenants	Deployed in Roland Park, Guilford, Homeland, Bolton Hill, Forest Park, Northwood
6	1917–1918	Preston's proposed mass quarantine plan	Mayor Preston proposed to move 90,000 Negroes to the county with health as pretext
7	1918–1920s	*Baltimore Sun* propaganda and protective associations	*Baltimore Sun* primed White neighborhood groups to fight the "Negro Invasion"
8	1920s–1940s	Pro-segregation lobbying by White churches	White churches on the city's west and east sides fought the "Negro Invasion"
9	1925	Intimidation and threat of violence	Ku Klux Klan marched in Hampden; would become a reputed home of KKK members
10	1937–1968	HOLC Residential Security Map	Using Form NS-8, White real estate agents plus state assessors helped crystallize segrenomics
11	1937–1954	Housing Authority of Baltimore City segregated public housing	HABC placed family developments in Black neighborhoods and segregated tenants by race

12	1943	White resistance against Black public housing	Whites in Armistead Gardens protested and defeated Negro wartime public housing
13	1959	Mount Washington zoning	Mount Washington residents lobbied successfully for exclusive zoning
14	1954–1995	HABC intensifies racial segregation	HABC employed a controlled desegregation plan and placed scatter sites in Black areas
15	1996–present	Noncompliance with the 1968 Fair Housing Act's mandate to "affirmatively further fair housing"	Maintaining segregating zoning codes (Mount Washington), approving large development without inclusionary upzoning (Port Covington), no HOME Act to stop source of income discrimination (White L), most HABC Housing Choice Vouchers holders live in the Black Butterfly and very few live in the White L

Note: HOLC = Home Owners' Loan Corporation.

D: Tools and Tactics of Serial Forced Displacement in Baltimore

Wave	Time Frame	Displacement Name	Details and Description of Black Community Displacement
1	1650s–1820s	Trans-Atlantic Slave Trade	Baltimore's port served as disembarkation for ships in the slave trade (approximately 5,000)
2	1820s–1861	Domestic American Slave Trade	Shipped 30,000 enslaved Black people from Baltimore's port to Deep South
3	Mid-1880s	Displacement by the Baltimore and Ohio Railroad	The railroad displaced 100 Black families to expand railroad yards in South Baltimore
4	1880s–1910s	Black churches displaced	Black churches displaced from downtown
5	1914–1919	Preston Gardens	Displacement of Black people and Black churches from Gallows Hill
6	1930s–1940s	Slum clearance for public housing	Slum clearance to build segregated public housing; displaced 1,863 Black families
7	1951–1975	Urban renewal / public housing	BRA, BURHA, then DHCD with HABC displaced 10,599 Black households
8	1951–1975	Displacement by highways	"Highway to Nowhere" (US-40) displaced 960 Black families, also I-83 and I-395; 1,832 households total

9	1987, 1995-2001	HABC's HOPE VI demolitions	Demolished 4,051 units occupied by Black families in eight public housing developments across city
10	2000s-2010s	JHMI/EBDI displacement	Uprooted 742 Black families in Middle East community for biopark expansion
11	2000s-2010s	Mass school closures and Black teacher pushout	BCPSS closed 84 schools mostly in Black neighborhoods since 2000 and the Black teacher workforce was reduced by nearly 50% since 2005
12	2000s-2010s	HABC demolitions for redevelopment	Demolition of Black apartments or public housing—Pall Mall, Madison Park North, Somerset Courts
13	2000-2010s	Mass foreclosures and evictions	Due to subprime lending, reverse mortgages, and tax lien foreclosures; mass rental evictions
14	2000-2010s	Displacement by public subsidy	Project Create Opportunities for Renewal and Enterprise (CORE), Neighborhood Impact Investment Fund, Live Near Your Work

Note: Displacement Waves 1-10 are found in Track 3 in the section entitled "The Scope of Baltimore's Displacement." Displacement Waves 11-14 are discussed in Track 4 in the section entitled "Contemporary Resource Removal and Forced Uprootings." BCPSS = Baltimore City Public School System; BRA = Baltimore Redevelopment Agency; BURHA = Baltimore Urban Renewal and Housing Agency; DCHD = Department of Housing and Community Development, and HABC = Housing Authority of Baltimore City.

E: BMORE Caucus List of Demands for Baltimore City Public Schools

During their local Black Lives Matter Week of Action in February 2018, the Baltimore Movement of Rank-and-File Educators Caucus—or BMORE Caucus— and Baltimore Algebra Project wrote a list of demands that capture many of these same ideas. For their local demands, they asserted what is needed to make Black students, educators, and schools matter by writing the following:

Black students matter!

1. *Mandate Black History/Ethnic Studies K-12.* As an initial step, prepare educators by mandating Professional Development for teachers on Culturally Responsive Pedagogy. Fund time, resources, and staff for Black History/Ethnic Studies. Expand the curriculum audit to all courses. Involve educators and students to create a definition, rationale and curriculum framework for Black History/Ethnic Studies in Baltimore. Empower educators from historically oppressed groups to be the leaders of these spaces.

2. *Implement Restorative Practices* with fidelity and community engagement. Fund full-time restorative justice positions in each RP school. Allocate at least

$100,000 for each non-charter RP school. Draft a new or revised policy, regulation or guideline that specifically defines and guides RP work. Create a Restorative Practices Steering Committee that meets monthly and includes teachers, parents, students, administrators, partners, practitioners and advocates. Give the Restorative Practices Steering Committee the authority to: define tiers of RP; review resources; create easy-to-use online spaces for the sharing of RP resources; participate in the creation, assessment and revision of the RP practices policy/plan.

Black educators matter!

3. *Prioritize Black educator recruitment and retention.* Set a target for every new class of teachers to be 75% teachers of color with at least 60% of incoming teachers being African American. Publish a long-term plan for meeting the 75% and 60% targets. Publish a comprehensive study about the decline in black educators in Baltimore City since 2000. Black male educators are the most underrepresented demographic in the teaching force, and yet provide irreplaceable role modeling and support for all of our students, regardless of their demographic characteristics. Hire more Black men. Prioritize graduates from local HBCUs above recruits from alternative certification programs. Encourage and prepare Baltimore City youth to enter the teaching profession. Work with high schools to create an education-careers vocational track with internships in Baltimore City schools. Set a goal of 50% gender equity for the high school program. Engage in a PR campaign that encourages Baltimore City residents to become educators. Set up a intergenerational workgroup of Baltimore Black educators to make recommendations to the district for increasing retention of black educators currently in the classroom.

Black schools matter!

4. *Ensure racial equity in funding.* At the state level, advocate that the Kirwan Commission recommend reparations for the $3 billion dollars of historical underfunding of Baltimore City. Advocate for Delegate Mary Washington's casino lockbox bill, which ensures an IMMEDIATE restoration of the promised casino funds. On the citywide level, allocate Fair Student Funding in a way that addresses structural barriers to achievement. Create and publish a priority list for the Capital budget for infrastructure. Include racial equity block grants as part of state and city funding formulas (Kirwan Commission and Fair Student Funding). Institute a moratorium on school closures. Do not accept school closures as a compromise in order to gain additional 21st Century Building funds. Implement restorative justice for black communities that have been targeted for school closure.

F: Tracking Racial Equity Impact with Community Equity Metrics

Baltimoreans can measure and track the impact of racial equity work to ensure that our words produce real results and not simply rhetoric. My 2016-2017 Community Needs Solutions students and I created a beta version of Community

Equity Metrics (CEMs) for Baltimore City to do just this.* The digital power map we created can be found online at equitybaltimore.org. There are seven domains to our CEMs, which are designed to capture the past actions and the current status with respect to seven domains for the City of Baltimore. The seven domains along with the measures we selected for our CEMs currently include:

- *Education*—kindergarten readiness, eighth-grade reading proficiency, percentage of residents with a bachelor's degree
- *Community economic development*—banks per 1,000 people, unemployment rate, and median annual household income
- *Housing*—vacancy rate, foreclosure rate, public housing siting, median price of homes sold
- *Health*—health professional availability, liquor outlet density, lead poison violation rate
- *Transit*—percentage of people who walk to work, travel at least 45 minutes to work, and direct access to MTA light rail, Charm City Circulator, Zipcar stations, and bike share stations
- *Planning*—color status of Community Statistical Areas in the 1937 Residential Security Map, presence of a community benefits district
- *Public safety*—crime per 1,000 residents, violent crime rate, Baltimore Police Department reported stops, Stingray usage

Each of these seven domains is constructed using several metrics and indicators to create seven equity metrics that are then added together to compute a total CEM for each of Baltimore's 55 Community Statistical Areas.

G: Historical Trauma, Baltimore Apartheid Syllabus

This syllabus was compiled to highlight the impacts of ongoing historical trauma in Baltimore's Black Butterfly communities. As such, this is *not* a syllabus of the complete history of Baltimore per se. What this syllabus attempts to capture most is how multiple systems in Baltimore were created and various systems continue to proliferate structural disadvantage in Black Butterfly neighborhoods. Systems analyses here include education, real estate and housing, food and water, philanthropy, industry, transportation, public health, urban renewal, economic development, corrections, and police.

1. Michelle Sotero (2006). "A Conceptual Model of Historical Trauma: Implications for Public Health Practice and Research." *Journal of Health Disparities Research and Practice* 1 (1): 93–108.
2. Fatima Jackson, Latifa Jackson, Zainab ElRadi Jackson (2018). "Developmental Stage Epigenetic Modifications and Clinical Symptoms Associated with the Trauma and Stress of Enslavement and Institutionalized Racism." *Journal of Clinical Epigenetics* 4 (11).
3. Ralph Clayton (2004). *Cash for Blood: The Baltimore to New Orleans Domestic Slave Trade*. Heritage Books; Clayton (1993). *Slavery, Slaveholding, and the Free*

*Seven amazing 2016–2017 Morgan State University public health students helped create the seven Community Equity Metrics—Kerri, Adedoyin, Beatrice, Madiha, Mary, Omolola, and Shenika.

Black Population of Antebellum Baltimore. Heritage Books. Seminal works for understanding how both slavery and the slave trade functioned in Baltimore and served as the foundation for Baltimore's growth and development.

4. Bettye Thomas (1976). "Public Education and Black Protest in Baltimore 1865-1900." *Maryland Historical Society Magazine* 71 (3): 381-391. Excellent history of Black Baltimoreans' fight for racial equity in public education both during and after slavery.

5. Dennis Patrick Halpin (2019). *A Brotherhood of Liberty: Black Reconstruction and its Legacies in Baltimore, 1865-1920.* University of Pennsylvania Press. Absolutely critical history of Baltimore's Black community activism taking place during Black Reconstruction and as Baltimore Apartheid was being erected by White Baltimoreans.

6. Staff writer (1910). "Baltimore Tries Drastic Plan of Race Segregation." *New York Times Magazine.* Amazing time capsule of Baltimore when White Baltimoreans passed the first residential racial zoning law in American history and how Black Baltimore fought back.

7. William Ashbie Hawkins (November 1911). "A Year of Segregation in Baltimore." *The Crisis* (published by the NAACP), page 27; Staff correspondent (February 22, 1916). "How Segregation Law in Baltimore Operates after Being Annulled 3 Times." *St. Louis Post-Dispatch.* Both articles discuss the situation in Baltimore after the city's groundbreaking racial zoning laws were enacted during the 1910s.

8. Garrett Power (1983). "Apartheid Baltimore Style: The Residential Segregation Ordinances of 1910-1913." *Maryland Law Review* 42 (2): 289-328.

9. Elizabeth Evitts Dickinson (2014). "Roland Park: One of America's First Garden Suburbs, and Built for Whites Only." *Johns Hopkins Magazine.*

10. Unknown [although likely William T. Howard] (March 16, 1917). "What Can Be Done to Improve the Living Conditions of Baltimore's Negro Population." *Baltimore Municipal Journal* 5(5). Original journal is held at the George Peabody Library.

11. Garrett Power (2004). "*Meade v. Dennistone*: The NAACP's Test Case to '. . . Sue Jim Crow Out of Maryland with the Fourteenth Amendment.'" *Maryland Law Review* 63 (4): 773-810.

12. Corey Henderson (2017). "The Reverberating Influence of Historical Trauma on the Health of African Americans in Baltimore City." PhD diss., Morgan State University. Brilliant work extending the Sotero model of historical trauma and applying the model to Black Lives in Baltimore City. Also analyzes the nature of historical trauma for Black Baltimoreans who lived in Baltimore during Jim Crow and their experience in the age of desegregation.

13. Samuel K. Roberts (2009). *Infectious Fear: Politics, Disease, and the Health Effects of Segregation.* University of North Carolina Press. In-depth examination of how Baltimore's racial segregation intensified epidemics of tuberculosis, yellow fever, and cholera among the city's Black residents. Also details the racism endemic in medicine and public health.

14. Harold A. McDougall (1993). *Black Baltimore: A New Theory of Community.* Temple University Press. A work that gives great detail to the history of Black Baltimoreans especially before, during, and after the 1968 Holy Week Uprising.

15. Antero Pietila (2010). *Not in My Neighborhood: How Bigotry Shaped a Great American City.* Ivan R. Dee. Historical narrative outlining racial segregation in Baltimore.

16. Karl Taeuber (2003). "Public Housing and Racial Segregation in Baltimore." Plaintiff's Exhibit No. 2, and Arnold Hirsch (2003). "Public Policy and Residential Segregation in Baltimore, 1900–1968." Plaintiff's Exhibit No. 3. *Thompson v. HUD Court Files.* Case Number MJG 95-309. University of Baltimore, Langsdale Library Special Collections. Both works delve into the history of racial segregation perpetuated by the Housing Authority of Baltimore City.

17. Emily Lieb (2018). "'Baltimore Does Not Condone Profiteering in Squalor': The Baltimore Plan and the Problem of Housing-Code Enforcement in an American City." *Planning Perspectives* 33 (1): 75–95, 78. Great analysis of Baltimore's policy implementation of slum clearance and urban renewal.

18. Staff writer (1978). "Urbanologist Scores Baltimore: Excerpts from an AFRO Interview with Dr. Homer Favor." *Baltimore Afro-American*, October 3. Amazing interview that proves very prophetic regarding coming displacement and the White return to the city.

19. Thomas LaVeist et al. (2011). "Place, Not Race: Disparities Dissipate In Southwest Baltimore When Blacks and Whites Live under Similar Conditions." *Health Affairs* 30 (10): 1880–1887.

20. Marisela Gomez (2013). *Race, Class, Power, and Organizing in East Baltimore: Rebuilding Abandoned Communities in America.* Lexington Books. Covers the forced displacement of the Middle East community by the City, Johns Hopkins medical campus, the East Baltimore Development Initiative, and the Annie E. Casey Foundation.

21. Bradford Van Arnum (2014). *Recreation Center Closings in Baltimore: Reconsidering Spending Priorities, Juvenile Crime, and Equity.* Citizens Planning and Housing Association.

22. Lawrence Brown (2015). "Down to the Wire: Disinvestment and Displacement in Baltimore City." In *The 2015 State of Black Baltimore: Separate, Still Unequal*. Greater Baltimore Urban League; Brown (2016). "Two Baltimores: The White L vs. the Black Butterfly." *Baltimore City Paper*; Nicole Fabricant (2018). "Black Neighborhoods Matter." *New Politics.*

23. Douglass Massey and Jonathan Tannen (2015). "A Research Note on Trends in Black Hypersegregation." *Demography* 52 (3): 1025–1034. Seminal article on hypersegregation, how it is defined, and its effects on redlined Black neighborhoods.

24. National Community Reinvestment Coalition (2015). *Home Mortgages and Small Business Lending in Baltimore and Surrounding Areas.* Details ongoing redlining in Baltimore from 2011 to 2013 with terrific maps illustrating bank redlining.

25. Alec MacGillis (2016). "The Third Rail." *Places Journal.* Article illuminating transit apartheid in Baltimore. "In Baltimore, public investment—and disinvestment—in transportation have figured greatly in the persistence of racial and economic inequality."

26. Lester Spence (2015). *Knocking the Hustle: Against the Neoliberal Turn in Black Politics.* Punctum Books; Audrey G. McFarlane (2009). "Operatively White? Exploring the Significance of Race and Class through the Paradox of Black Middle-Classness." *Law and Contemporary Problems* 72:163–196; Jared Ball. These works are essential for understanding how Black political (mis)leadership in Baltimore perpetuates racial inequity.

27. David Dudley, ed. (2015). "Fix the City. Urbanite: Truth, Reconciliation, and Baltimore." *Urbanite Magazine*. Great series of short pieces on solutions for Baltimore. Published months after the 2015 uprising.

28. Andrea K. McDaniels (2015). "Stress of Baltimore Unrest Could Stay with Residents for Awhile." *Baltimore Sun*; McDaniels (2014). "Collateral Damage." *Baltimore Sun*. Examines the impacts of violence on children, caregivers, and victims' relatives in Upton and other communities; McDaniels (2015). "When Violence Leads to Sleep Problems in Children." *Baltimore Sun*.

29. Erica Green (2013). "Henderson-Hopkins School Divides East Baltimore Community." *Baltimore Sun*; Green (2015). "City Students Turn to Writing to Process Baltimore Unrest." *Baltimore Sun*; Green (2017). "Bridging the Divide: Within Integrated Schools, De Facto Segregation Persists." *Baltimore Sun*.

30. Molly Rath (2007). "100 Years: The State Takes Over City Schools." *Baltimore Magazine*.

31. Talia Richman (2018). "As Baltimore Prepares to Close More Schools, Many Worry about the Communities They Anchor." *Baltimore Sun*. For a deeper understanding of the issue of school closures in Black neighborhoods, please read Eve Ewing (2018). *Ghosts in the Schoolyard: Racism and School Closings on Chicago's South Side*. University of Chicago Press. Although Ewing's book covers Chicago, many of the issues with massive school closures apply to Baltimore and the dynamics are the same. Also read Ebony M. Duncan-Shippy. (2019). *Shuttered Schools: Race, Community, and School Closures in American Cities*. Information Age Publishing.

32. Timothy Wheeler and Luke Broadwater (2015). "Lead Paint: Despite Progress, Hundreds of Maryland Children Still Poisoned." *Baltimore Sun*; Luke Broadwater (2016). "Advocates Say Lead Paint Industry Should Be Held Liable in Poisoning of Baltimore Children." *Baltimore Sun*.

33. Johns Hopkins Center for a Livable Future (2015). *Mapping Baltimore City's Food Environment: 2015 Report*. City of Baltimore. Contains fantastic maps highlighting the way in which food apartheid is concentrated in the Black Butterfly.

34. The Thurgood Marshall Institute (2019). *Water/Color: A Study of Race & the Water Affordability Crisis in America's Cities*. NAACP Legal Defense and Educational Fund. Great background on water affordability with a Baltimore focus located on pages 33–36.

35. Mark Puente (2014). "Undue Force." *Baltimore Sun*; Justin Fenton (2019). "Cops and Robbers" (investigative series on the Baltimore Police Department's Gun Trace Task Force who were caught selling drugs, robbing residents, and operating a criminal enterprise). *Baltimore Sun* and Pulitzer Center.

36. Department of Justice (2016). *Investigation of the Baltimore City Police Department*. Civil Rights Division of the United States Department of Justice. Hard-hitting report detailing the systemic abuses and misconduct of the Baltimore Police Department in the aftermath of the April 27, 2015, Uprising.

37. Amanda Petteruti, Aleks Kajstura, Marc Schindler, Peter Wagner, and Jason Ziedenberg (2015). *The Right Investments? Corrections Spending in Baltimore City*. Justice Policy Institute and Prison Policy Initiative. According to the authors, "25 communities account for 76 percent of the money spent on incarcerating people from Baltimore for a total of $220 million" (p. 13).

38. Doug Donovan and Jean Marbella (2016). "Dismissed: Tenants Lose, Landlords Win in Baltimore's Rent Court." *Baltimore Sun*. Investigative series on Baltimore's rental eviction crisis.

39. Anonymous Collective (2017). *The Baltimore Black Paper*. Details how Baltimore developed to the point it is today, analyzes multiple systems in the city, and discusses where it needs to go with emphasis on racial equity; Baltimore Black Worker Center Research Team (2018). *The State of Black Workers in Baltimore*. Baltimore Black Worker Center; Jing Li and Richard Clinch (2018). *Analysis of Patterns of Employment by Race in Baltimore City and the Baltimore Metropolitan Area*. Associated Black Charities.

40. Oscar Perry Abello (2017). "Baltimore Reckons with Its Legacy of Redlining." Next City. Details a study of inequitable spending in majority White neighborhoods vs. majority communities of color as it relates to dollars spent from the city's capital budget. The study was led by Delegate Stephanie Smith.

41. Madeleine Pill (2018). "The Austerity Governance of Baltimore's Neighborhoods: 'The Conversation May Have Changed but the Systems Aren't Changing.'" *Journal of Urban Affairs*. Special issue. Breaks down how Baltimore's philanthropic and large corporate entities drive the city's development agenda and how they promised changes after the April 27, 2015, Uprising. Very few actually delivered.

42. Nicole Fabricant (2018). "Environmental Justice Movement in South Baltimore: United Workers Take on Multiple Crises of Capitalism." *New Politics*.

43. Brett Theodos, Eric Hangen, and Brady Meixell (2019). *"The Black Butterfly": Racial Segregation and Investment Patterns in Baltimore*. Urban Institute.

44. Angel King Wilson (2019). *Am I Doing This Right?* Silent Books. A vital, short memoir of a young Black woman born and raised in West Baltimore. She touches on her experiences in Baltimore with education, water tainted with toxic lead, lead paint, redlining, and more.

45. Ron Cassie (2019). "Hell and High Water." *Baltimore Magazine*. Seminal article on the current and coming climate change in Baltimore City and its racially inequitable impacts.

46. Lawrence Lanahan (2019). *The Lines between Us: Two Families and a Quest to Cross Baltimore's Racial Divide*. New Press. Among other things, it provides an account of Baltimore during the April 2015 Uprising, the Sagamore TIF debate, and ongoing struggle for fair housing and desegregating Baltimore City.

47. D. Watkins (2019). *We Speak for Ourselves: A Word from Forgotten Black America*. Powerful reflections and analysis from a young Black man born and raised in East Baltimore.

48. P. Nicole King, Kate Drabinski, and Joshua Clark Davis (2019). *Baltimore Revisited: Stories of Inequality and Resistance in a U.S. City*. Rutgers University Press. Tremendous collection of essays and chapters covering multiple issues and highlighting multiple communities in Baltimore.

49. National Nurses United (2019). *Burdening Baltimore: How Johns Hopkins Hospital and Other Not-for-Profit Hospitals, Colleges, and Universities Fail to Pay Their Fair Share*. A critical examination of how nonprofits in Baltimore escape paying their taxes and contributing more to the economic health of the city.

50. Brentin Mock (2019). "Are Reparations Baltimore's Fix for Redlining, Investment Deprivation?" CityLab.

H: Online Mapping and Data Web Tools for Analyzing Baltimore and American Apartheid

1. City of Baltimore. "Open Budget Baltimore." Great for analyzing budget allocations in Baltimore City.
2. Robert K. Nelson, LaDale Winling, Richard Marciano, Nathan Connolly, et al., "Mapping Inequality." In *American Panorama: An Atlas of United States History*, edited by Robert K. Nelson and Edward L. Ayers (Richmond, VA: University of Richmond, 2015). Tremendous mapping tool for Baltimore's redlining or Residential Security Map that also contains pivotal area descriptions.
3. Digital Scholarship Lab. "Renewing Inequality: Family Displacements through Urban Renewal—1950-1966." In Nelson and Ayers, *American Panorama*.
4. Liam Hogan. *Collective Punishment: Mob Violence, Riots, and Pogroms against African American Communities*. https://medium.com/@Limerick1914/collective -punishment-mob-violence-riots-and-pogroms-against-african-american -communities-e1a801c41aa4.
5. Dustin Cable. "The Racial Dot Map." Cooper Center at the University of Virginia. Mapping resource for visually examining America's racial demographics as it existed in 2010.
6. National Community Revitalization Coalition. "Redlining Dashboard."
7. Urban Institute. "An Interactive View of the Housing Boom and Bust." Zoom in to Baltimore and get see where foreclosures and mortgage originations occur in Baltimore between 2000 and 2015.
8. Luke Broadwater. "Baltimore TIFs and PILOTs." Google Map.
9. *Baltimore Business Journal* (BBJ). "Crane Watch." Digital map on BBJ's platform to track development in and near Baltimore City.
10. Renee Hatcher, Lawrence Brown, Joseph Fioramonti. "Equity Baltimore." Web tool with solutions for redlined communities and a powermap highlighting inequity by Community Statistical Areas in Baltimore.

I: Baltimore's Opioid Overdoses and Homicides (2007–2018)

Year	Alcohol	Methadone	Pharma-ceutical Drug Overdose	Heroin	Fentanyl	Cocaine	Homicides	Total OD Deaths
2007	56	80	95	202	3	106	282	287
2008	41	47	60	107	2	57	233	184
2009	54	50	63	151	4	72	240	239
2010	39	53	61	93	4	45	224	172
2011	44	65	82	76	2	48	197	167
2012	71	54	74	131	4	59	219	225
2013	86	57	86	150	12	47	235	246
2014	86	54	84	192	72	82	211	305

Year	Alcohol	Methadone	Pharma-ceutical Drug Overdose	Heroin	Fentanyl	Cocaine	Homicides	Total OD Deaths
2015	114	78	105	260	120	93	344	393
2016	222	82	113	454	419	202	318	694
2017	198	87	123	380	573	285	343	761
2018	187	85	128	286	758	388	309	888

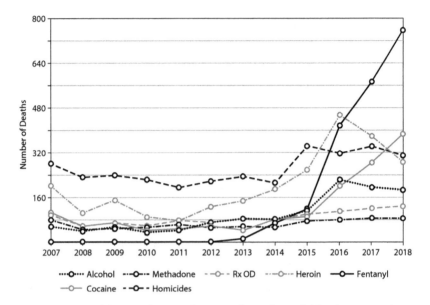

Figure I.1. Baltimore City Overdose Deaths and Homicides (2007–2018)

Notes

Introduction to Racial Equity

1. Harry A. Ezratty, *Baltimore in the Civil War: The Pratt Street Riot and a City Occupied* (Charleston: History Press, 2013), 51.
2. Ezratty, *Baltimore in the Civil War,* 75.
3. Cheryl Janifer LaRoche, *Free Black Communities and the Underground Railroad: The Geography of Resistance* (Urbana: University of Illinois Press, 2004). LaRoche explains: "From the earliest moments of the African diaspora, men and women fled slavery to reject their condition. . . . Maroon communities functioned as the diaspora's first free Black settlements. Whether in midwestern hills, the Great Dismal Swamp, the Florida bayou, or the remote regions of Cuba, Brazil, or Jamaica, communities of escaped [formerly enslaved people] proclaimed their right to be free. Maroon communities began the progression to free Black settlements and the Underground Railroad" (103). Underground Railroad resistance was often led and organized by Black churches—especially African Methodist Episcopal (AME), AME Zion, and Baptist churches. The Underground was also organized by Black Freemasons and free Black communities such as Rocky Forge and Miller Grove in Illinois, Lick Creek in Indiana, and Poke Patch in Ohio. See also Richard Price, "Maroons: Rebel Slaves in the Americas," in *1992 Festival of American Folklife* (Washington, DC: Center for Folklife and Cultural Heritage of the Smithsonian Institution, 1992), https://folklife.si.edu /resources/maroon/educational_guide/23.htm.
4. Liam Hogan, "Collective Punishment: Mob Violence, Riots, and Pogroms against African American Communities (1824-1974)," 2015, accessed June 19, 2018, https://collectivepunishment.wordpress.com.
5. Robert K. Nelson, LaDale Winling, Richard Marciano, Nathan Connolly, et al., "Mapping Inequality: Redlining in New Deal America, 1935-1940," *American Panorama: An Atlas of United States History,* ed. Robert K. Nelson and Edward L. Ayers, University of Richmond, 2017, https://dsl.richmond .edu/panorama/redlining/.
6. Christina Caron and Liam Stack, "Maryland House of Delegates Censures Mary Ann Lisanti for Using Racist Slur," *New York Times,* February 28, 2019, https://www.nytimes.com/2019/02/28/us/politics/mary-ann-lisanti-racism .html; Lawrence Brown, "The Problem with Delegate Lisanti's 'Nigger District,'" *Baltimore Beat,* March 6, 2019, http://baltimorebeat.com/2019 /03/06/the-problem-with-delegate-lisantis-nigger-district/. Lisanti was censured but not expelled by her colleagues in the Maryland General Assembly.

7. Donald Trump (@realDonaldTrump), "As proven last week during Congressional tour, . . ." Twitter, July 27, 2019, 7:14 a.m., https://twitter.com/realDonaldTrump/status/1155073964634517505.

8. "In a series of studies, Bonam has found that white Americans hold ironclad stereotypes about black neighborhoods—even when they display little or no animus toward black people. They're likely to infer from the presence of a black family that a neighborhood is 'impoverished, crime-ridden, and dirty,' though they make none of those assumptions about an identical white family in the same house. They'll knock the value of a house down by \$20,000, or nearly 15 percent, if they believe the neighborhood is black." Henry Grabar, "Black Space, White Blindness," *Slate*, September 18, 2018, https://slate.com/business/2018/09/black-neighborhoods-white-racism.html.

9. Jones and Jackson describe discursive redlining as an everyday practice warning others to avoid entire neighborhoods and discourage people who live in advantaged areas from building relationships with people in redlined Black neighborhoods. They also describe discursive redlining as crucial to efforts to police and uproot Black people described as "ghetto." Nikki Jones and Christina Jackson, "'You Just Don't Go Down There': Learning to Avoid the Ghetto in San Francisco," in *The Ghetto: Contemporary Global Issues and Controversies*, ed. Ray Hutchinson (n.p.: Routledge, 2019), 85–86.

10. Camilla Hawthorne, "Black Matters Are Spatial Matters: Black Geographies for the Twenty-First Century, *Geography Compass* 13, no. 11 (July 2019): 3, https://doi.org/10.1111/gec3.12468.

11. "Spatial racism refers to patterns of metropolitan development in which some affluent whites create racially and economically segregated suburbs or gentrified areas of cities, leaving the poor—mainly African Americans, Hispanics and some newly arrived immigrants—isolated in deteriorating areas of the cities and older suburbs." Francis Cardinal George, *Dwell in My Love: A Pastoral Letter on Racism (Tenth Anniversary 2001-2011)* (Chicago: Archdiocese of Chicago, 2011), 12, http://legacy.archchicago.org/Cardinal/pdf/DwellInMyLove_10thAnniversary.pdf.

12. "Spatial equity can . . . be defined as both a process and an outcome. As process, it involves the redistribution of the overall resources and development opportunities and/or the optimization of . . . locally existing resources and development opportunities. . . . As an outcome, it envisions [a] region or area where such redistribution or optimization is achieved and sustained." J. Buhangin, "Spatial Equity: A Parameter for Sustainable Development in Indigenous Regions," in *The Sustainable City VIII: Urban Regeneration and Sustainability*, ed. S. S. Zubir and C. A. Brebbia (Southampton, UK: WIT Press, 2013), 1343.

13. According to Alice Dalton and colleagues, spatial equity involves a consideration of access to amenities and proximity to disamenities as it relates to health. They write that spatial equity "emphasises the importance of understanding how need and provision vary spatially so that interventions can be located to serve . . . high-need yet often overlooked populations. . . . Spatial equity is the first step in a process towards reducing health inequality via structural or area-based interventions." Alice M. Dalton, Andrew Jones, David Ogilvie, Mark Petticrew, Martin White, and Steven Cummins, "Using Spatial Equity Analysis in the Process Evaluation of Environmental Interven-

tions to Tackle Obesity: The Healthy Towns Programme in England," *International Journal for Equity in Health* 12, no. 43 (2013): 2.

14. Mindy Thompson Fullilove, Lourdes Hernández-Cordero, and Robert E. Fullilove, "The Ghetto Game: Apartheid and the Developer's Imperative in Postindustrial American Cities," in *The Integration Debate: Competing Futures for American Cities*, ed. Chester Hartman and Gregory D. Squires (New York: Routledge Taylor & Francis Group, 2009), 199–212.

15. Douglass Massey and Jonathan Tannen, "A Research Note on Trends in Black Hypersegregation," *Demography* 52, no. 3 (2015): 1025–1034.

16. Dawn Phillips, Lois Flores, and Jamila Henderson, "Development without Displacement," Causa Just :: Just Causa, 2014, https://cjjc.org/wp-content/uploads/2015/11/development-without-displacement.pdf.

17. Michelle Sotero, "A Conceptual Model of Historical Trauma: Implications for Public Health Practice and Research," *Journal of Health Disparities Research and Practice* 1, no. 1 (Fall 2005): 93–108. Maria Yellow Horse Brave Heart defined historical trauma as "collective and cumulative emotional wounding across generations that results from massive cataclysmic events—Historically Traumatic Events." However, Kirmayer and colleagues argued that "studies of historical trauma must be balanced by analyses of how political and economic dynamics interact with community wellbeing." Laurence J. Kirmayer, Joseph P. Gone, and Joshua Moses, "Rethinking Historical Trauma," *Transcultural Psychiatry* 51, no. 3 (2014): 299–319, 312.

18. Massey and Tannen, "A Research Note," 1025–1034.

19. Nelson et al., "Mapping Inequality."

20. Jessica Trounstine, *Segregation by Design: Local Politics and Inequality in American Cities* (Cambridge: Cambridge University Press, 2018), 150–155.

21. Mindy T. Fullilove and Rodrick Wallace, "Serial Forced Displacement in American Cities, 1916–2010," *Journal of Urban Health: Bulletin of the New York Academy of Medicine* 88, no. 3 (2011): 381–389.

22. Noliwe Rooks, *Cutting School: Privatization, Segregation, and the End of Public Education* (New York: New Press, 2018), 2.

23. Van Jones, "'This Was a Whitelash': Van Jones' Take on the Election Results," CNN, November 11, 2016, https://www.cnn.com/2016/11/09/politics/van-jones-results-disappointment-cnntv/index.html.

24. Samuel Stein, *Capital City: Gentrification and the Real Estate State* (London: Verso, 2019), 5. According to Stein: "The real estate state is not new, nor is it all-encompassing. Like the carceral state, the warfare state, the welfare state or administrative state, it is an expansion of government—a component, a bloc, a manifestation, a tendency—that has been around in one form or another for as long as states and private property have existed."

Track 1. The Trump Card

1. This chart was developed using 2010 US Census Bureau data.

2. Andrew Flowers, "Where Trump Got His Edge," FiveThirtyEight, November 11, 2016, https://fivethirtyeight.com/features/where-trump-got-his-edge/.

3. Douglass Massey and Jonathan Tannen, "A Research Note on Trends in Black Hypersegregation," *Demography* 52, no. 3 (2015): 1025–1034.

4. It also provides the spatial dynamics that give rise to electoral gerrymandering.

5. Mindy Fullilove, Lourdes Hernández-Cordero, and Robert E. Fullilove define American Apartheid as "both a system of separation and of serial forced displacement." Put another way, American Apartheid is the combination of government-enforced racial segregation and serial forced displacement. Fullilove et al., "The Ghetto Game: Apartheid and the Developer's Imperative in Postindustrial American Cities," in *The Integration Debate: Competing Futures for American Cities*, ed. Chester Hartman and Gregory D. Squires (New York: Routledge Taylor & Francis Group, 2009), 199–21.

6. Jon Huang, Samuel Jacoby, Michael Strickland, and K. K. Rebecca Lai, "Election 2016: Exit Polls," *New York Times*, November 8, 2016, https://www .nytimes.com/interactive/2016/11/08/us/politics/election-exit-polls.html.

7. Daniel Cox, Rachel Lienesch, and Robert P. Jones, *Beyond Economics: Fears of Cultural Displacement Pushed the White Working Class to Trump* (Washington, DC: Public Religion Research Institute & The Atlantic Report, 2017), https://www.immigrationresearch.org/report/other/beyond-economics -fears-cultural-displacement-pushed-white-working-class-trump-prrithe-a.

8. Emily Flitter and Chris Kahn, "Trump Supporters More Likely to View Blacks Negatively—Reuters/Ipsos Poll," Reuters, June 28, 2016, https:// www.reuters.com/article/us-usa-election-race/exclusive-trump-supporters -more-likely-to-view-blacks-negatively-reuters-ipsos-poll-idUSKCN0ZE2SW.

9. Sean McElwee and Jason McDaniel, "Economic Anxiety Didn't Make People Vote Trump, Racism Did," *The Nation*, May 8, 2017, https://www.thenation.com /article/economic-anxiety-didnt-make-people-vote-trump-racism-did/. See also Michael Scherer, "White Identity Politics Drives Trump, and the Republican Party under Him," *Washington Post*, July 16, 2019, https://www.washingtonpost .com/politics/white-identity-politics-drives-trump-and-the-republican-party -under-him/2019/07/16/a5ff5710-a733-11e9-a3a6-ab670962db05_story.html.

10. Gus T. Renegade, *Dr. Frances Cress Welsing: Donald J. Trump and the Reconstruction of White Supremacy*, 2017, available at Academia.edu.

11. Some such decisions include:

- Parents Involved v. Seattle School District (2007)—helped stop school desegregation and undermine Brown v. Board of Education's aim.
- Rocco v. DeStefano (2009)—weakened the disparate impact clause of Title VII of the 1964 Civil Rights Act; gives rise to reverse discrimination claims.
- King v. Burwell (2012)—or what I call the Neo-Confederate Nullification of the Affordable Care Act (ACA) gave states the right to opt out of the Medicaid expansion of the ACA, thereby weakening the viability of exchanges and denying millions of Black people health care coverage.
- Shelby v. Holder (2013)—gutted the enforcement mechanism of the 1965 Voting Rights Act so that states no longer had to submit their changes to election laws and procedures to the DOJ for review/approval. This helped Southern states close at least 868 polling sites after 2012 and introduce voter restrictions and voter ID laws.
- Texas DCHA v. Inclusive Communities (2015)—upheld disparate impact claims but makes it harder to file cases alleging discriminatory impact. Must now identify a specific policy and show that the policy is the cause of the disparity. Weakens the 1968 Fair Housing Act.

- Utah v. Strieff (2016)—enhances police powers, expands stop-and-frisk and weakened the Fourth Amendment because an unlawful search can now produce evidence to be used at trial. Strengthens Illinois v. Wardlow (2000).

12. Matt Ford, "Justice Sotomayor's Ringing Dissent," *The Atlantic*, June 16, 2016, https://www.theatlantic.com/politics/archive/2016/06/utah-strieff -sotomayor/487922/.

13. Glenn Kessler, "When Did McConnell Say He Wanted to Make Obama a 'One-Term President'"?, *Washington Post*, September 25, 2012, https://www .washingtonpost.com/blogs/fact-checker/post/when-did-mcconnell-say-he -wanted-to-make-obama-a-one-term-president/2012/09/24/7.

14. Lawrence Brown, "Yes We Did: Assessing Black Progress during the Obama Era," *Abernathy*, January 20, 2017, https://abernathymagazine.com/black -progress-obama-era/.

15. Michelle Sotero, "A Conceptual Model of Historical Trauma: Implications for Public Health Practice and Research," *Journal of Health Disparities Research and Practice* 1, no. 1 (2006): 93–108.

16. Sarah Malotane, "Restorative Justice as a Tool for Peacebuilding: A South African Case Study" (PhD diss., University of KwaZulu Natal, 2012), 63.

17. David Pierce, "Officer Shot during West Baltimore Traffic Stop," WBAL, December 16, 2014, http://www.wbaltv.com/article/officer-shot-during -west-baltimore-traffic-stop/7090851.

18. Ryan's rhetoric elided the fact that lynch mobs in American history were decidedly and demographically White in racial composition while the victims of White American lynch mobs were decidedly Black women, men, boys, and girls.

19. Lara Putnam, Erica Chenoweth, and Jeremy Pressman. "The Floyd Protests Are the Broadest in U.S. History—and Are Spreading to White, Small-Town America," *Washington Post*, June 6, 2020, https://www.washingtonpost.com /politics/2020/06/06/floyd-protests-are-broadest-us-history-are-spreading -white-small-town-america/.

20. @Creosotemaps, "Black Lives Matter Protests 2020," Creosote Maps, June 14, 2020, https://www.creosotemaps.com/blm2020/. See also Audra D. S. Burch, Weiyi Cai, Gabriel Gianodoli, Morrigan McCarthy, and Jugal K. Patel, "How Black Lives Matter Reached Every Corner of America," *New York Times*, June 13, 2020, https://www.nytimes.com/interactive/2020 /06/13/us/george-floyd-protests-cities-photos.html.

21. Anne Helen Petersen, "Why the Small Protests in Small Towns across America Matter," BuzzFeed, June 3, 2020, https://www.buzzfeednews.com /article/annehelenpetersen/black-lives-matter-protests-near-me-small -towns.

Track 2. *This Is America*

1. The Schomburg Center in Black Culture, Howard Dodson, and Sylvaine A. Diouf, *The Abolition of the Slave Trade* (New York Public Library), 2005, http://abolition.nypl.org/essays/us_slave_trade/.

2. Schomburg Center in Black Culture et al., *In Motion*, 26.

3. Marimba Ani, *Let the Circle Be Unbroken: The Implications of African Spirituality in the Diaspora* (New York: Nkonimfo Publications, 2004).

4. W. E. B. Du Bois, *Black Reconstruction in America 1860–1880* (New York: Free Press, 1935), 42–45. See also Schomburg Center et al., *In Motion*, 45.

5. Schomburg Center et al., *In Motion*, 45.

6. Frederick Douglass, "What to the Slave Is the Fourth of July?" (speech, Corinthian Hall, Rochester, NY, July 5, 1852).

7. Ralph Clayton, *Cash for Blood: The Baltimore to New Orleans Domestic Slave Trade* (n.p.: Heritage Books, 2002).

8. James Cox, "Corporations Challenged by Reparations Activists," *USA Today*, February 21, 2002, http://usatoday30.usatoday.com/money/general/2002/02/21/slave-reparations.htm. Medical doctors were involved in the examination of enslaved people for slave traders and enslavers.

9. According to Daina Ramey Berry, "Medical examiners aided enslavers, insurance companies, and traders to determine an enslaved person's health—including bodily integrity and perceived mental stability—which had a direct relationship to his or her appraised and market values. . . . Healthy enslaved people were poked, prodded, and examined. At some sales, for privacy during a more physical exam, they were taken behind a curtain or into a 'little room,' but one wonders for whom this privacy was reserved." Berry, *The Price for Their Pound of Flesh: The Value of the Enslaved, from Womb to Grave, in the Building of a Nation* (Boston: Beacon Press, 2017), 70–71.

10. Craig Steven Wilder, *Ebony and Ivy: Race, Slavery, and the Troubled History of America's Universities* (New York: Bloomsbury Press, 2013).

11. Du Bois, *Black Reconstruction in America*, 4.

12. Du Bois, *Black Reconstruction in America*, 42.

13. Dale E. Watts, "How Bloody Was Bleeding Kansas? Political Killings in Kansas Territory, 1854–1861," *Kansas History: A Journal of the Central Plains* 18, no. 2 (1995): 129. For W. E. B. Du Bois, the Civil War starts in Kansas: "Then came this battle called the Civil War, beginning in Kansas in 1854, and ending in the presidential election of 1876—twenty awful years. The slave went free; stood a brief moment in the sun; then moved back again toward slavery. The whole weight of America was thrown to color caste" (Du Bois, *Black Reconstruction in America*, 30). Regarding the Civil War beginning in Kansas, Du Bois wrote: "The two forces met in Kansas, and in Kansas civil war began" (29).

14. Roger Taney, 1857. *The Dred Scott Decision: Opinion of Chief Justice Taney*, 60 US 393 (1857).

15. Taney, *The Dred Scott Decision*.

16. Du Bois, *Black Reconstruction in America*, 28–30.

17. National Park Service, "The Pratt Street Riot," National Park Service, 2019, https://www.nps.gov/articles/the-pratt-street-riot.htm.

18. Thomas B. Allen, *Harriet Tubman, Secret Agent: How Daring Slaves and Free Blacks Spied for the Union during the Civil War* (Washington, DC: National Geographic Society, 2009), 134, 139.

19. Schomburg Center for Research in Black Culture, Photographs and Prints Division, New York Public Library, "Our ticket, Our Motto: This is a White Man's Country; Let White Men Rule," campaign badge supporting Horatio Seymour and Francis Blair, Democratic candidates for President and Vice-President of the Unites States, 1868, New York Public Library Digital Collections, 2019, https://digitalcollections.nypl.org/items/62a9d0e6-4fc9-dbce-e040-e00a18064a66.

20. Black economic districts were built in cities such as Hayti in Durham, NC; Greenwood in Tulsa, OK; Sweet Auburn Avenue in Atlanta, GA. Black cities were built in places such as Rosewood, FL; Seneca Village, NY; and Freedman's Town in Houston, TX. Brandee Sanders, "History's Lost Black Towns," *The Root*, January 27, 2011, https://www.theroot.com/historys-lost-black-towns -1790868004. See also DeNeen Brown, "All-Black Towns across America: Life Was Hard but Full of Promise," *Washington Post*, March 27, 2015, https://www .washingtonpost.com/lifestyle/style/a -list-of-well-known-black-towns/2015 /03/27/9f21ca42-cdc4-11e4-a2a7-9517a3a70506_story.html.

21. Douglas Egerton, *The Wars of Reconstruction: The Brief, Violent History of America's Most Progressive Era* (London: Bloomsbury Press, 2015).

22. According to the National Endowment for the Humanities: "By 1873, many white Southerners were calling for 'Redemption'—the return of white supremacy and the removal of rights for blacks—instead of Reconstruction. This political pressure to return to the old order was oftentimes backed up by mob and paramilitary violence, with the Ku Klux Klan, the White League, and the Red Shirts assassinating pro-Reconstruction politicians and terrorizing Southern blacks." National Endowment for the Humanities. "Reconstruction vs. Redemption," NEH, February 11, 2014, https://www.neh.gov/news/reconstruction-vs -redemption.

23. Equal Justice Initiative, *Reconstruction in America: Racial Violence after the Civil War, 1865–1876* (Montgomery, AL: EJI, 2020). The report provides additional context to the tally of racial terror lynchings. The authors write that "the Equal Justice Initiative has documented more than 2,000 Black victims killed during the Reconstruction era, from 1865 to 1876. This is a staggering figure compared to the more than 4,400 victims documented for the 74-year era of racial terror lynching that spans 1877 to 1950. It is an even more horrific figure considering the thousands of additional victims who may be documented in other records, or who are undocumented and forever lost to history" (44).

24. Equal Justice Initiative, *Lynching in America: Confronting the Legacy of Racial Terror* (Montgomery, AL: EJI, 2015).

25. Equal Justice Initiative, *Lynching in America.*

26. Ida B. Wells lifted up Black women as victims of lynchings: "The women of the race have not escaped the fury of the mob. In Jackson, Tennessee, in the summer of 1886, a white woman died of poisoning. Her black cook was suspected, and as a box of rat poison was found in her room, she was hurried away to jail. When the mob had worked itself to the lynching pitch, she was dragged out of jail, every stitch of clothing torn from her body, and she was hung in the public court-house square in sight of everybody. Jackson is one of the oldest towns in the State, and the State Supreme Court holds its sittings there; but no one was arrested for the deed—not even a protest was uttered. The husband of the poisoned woman has since died a raving maniac, and his ravings showed that he, and not the poor black cook, was the poisoner of his wife. A fifteen year old Negro girl was hanged in Rayville, Louisiana, in the spring of 1892, on the same charge of poisoning white persons. There was no more proof or investigation of this case than the one in Jackson. A Negro woman, Lou Stevens, was hanged from a railway bridge in Hollendale, Mississippi, in 1892. She was charged with being accessory to the murder of her white paramour, who had shamefully abused her." Ida B. Wells, "Lynch

Law in All Its Phases" (Boston Monday Lectureship, 1893); see also Shirley Wilson Logan, "Lynch Law in All Its Phases," Voices of Democracy: The U.S. Oratory Project, vol. 2, 56–58, 2007, https://voicesofdemocracy.umd.edu /wp-content/uploads/2010/07/logan-wells.pdf.

27. Liam Hogan, "Mob Violence, Riots, and Pogroms against African American Communities," Collective Punishment, 2015, https://collectivepunishment .wordpress.com.

28. Schomburg Center for Research in Black Culture, *In Motion: The African American Migration Experience* (Washington DC: National Geographic, 2005), 45; see also Hogan, "Mob Violence, Riots and Pogroms."

29. Ida B. Wells, *Crusade for Justice: The Autobiography of Ida B. Wells* (Chicago: University of Chicago Press, 1970).

30. James Loewen, *Sundown Towns: A Hidden Dimension of American Racism* (Touchstone: New York, 2006).

31. Matt Novak, "Oregon Was Founded as a Racist Utopia," Gizmodo, 2015, https://gizmodo.com/oregon-was-founded-as-a-racist-utopia-1539567040; see also Natasha Geiling, "How Oregon's Second Largest City Vanished in a Day," Smithsonian.com, February 18, 2015, https://www.smithsonianmag .com/history/vanport-oregon-how-countrys-largest-housing-project -vanished-day-180954040/#vBzkM6RPQbSCcqKY.99.

32. Geiling, "How Oregon's Second Largest City Vanished."

33. The History Channel, *Aftershock: Beyond the Civil War*, 2006.

34. Edward Blum, *W. E. B. Du Bois: American Prophet* (Philadelphia: University of Pennsylvania Press, 2007).

35. In fact, Black people became linked with their neighborhood characteristics in the minds of White Americans. As Jessica Trounstine argues: "Above all else, whites feared that integration would jeopardize their single largest investment: the value of their home, as well as the quality of their neighbor- hood. Blacks were seen as undesirable neighbors, in part, because the features of their neighborhoods became associated with individual members of the racial group." Trounstine, *Segregation by Design: Local Politics and Inequality in American Cities* (Cambridge: Cambridge University Press, 2018), 31; see also Lawrence Brown, "Collective Punishment Reveals White Supremacist Theology," *Journal of Southern Religion* 17 (2015), http://jsreligion.org/issues /vol17/Brown.html.

36. In a May 1911 article in *The Crisis*, W. E. B. Du Bois described how cities' policies caused poor physical conditions in Black neighborhoods: "If, for instance, you go to an ordinary Southern town you are shown the Negro districts; the streets are unpaved; sidewalks are in a dilapidated condition; the drainage is bad; the garbage is not cared for, and the houses are dilapidated. Now, without doubt, part of this condition can be charged to the colored dwellers, but much of it is due to the deliberate refusal of the city to spend any public money on city improvements in the Negro district or to properly police this district." W. E. B. Du Bois, "Violations of Property Rights," *The Crisis: A Record of the Darker Races* 2, no. 1 (1911): 28–32, 31.

37. Trounstine, *Segregation by Design*, 2, 29–32.

38. Trounstine, *Segregation by Design*, 1–2.

39. Douglas Blackmon, *Slavery by Another Name: The Re-enslavement of Black Americans from the Civil War to World War II* (New York: Anchor, 2009).

40. Schomburg Center for Research in Black Culture, *In Motion,* 45. See also Stephen Meyer Grant, *As Long as They Don't Move Next Door: Segregation and Racial Conflict in American Neighborhoods* (Lanham, MD: Rowman & Littlefield, 2000).

41. Pete Daniel, *Dispossession: Discrimination against African American Farmers in the Age of Civil Rights* (Chapel Hill: University of North Carolina Press, 2015). See also Andrew Kahrl, *The Land Was Ours: How Black Beaches Became White Wealth in the Coastal South* (Chapel Hill: University of North Carolina Press, 2016).

42. National Commission on Urban Problems, 1968. *Building the American City: Report to the Congress and the President of the United States* (Washington, DC: Government Printing Office). See also Mark Rose and Raymond Mohl, *Interstate: Highway Politics and Policy since 1939* (Knoxville: University of Tennessee Press, 2012); Michelle Alexander, *The New Jim Crow: Mass Incarceration in the Age of Colorblindness* (New York: New Press, 2012).

43. Mindy Fullilove and Roderick Wallace, "Serial Forced Displacement in American Cities, 1916–2010," *Journal of Urban Health* 88, no. 3 (2011): 381–389. For the neoliberal dismantling of public housing in the aftermath of Hurricane Katrina, see John Arena, *Driven from New Orleans: How Nonprofits Betray Public Housing and Promote Privatization* (Minneapolis: University of Minnesota Press, 2012). For the dismantling of public housing, see Edward Goetz, *New Deal Ruins: Race, Economic Justice, and Public Housing Policy* (Ithaca, NY: Cornell University Press, 2013). For the permanent closings of Black public school, see Journey for Justice Alliance, *Death by a Thousand Cuts: Racism, School Closures, and Public School Sabotage*, Organizational report, May 2014. See also Eve Ewing, *Ghosts in the Schoolyard: Racism and School Closings on Chicago's South Side* (Chicago: University of Chicago Press, 2018).

44. Robert V. Haynes, "Houston Riot of 1917," Texas State Historical Society, 2010, https://tshaonline.org/handbook/online/articles/jch04.

45. Cameron McWhirter, *Red Summer: The Summer of 1919 and the Awakening of Black America* (New York: Henry Holt, 2011).

46. Raymond Mohl, "Race and Housing in the Postwar City: An Explosive History," *Journal of the Illinois State Historical Society* 94, no. (2001): 8–30, 16. See also Walter Rucker and James Nathaniel Upton, *The Encyclopedia of American Race Riots*, vols. 1 and 2 (Westport, CT: Greenwood Press, 2007).

47. Ida B. Wells-Barnett, *The Arkansas Race Riot* (Aquila Press reprint, 1920), 68–69.

48. Wells-Barnett, *The Arkansas Race Riot.* In her pamphlet, Wells-Barnett highlighted the Black economic organizing that provoked the white supremacist mob violence in Elaine, Arkansas: "The lodge employed Mr. Braxton, a white lawyer, to represent the members in their effort to secure the market price for their cotton, to arrange for better contracts, to adjust their accounts with the landowners and to generally safeguard their interests. This labor movement among colored farmers did not please the white landowners and the proposal of the farmers to act through a white lawyer constituted a menace to the profiteering practices of the white people of the neighborhood. The dissatisfaction of the white people found expression at first in the gentle hints that the Negroes were making a mistake; these were followed by warnings to colored people to let that lodge business alone. . . . Then came the tragedy such as no labor movement in this country has ever witnessed" (68). Just as with the lynchings of the three Black owners of

Peoples Grocery store in Memphis, Tennessee, in 1892, the motivations of white supremacist terrorist attacks were often rooted in the economic destruction of Black neighborhoods or cooperative economic efforts.

49. Herbert Shapiro, *White Violence and Black Response: From Reconstruction to Montgomery* (Amherst: University of Massachusetts Press, 1988), 226–250.

50. Mohl, "Race and Housing in the Postwar City," 17–21.

51. One reason it is important to recount the legacy of white supremacist urban violence is that it serves as an important corrective to the false narrative that white supremacist violence against Black people was relegated to the Deep South or to rural areas (usually in the form of lynchings). The violence of the Red Summer in over 25 cities and postwar white supremacist urban violence in cities from Los Angeles to Atlanta reveals that white supremacist violence took place in the West, Midwest, and North in large urban centers.

52. Ira Katznelson, *When Affirmative Action Was White: An Untold History of Racial Inequality in Twentieth-Century America* (New York: W. W. Norton, 2005).

53. National Commission on Urban Problems, *Building the American City,* 99.

54. Katznelson, *When Affirmative Action Was White.* See also National Commission on Urban Problems, *Building the American City*; Mohl, "Race and Housing in the Postwar City," 12.

55. National Commission on Urban Problems, *Building the American City,* 97 (FHA home loans), 99 (FHA home improvement loans), 103 (Veterans Administration), and 105 (Fannie Mae).

56. Certainly, Black veterans did receive some of these loans. I did not subtract this amount from the $184.8 billion estimate since dollars allocated to homebuyers by race was not tracked at the time. Thus, the $184.8 billion and $1.4 trillion are not precise nor are they meant to be exact. The numbers are meant to give a rough idea of the vast resources committed to funding White suburbs. The numbers could certainly be higher if the amount of spending on programs such as urban renewal or the amount of money suburban homeowners received from the mortgage interest deduction were included. The expenditures to support the White flight and suburban housing affirmative action package could come close to $2 trillion in 2019 spending.

57. Katznelson, *When Affirmative Action Was White,* 163–164.

58. National Commission on Urban Problems, *Building the American City,* 101.

59. National Commission on Urban Problems, *Building the American City.* According to the commission: "FHA almost never insured mortgages on homes in slum districts, and did so very seldom in the gray areas which surrounded them. Even middle class residential districts in the central cities were suspect, since there was always the prospect that they, too, might turn as Negroes and poor whites continued to pour into the cities, and as middle and upper-middle income whites continued to move out" (100).

60. In his book *Dispossession*, Pete Daniels summarizes the scope of Black land dispossession: "In the quarter century after 1950, over half a million African American farms went under, leaving only 45,000. In the 1960s alone, the black farm count in ten southern states (minus Florida, Texas, and Kentucky) fell from 132,000 to 16,000, an 88 percent decline. . . . The civil rights and equal opportunity laws of the mid-1960s prompted USDA bureaucrats to embrace equal rights rhetorically even as they intensified discrimination. This passive nullification, voicing agreement with equal rights while continu-

ing or intensifying discrimination, did not rely on antebellum intellectual arguments or confrontation but instead thrived silently in the offices of biased employees."

61. Krista Michelle Jones, "'It Was Awful, but It Was Politics': Crittenden County and the Demise of African American Political Participation" (master's thesis, University of Arkansas, 2002).

62. N. Tasmin Din and Brian Hilburn, "The Murder of Isadore Banks," Civil Rights and Restorative Justice Project, 2011, https://repository.library .northeastern.edu/downloads/neu:m042w3682?datastream_id=content.

63. Staff writer, "Bare 2 Angles in Torch Slaying of Farmer: The Gruesome Work of Fiends," *Tri-State Defender*, June 19, 1954. See also Din and Hilburn, "The Murder of Isadore Banks."

64. White supremacist violence often targeted Black cooperatives, businesses, or labor organizing efforts, including Peoples Grocery (Shelby County, Tennessee), Grant Co-Op Gin (Crittenden County, Arkansas), Progressive Farmers and Householders Union of America (Philips County, Arkansas), Sharecroppers' Union (Tallapoosa County, Alabama), and Southern Tenants Farmers' Union (northeast Arkansas and southeast Missouri). Successful Black economic districts or landowners were also targeted by white supremacist violence, including Black Springfield's economic district (Springfield, Illinois), Black landowners (Crittenden County, Arkansas, in 1888 and 1954), and Greenwood economic district (Tulsa, Oklahoma). This historical analysis reveals the ways in which Black Southerners were incredibly organized and cohesive in creating economic efforts so successful that they elicited jealousy and vindictiveness among their White Southern counterparts. Their economic acumen reveals that Black sharecroppers and farmers were agents of their own destiny—when not disturbed. They organized and created unions, cooperatives, and business districts that were quite successful (or posed the threat of success) until they were destroyed or undermined by white supremacists who were acting to eliminate successful or potentially viable economic competitors. In her groundbreaking analysis of the cooperative economic efforts in African American history, Jessica Gordon Nembhard found that Black urban and rural communities were avid practitioners of cooperative economics and pooling resources. The reason for their demise and near erasure from Black historical memory is clear according to Nembhard. "Many if not all of these efforts were targeted for destruction by White supremacists, unsympathetic (often fearful) Whites, and/or White economic competitors (the plantation bloc and/or corporatists)." Jessica Gordon Nembhard, *Collective Courage: A History of African American Cooperative Economic Thought and Practice* (University Park: Pennsylvania State University Press, 2014), 29.

65. Danielle L. McGuire, *At the Dark End of the Street: Black Women, Rape, and Resistance—a New History of the Civil Rights Movement from Rosa Parks to the Rise of Black Power* (New York: Vantage Books, 2010), xviii. McGuire writes: "The rape of black women by white men continued, often unpunished, throughout the Jim Crow era. As Reconstruction collapsed and Jim Crow arose, white men abducted and assaulted black women with alarming regularity. White men lured black women and girls away from home with promises of steady work and better wages; attacked them on the job; abducted them at gunpoint while traveling to or from home, work, or church; raped

them as a form of retribution or to enforce rules of racial and economic hierarchy; sexually humiliated and assaulted them on streetcars and buses, in taxicabs and trains, and in other public spaces."

66. DeNeen L. Brown, "How Recy Taylor's Brutal Rape Has Become a Symbol of #MeToo and #TimesUp." *Washington Post,* January 30, 2018, https://www .washingtonpost.com/news/retropolis/wp/2017/11/27/the-gang-rape-was -horrific-the-naacp-sent-rosa-parks-to-investigate-it/?utm_term=.a16a52713a96.

67. This includes students from HBCUs such as Morgan State University, Shaw University, and Howard University. Morgan College (as it was then known) produced the first fully formed student-led Civil Rights Movement to defeat Jim Crow that lasted from the late 1940s to 1963. Morgan College students would help desegregate multiple establishments in the Northwood Plaza. Shaw University would be the site where the Student Nonviolent Coordinating Movement (SNCC) would be born under the tutelage of the great organizer Ella Baker in April 1960—sparking sit-ins, Freedom Rides, and voter registration campaigns that would topple Jim and Jane Crow in the Deep South. One of SNCC's premiere organizers, Stokely Carmichael (who would later become Kwame Ture) was a student and graduate of Howard University.

68. They were joined by a good number of allied White students from Johns Hopkins University and Goucher College.

69. Peter Levy, *The Great Uprising: Race Riots in Urban America during the 1960s* (Cambridge: Cambridge University Press, 2017), 9. According to Levy, there were 8 uprisings in 1964, 5 uprisings in 1965, 21 uprisings in 1966, 233 uprisings in 1967, 360 uprisings in 1968, 131 uprisings in 1969, 67 uprisings in 1970, and 46 uprisings in 1971.

70. Jeffrey O. G. Ogbar, "The FBI's War on Civil Rights Leaders," *Daily Beast,* January 16, 2017, https://www.thedailybeast.com/the-fbis-war-on-civil-rights -leaders; Nathan Blackstock, *COINTELPRO: The FBI's Secret War on Political Freedom* (New York: Pathfinder Press, 1988); Huey P. Newton, *War against the Panthers: A Study of Repression in America* (London: Writers and Readers Press, 2000).

71. Elizabeth Hinton, "'A War within Our Own Boundaries': Lyndon Johnson's Great Society and the Rise of the Carceral State," *Journal of American History* 102, no. 1 (2015): 100–112.

72. Tom LoBianco, "Report: Aide Says Nixon's War on Drugs Targeted Blacks and Hippies," CNN, March 24, 2016, https://www.cnn.com/2016/03/23/politics /john-ehrlichman-richard-nixon-drug-war-blacks-hippie/index.html.

73. Ashley Farmer, *Remaking Black Power: How Black Women Transformed an Era* (Chapel Hill: University of North Carolina Press, 2017). See Keeanga-Yamahtta Taylor, *How We Get Free: Black Feminism and the Combahee River Collective* (Chicago: Haymarket Books, 2017). See also Rhonda Williams, *The Politics of Public Housing: Black Women's Struggles against Urban Inequality* (New York: Oxford University Press, 2004).

74. R. D. G. Kelley, "Kickin' Reality, Kickin' Ballistics: Gangsta Rap and Postindustrial Los Angeles," in *Droppin' Science: Critical Essays on Rap Music and Hip Hop Culture,* ed. W. E. Perkins, 117–158 (Philadelphia: Temple University Press, 1996). See also Ernest Allen Jr., "Making the Strong Survive: The Contours and Contradictions of Message Rap," in Perkins, *Droppin' Science,* 159–191.

75. Fullilove and Rodrick, "Serial Forced Displacement in American Cities," 381–389.

76. Appendix B contains a listing of multiple systems, policies, and practices that have extracted wealth from Black bodies, people, and neighborhoods throughout the course of American history.

77. Steven Yaccino, Michael Schwirtz, and Marc Santora, "Gunman Kills 6 at a Sikh Temple Near Milwaukee," *New York Times*, August 5, 2012, https://www .nytimes.com/2012/08/06/us/shooting-reported-at-temple-in-wisconsin .html.

78. Alan Blinder and Kevin Sack, "Dylann Roof Is Sentenced to Death in Charleston Church Massacre," *New York Times*, January 10, 2017, https:// www.nytimes.com/2017/01/10/us/dylann-roof-trial-charleston.html.

79. Lawrence Brown, "This Is American Terrorism: White Supremacy's Brutal, Centuries-Long Campaign of Violence," *Salon*, June 19, 2015, https://www .salon.com/2015/06/19/this_is_american_terrorism_white_supremacys _brutal_centuries_long_campaign_of_violence/.

80. Barbara Ransby situates the election of Trump as a response to the Black Lives Matter Movement/Movement for Black Lives [BLMM/M4BL]. She argues: "The election of racist and misogynist demagogue Donald Trump as the forty-fifth president of the United States in November 2016 represented an indirect backlash against the radical antiracism of BLMM/M4BL. This new administration in Washington, with all of its belligerence and appeals to white nationalists, also challenged and impacted the movement in unexpected ways, catapulting it into a new phase of activity focused on broad-based united front and coalition work." See Ransby, *Making All Black Lives Matter: Reimagining Freedom in the 21st Century* (Oakland: University of California Press, 2018), 8–9.

81. Some Trump administration policies and actions include (1) executive order instituting a ban on travel from 7 countries; (2) repeated attempts to repeal the Patient Protection and Affordable Care Act (PPACA); (3) signing a $1.5 trillion tax cut to huge gains for the wealthy, which also undermined the PPACA by eliminating the individual mandate; (4) rolling back the enforcement mechanisms of the 1977 Community Reinvestment Act; (5) postponing the implementation of the 2015 HUD Affirmatively Furthering Fair Housing policy until after 2020 and suspending HUD's 2016 rule for Small Area Fair Market Rent (although a federal court reinstated it); and (6) separating children from their families seeking asylum after fleeing countries with high levels of violence in Central America.

82. Ali Vitali, Kasie Hunt, and Frank Thorp V, "Trump Referred to Haiti and African Nations as 'Shithole' Countries," *NBC News*, January 11, 2018, https://www.nbcnews.com/politics/white-house/trump-referred-haiti -african-countries-shithole-nations-n836946.

83. Debbie Lord, "What Happened at Charlottesville: Looking Back on the Anniversary of the Deadly Rally," *Atlanta Journal-Constitution*, August 10, 2018, https://www.ajc.com/news/national/what-happened-charlottesville -looking-back-the-anniversary-the-deadly-rally/fPpnLrbAtbxSwNI9BEy93K/.

84. Jason Wilson, "Exclusive: Video Shows Portland Officers Made Deal with Far-Right Group Leader," *The Guardian*, March 1, 2019, https://www

.theguardian.com/us-news/2019/mar/01/exclusive-video-shows-portland
-officers-made-deal-with-far-right-group-leader.

85. US Department of Justice, *Multiple White Supremacist Gang Members among 54 Defendants Charged in RICO Indictment* (Washington, DC: Department of Justice, Office of Public Affairs), February 12, 2019, https://www.justice .gov/opa/pr/multiple-white-supremacist-gang-members-among-54 -defendants-charged-rico-indictment.

86. Leila Fidel, "Civil Rights and Faith Leaders to FBI: Take White Nationalist Violence Seriously," National Public Radio, March 20, 2019, https://www.npr .org/2019/03/20/705123229/civil-rights-and-faith-leaders-to-fbi-take-white -nationalist-violence-seriously.

87. Ayal Feinberg, Regina Branton, and Valerie Martinez-Ebers, "Counties That Hosted a 2016 Trump Rally Saw a 226 Percent Increase in Hate Crimes," *Washington Post*, March 22, 2019, https://www.washingtonpost.com/politics /2019/03/22/trumps-rhetoric-does-inspire-more-hate-crimes/.

88. Andrew Blake, "White Supremacists Pose 'Persistent, Pervasive' Threat, FBI Chief Says," *Washington Times*, April 4, 2019, https://www.washingtontimes .com/news/2019/apr/4/christopher-wray-fbi-director-says-white-supremaci/.

89. Mitch Smith, Rick Rojas, and Campbell Robertson, "Dayton Gunman Had Been Exploring 'Violent Ideologies,' F.B.I. Says," *New York Times,* August 5, 2019, https://www.nytimes.com/2019/08/06/us/mass-shootings.html.

90. Writing on his Twitter account on August 4, Republican Senator Ted Cruz stated: "As the son of a Cuban immigrant, I am deeply horrified by the hateful anti-Hispanic bigotry expressed in the shooter's so-called 'manifesto.' This ignorant racism is repulsive and profoundly anti-American. We must speak clearly to combat evil in any form it takes. What we saw yesterday was a heinous act of terrorism and white supremacy." Jim Banks and Tim Scott also made statements condemning white supremacy in response to the El Paso massacre. Rebecca Morin, "Red Flag Laws, Mental Health Concerns: How the GOP Is Responding to the El Paso, Dayton Shootings," *USA Today*, August 6, 2019, https://www.usatoday.com/story/news/politics/2019/08/05/el-paso -dayton-shootings-how-trump-mcconnell-gop-responding/1925610001/.

91. Cedar Attanasio, Jake Bleiberg, and Paul J. Weber, "Police: El Paso Shooting Suspect Said He Targeted Mexicans," Associated Press, August 9, 2019, https://www.apnews.com/456c0154218a4d378e2fb36cd40b709d.

92. Editorial Board, "We Have a White Nationalist Terrorism Problem," *New York Times*, August 4, 2019, https://www.nytimes.com/2019/08/04/opinion /mass-shootings-domestic-terrorism.html.

93. Tim Hains, "Princeton Professor Eddie Glaude: Trump's Anti-Immigration Rhetoric Has Led America into 'Cold Civil War.'" Real Clear Politics, August 4, 2019, https://www.realclearpolitics.com/video/2019/08/04/eddie_glaude _trumps_immigration_rhetoric_has_led_american_in_a_cold_civil_war.html. Glaude argued on NBC's *Meet the Press*: "What happens, when we use language, like infestation, children—you used this, Governor—children carrying, perhaps, disease across the border? What happens? You set the stage for people who are even more on the extreme to act violently. We are in a cold civil war. We are in a cold civil war. And there are some people who bear the burden of it."

94. Ashraf Khalil, Aaron Morrison, and Jim Vertuno, "US Heads into a New Week Shaken by Violence and Pandemic," June 1, 2020, *AP News*, https://

www.kxan.com/news/newsfeed-now-protests-across-america-morning
-update-june-1-2020/.
95. Jeff Chang, *We Gon' Be Alright: Notes on Race and Resegregation* (New York: Picador, 2016), 70–71.
96. Lauren Camera, "The Quiet Wave of School District Secessions," *US News and World Report*, May 2017, https://www.usnews.com/news/education-news /articles/2017-05-05/the-quiet-wave-of-school-district-secessions.

Track 3. The "Negro Invasion"

1. See appendix C.
2. Bettye Thomas, "Public Education and Black Protest in Baltimore 1865–1900," *Maryland Historical Society Magazine* 71, no. 3 (1976): 381–391.
3. Dennis Patrick Halpin, *A Brotherhood of Liberty: Black Reconstruction and Its Legacies in Baltimore, 1865–1920* (Philadelphia: University of Pennsylvania Press, 2019), 101.
4. David S. Bogan, "Precursors of Rosa Parks: Maryland Transportation Cases Between the Civil War and the Beginning of World War I," *Maryland Law Review* 63, no. 1 (2004): 721–751. In her article, Bettye Thomas highlighted the education advocacy of Black clergy such as Rev. Harvey Johnson, the pastor of Union Baptist Church for over 50 years (1872–1923). "On June 22, 1885, Harvey Johnson and five other influential Baptist ministers organized the Brotherhood of Liberty. During the fall of 1885 the brotherhood held its first public meeting with Frederick Douglass as the main speaker. Among the various topics considered during the three-day meeting was the question of black teachers in public schools and equal facilities for black children. The brotherhood established a Committee on Education that was to be responsible for pressuring the school board, the mayor, and the city council into recognizing its legitimate demands for teachers and better schools. This committee was instrumental in establishing the Maryland Educational Union which was directed mainly by the brotherhood." Thomas, "Public Education and Black Protest in Baltimore," 385. Union Baptist Church would move to its present location from the midtown area to West Baltimore after the Great Fire of 1904. Stefan Goodwin and Dean R. Wagner, "National Registry of Historical Places: Registration Form" (US Department of the Interior, National Park Service, 2009), sec. 8, p. 2.
5. Halpin, *A Brotherhood of Liberty*, 92–113.
6. Although the ordinance appeared race neutral on the surface, it was decidedly racist in execution. The law blocked both Black and White homebuyers from purchasing property in blocks that were predominated by the other race. This appears to be equally exclusionary until one realizes that Baltimore was over 80% White in population in 1910, and, therefore, most city blocks would have been majority White, thereby restricting Black homebuyers only to the streets where they were the majority.
7. Staff writer, "Baltimore Tries Drastic Plan of Race Segregation: Strange Situation Which Led the Oriole City to Adopt the Most Pronounced 'Jim Crow' Measure on Record," *New York Times Magazine*, December 25, 1910. See first column and the fourth full paragraph from the bottom.
8. Christopher Silver, "The Origins of Racial Zoning in American Cities," in *Urban Planning and the African American Community: In the Shadows*, ed.

June Manning Thomas and Marsha Ritzdorf (Thousand Oaks, CA: Sage Publications, 1997).

9. This was just days after the first comprehensive residential racial zoning ordinance in the United States targeting African Americans was passed by the Baltimore City Council and signed by Mayor John Barry Mahool on December 20, 1910.

10. Staff writer, "Baltimore Tries Drastic Plan of Race Segregation."

11. William Ashbie Hawkins, "A Year of Segregation in Baltimore," *The Crisis*, November 1911, 27. See also Garrett Power, "Apartheid Baltimore Style: The Residential Segregation Ordinances of 1910–1913," *Maryland Law Review* 42, no. 2 (1983): 289–329, 297–298.

12. Morgan State University, "A Brief History of Morgan State University," Morgan State University, 2019, https://www.morgan.edu/about/history .html. Morgan College was originally known as the Centenary Biblical Institute. The name was changed to Morgan College in 1890. Morgan College was located in West Baltimore until 1917 when it moved to Northeast Baltimore adjacent to the Lauraville community. With respect to George McMechen's educational background, see "Baltimore Tries Drastic Plan of Race Segregation" (see n. 7).

13. Staff writer, "Baltimore Tries Drastic Plan of Race Segregation."

14. Staff writer, "Baltimore Tries Drastic Plan of Race Segregation," seventh column, below picture. See also Hawkins, "A Year of Segregation in Baltimore," 27–30.

15. Staff correspondent, "How Segregation Law in Baltimore Operates after Being Annulled 3 Times," *St. Louis Post-Dispatch*, February 22, 1916. Perhaps the *St. Louis Post-Dispatch* writer correctly predicted a race war in nearby East St. Louis, which would witness explosive violence in 1917. In 1919, white supremacist urban violence was unleashed during the Red Summer in over 25 cities across the nation.

16. Lawrence Brown, "Collective Punishment Reveals White Supremacist Theology," *Journal of Southern Religion* 17 (2015), http://jsreligion.org /issues/vol17/Brown.html. In 1898, a group of white supremacist Democrats in Wilmington, North Carolina, carried out a violent coup d'état— overthrowing a mixed raced government, killing over 200 Black Wilmington residents, and caused a mass exodus of 2,100 Black residents. Eight years later, dozens of Black residents were killed after Atlanta newspapers printed false stories of Black men attacking White women. In 1908, the city of Springfield, Illinois, white supremacists destroyed the Black business district known as Levee and torched the Black neighborhood known as the Badlands. Two Black men were also lynched and approximately 2,000 Black residents fled the city to escape racial terror. Another instance of white supremacist violence took place in Slocum, Texas, in 1910. According to the Texas Historical Commission, "Beginning on the morning of July 29, 1910, groups of armed white men shot and killed African Americans. . . . The murders of eight men were re- corded. . . . Many African Americans fled and did not return." Other locations of white supremacist violence included Sabine County, Texas, in 1908; Anna, Illinois, in 1909; Forsyth County, Georgia, in 1912; and New Madrid, Missouri, in 1915. See Liam Hogan, "Mob Violence, Riots, and Pogroms against African American Communities," Collective Punishment, 2015, https:// collectivepunishment.wordpress.com.

17. Staff writer, "They Blocked Invasion; Residents of Locust Point Quickly Solved Negro Problem by Force and Moral Suasion," *Baltimore Sun*, October 8, 1910. Perhaps as an enduring legacy, the Community Statistical Area containing the Locust Point community remains 90% White today and contains the smallest percentage of Black residents in the entire city.

18. Eli Pousson, "1885-1929: Segregation and the Fourteenth Amendment," Baltimore Civil Rights Heritage, 2019, https://baltimoreheritage.github.io /civil-rights-heritage/overview/1885-1929/. The power of White media and cultural productions are important to consider given the type of books and movies that were circulating between 1900 and 1920. As writers for the Baltimore Civil Rights Heritage website note, theatrical plays such as *The Clansman* and movies such as *The Birth of a Nation* both appeared in Baltimore, noting that:

> Black Baltimoreans pushed back against racism in popular culture. When two advance agents for the notoriously racist play *The Clansman* arrived in Baltimore in March 1906, waiters at the Saint James Hotel located at the southwest corner of Charles and Centre Streets refused them service in protest reportedly with the encouragement of the "Constitutional League." *The Birth of a Nation*, D. W. Griffith's movie based on *The Clansman*, screened for the first time in Baltimore the evening of March 6, 1916, before a crowd at Ford's Theatre that "packed the house to its utmost limit." The 1871 theater on Fayette Street near Eutaw Street, hosted the show for seven weeks reportedly "beating all records for length of run and for receipts." The screening drew outrage from the writers at the *Baltimore Afro-American* newspaper who had been closely following the NAACP's national campaign to restrict the film's distribution. Two days after the opening night at Ford's, the newspaper reported that "yells of rage and screams of hate" elicited by the film "did not cease with the end of the show." The article quotes a "colored man" calling it "the most disgusting thing I have ever seen," and a white man coming out of a Saturday performance, saying, "I should like to kill all of the damn niggers in the United States."

19. The *New York Times Magazine* would use the language as well in their seminal December 25, 1910, article. A caption to one of the pictures states: "Lanvale Lot: Where the Negro Invasion Has Depreciated Values." One thing worth lifting up here is how demonizing language can influence discriminatory policy for immigrant and refugee populations. During the period of the first African American Great Migration from 1910 to roughly 1940, language such as "Negro Invasion" was used to advance residential racial segregation and build policy walls to keep Southern Black migrants and existing Black residents from moving into White neighborhoods. This pattern was repeated in the late 2010s by President Donald Trump as he repeatedly referred to the migration of Central American immigrants at the Southern border as an "invasion."

20. As Dennis Patrick Halpin argues: "Dashiell's reliance on 'police power' has been overlooked in previous analyses of Baltimore's segregation effort. Its invocation, however, was telling. Over the course of the previous decade, segregationists had steadily built the specious case that African Americans were inherently criminal. They used this contention to justify efforts to disenfranchise black voters, dole out harsher punishments to black defen-

dants, and control African Americans in the city's public spaces. By relying on 'police power,' the West Segregation Ordinance effectively expanded the roles that the police played as foot soldiers in the fight against integration." Halpin, *A Brotherhood of Liberty*, 156.

21. Staff correspondent, "How Segregation Law in Baltimore Operates" (see n. 15).
22. Staff writer, "In Hurry for Ordinance: Demand for Race Segregation Measure at Once Is Becoming Insistent," *Baltimore Sun*, August 8, 1913.
23. Staff writer, "Mayor in Sympathy: Disapproves Location of Negro College at Mt. Washington—Cannot Preside at Meeting," *Baltimore Sun*, September 28, 1913.
24. Letter by John Trainor to Baltimore mayor James Preston, James Preston Files—1913, Baltimore City Archives.
25. A dornick is a pebble, stone, or small boulder.
26. Staff writer, "Baltimore in Race War over Invasion of Negro: Whites Fight to Protect Home Districts from Black Residents," *St. Louis Star and Times*, October 23, 1913. "Then, again, Morgan College wants to locate out in Mount Washington. . . . Mount Washington is a high-class suburban development, next-door neighbor to Roland Park, which every one knows is the most unusual and beautiful residence tract in the nation." This highlights how Morgan College's attempted move was actually to Baltimore County as E. Cold Spring Lane was the northernmost boundary of the city until 1918.
27. Staff correspondent, "How Segregation Law in Baltimore Operates."
28. Historian Raymond Mohl elucidates the role of real estate agents further: "the real estate industry had a major stake in the process of residential change. Mainstream realtors, such as those associated with the National Association of Real Estate Boards (NAREB) sought to keep white neighborhoods white. As early as the 1920s, in response to the first 'great migration' of southern blacks to northern cities and subsequent housing pressures, NAREB and local real estate boards in Chicago, St. Louis, and elsewhere promoted race restrictive covenants to prevent black neighborhood 'invasions.'" Mohl, "Race and Housing in the Postwar City: An Explosive History," *Journal of the Illinois State Historical Society* 94, no. 1 (2001): 8-30, 14.
29. Staff writer, "Baltimore Tries Drastic Plan of Race Segregation."
30. Staff writer, "Baltimore Tries Drastic Plan of Race Segregation."
31. The policies passed by people who self-proclaim their friendliness toward Black people is an object lesson in the function of racist policies. Policymakers and government officials might actually be friendly people with friendly dispositions while passing and enforcing deeply discriminatory laws that have a disparate impact by race.
32. Staff writer, "Negro Segregation Plan May Be Tried in Baltimore," *New-York Tribune*, February 20, 1917.
33. Staff writer, "To Aid 90,000 Negroes Mayor Is Authorized to Name Housing Committee: Suburban Colony Proposed," *Baltimore Sun*, February 24, 1917.
34. Staff writer, "Fights Negro Invasion: Lauraville Is Up in Arms against Morgan College," *Baltimore Sun*, May 2, 1917. At this time, Lauraville was still a part of Baltimore County. It would not join the city until the following year after annexation.
35. Staff writer, "Fights Negro Invasion." According to the *Sun*, "delegations from Lauraville, Hamilton, Clifton Park, Montebello Park, and Northeast

Baltimore will meet at the doors of Morgan College . . . to present a resolution of protest." Additionally, the Northeast Baltimore Improvement Association pledged to assist the Lauraville Improvement Association in its fight.

36. Steven K. Ragsdale, "Diggs v. Morgan College: Morgan Expands to the County: Racial Segregation and Baltimore Housing" (University of Maryland Law School, Baltimore, 2017).

37. Court of Appeals of Maryland, Russell I. Diggs et al. v. Morgan College, October 29, 1918, 105 A., 157.

38. Garrett Power, "Meade v. Dennistone: The NAACP Test Case to '. . . Sue Jim Crow Out of Maryland with the Fourteenth Amendment.'" *Maryland Law Review* 63 (2004): 773–810, 790–791.

39. In fact, several cities continued to draft and enact racial zoning ordinances. When the courts would strike down these illegal ordinances, many cities simply turned to race-based urban planning and leaned on racially restrictive covenants to achieve practically the same effect of racial zoning. See Silver, "Origins of Racial Zoning in American Cities." Given the fact that the federal government would draft Residential Security Maps starting in the 1930s, I would argue that racial zoning continued in the guise of color-coding which communities (based on their racial demographics) would receive capital lending by banks (which were guaranteed by the federal government). NS Form-8 makes the racist underpinnings of the Residential Security Map clear.

40. Special correspondent, "Races Confer in Baltimore: Mayor and Prominent White Citizens Meet Representative Colored Men," *New York Age*, March 30, 1918.

41. The 1918 annexation added communities such as Howard Part, Dickeyville, Franklintown, and Beechfield to the west and added neighborhoods such as Greektown, Highlandtown, Waltherson, and Claremont to the east.

42. Elizabeth Evitts Dickinson, "Roland Park: One of America's Garden Suburbs, and Built for Whites Only," *The Hub: Johns Hopkins Magazine*, Fall 2014, https://hub.jhu.edu/magazine/2014/fall/roland-park-papers-archives/.

43. Power, "Meade v. Dennistone, 795.

44. Power, "Meade v. Dennistone," 797–799.

45. Staff writer, "New Segregation Plan: Mayor Begins Work of Securing a Special Ordinance," *Baltimore Sun*, July 2, 1918.

46. Samuel Roberts, *Infectious Fear: Politics, Disease, and the Health Effects of Segregation* (Chapel Hill: University of North Carolina Press, 2009).

47. Unknown [but likely Assistant Commissioner of Health William T. Howard], "What Can Be Done to Improve the Living Conditions of Baltimore's Negro Population," *Baltimore Municipal Journal* 5, no. 5 (March 16, 1971), 1, second column. Although the author of the article is not clearly indicated, given the issue of public health being discussed, it is likely that a health department official is the author, most likely Assistant Commissioner of Health William T. Howard given his articulated support for Mayor Preston's racial segregation plans elsewhere and that he published several articles in the *Baltimore Municipal Journal* later that year.

48. This was the case particularly as many Black people served as domestic workers for wealthier White Baltimoreans, with many even living in White households as "the help." The *Baltimore Municipal Journal*—published by the City of Baltimore—makes the explicit connection between Black domestic

workers and the threat to White health: "As the Mayor has pointed out, the evil effects of the negro race are not confined within their own numbers. With little if any knowledge of their home surrounding we call upon these people to serve us in our households, prepare our food, tend our children and perform countless other services wherein personal contact is a matter of course. Regardless of our efforts to maintain [a] sanitary and healthful environment for ourselves and families the insidious influence of slum conditions is carried into our very midst to defile and destroy." See Unknown [but likely Assistant Commissioner of Health William T. Howard], "What Can Be Done to Improve the Living Conditions of Baltimore's Negro Population."

49. Staff writer, "New Segregation Plan."

50. Garrett Power, "Apartheid Baltimore Style: The Residential Segregation Ordinances of 1910–1913," *Maryland Law Review* 42, no. 2 (1983): 289–329, 314–315.

51. Staff writer, "North Baltimoreans Fear Negro Invasion: Two Organizations Are Formed to Prevent Ingress and Protect Property Values," *Baltimore Sun*, January 21, 1921. The health commissioner was involved in enforcing racial segregation under Mayor William F. Broening just as the health commissioner was heavily involved under Mayor James Preston. This also shows here and in other instances how White public health professionals in the Baltimore City Health Department helped legitimize and codify residential racial segregation in Baltimore City.

52. Halpin, *A Brotherhood of Liberty*, 144.

53. Staff writer, "To Prevent Negro Invasion: Stricker Street Property Owners Organize," *Baltimore Sun*, February 24, 1919.

54. The deployment of white supremacist urban violence to stop Black homebuyers was not unique to Baltimore. White supremacists in Kansas City would bomb and damage seven homes of Black families between April 1910 and November 1911 with another pair of bombings taking place 4.5 years afterward. See Stephen Meyer Grant, *As Long as They Don't Move Next Door: Segregation and Racial Conflict in American Neighborhoods* (Lanham, MD: Rowman and Littlefield, 2000), 20. Philadelphia would see three days of white supremacist urban violence starting July 26, 1918, when a Black woman named Ardella Bonds moved to a majority White block (36). Chicago was also a hotbed of anti-Black violence to stop the "Negro Invasion." As Eve Ewing writes: "From 1917 to 1921, fifty-eight bombs struck the homes of black residents, of bankers who gave them mortgages, or of real estate agents who sold them property. As the Chicago Commission on Race Relations noted, these bombings caused two deaths and did $100,000 of damage, averaging one bombing every twenty days over three years and eight months." See Eve L. Ewing, *Ghosts in the Schoolyard: Racism and School Closings on Chicago's South Side* (Chicago: University of Chicago Press, 2018), 61.

55. Staff writer, "Color Line with Vengeance: Baltimore Citizens Violently Resent Invasion of Negro," *Nebraska State Journal*, March 8, 1922.

56. Staff writer, "Negro Invasions Fought in Two More Sections: Efforts Made to Eject Families from Madison and Shirley Avenue Houses," *Baltimore Sun*, February 2, 1923.

57. Letter to Baltimore mayor Howard Jackson on behalf of five White churches supporting racial segregation, The Howard Jackson Files—1924, Baltimore City Archives.

58. This was made exceedingly clear in Chicago. The Kenwood and Hyde Park Property Owners' Association formed to protect White homeowners' property values. They also published the *Property Owners' Journal*. On January 1, 1920, the journal published the following sentiment: "As stated before, every colored man who moves into Hyde Park knows that he is damaging his white neighbors' property. Therefore, he is making war on the white man. Consequently, he is not entitled to any consideration and forfeits his right to be employed by the white man. If employers should adopt a rule of refusing to employ Negroes who persist in residing in Hyde Park to the damage of the white man's property, it would soon show good results. The Negro is using the Constitution and its legal rights to abuse the moral rights of the white." See Chicago Commission on Race Relations, *The Negro in Chicago: A Study of Race Relations and a Race Riot* (Chicago, University of Chicago Press, 1922), 121.

59. Letter by Baltimore mayor Howard Jackson to Philip Pitt, The Howard Jackson Files—1924.

60. In January 1924, representatives from multiple neighborhood associations would beseech the mayor to allow them to serve on the committee, including the Madison Avenue Protective and Improvement Association and the Wyman Park Improvement Association, and so forth. There is some question as to whether the *Baltimore Sun* was jumping the gun when announcing "Committee to Plan Segregation Named." The beat writer wrote: "A committee to work out a plan for segregation, suggested by the Real Estate Board as a result a recent conference at the City Hall, was announced by Mayor Jackson." See staff writer, "Committee to Plan Segregation Named: Mayor Announces Those Selected to Represent Both Races," *Baltimore Sun*, January 17, 1924. In his paper on Meade v. Denniston, Garrett Power discussed the Committee on Segregation citing the Howard Jackson Files in the Baltimore City Archives. See Power, "Meade v. Denniston," 792. However, when I visited the Baltimore City Archives to verify the Committee on Segregation firsthand, I found letters from Jackson refuting the *Sun*'s report and arguing that he would not form such a committee. Hence, I concluded that, based on the available evidence, the *Sun* was attempting to apply media pressure to Mayor Jackson to form a segregation committee to work out a plan for voluntary segregation (where Black people would agree to not move into White neighborhoods). This approach somewhat mirrors Mayor James Preston's clandestine attempt to form a mixed race segregation committee that met in March 1918.

61. Staff writer, "Segregation of Negroes to Be Urged at Meeting: Lafayette Square Protective Association Will Discuss Invasion of Race," *Baltimore Sun*, April 22, 1924.

62. Staff writer, "Meeting Called to Fight against Negro Invasion: Greenmount Protection Association Also to Take Up Other Subjects," *Baltimore Sun*, October 13, 1924.

63. Staff writer, "Cedar Avenue 'Negro Invasion' Scare Ended by Investigation," *Baltimore Sun*, January 6, 1926.

64. Letter by Sister I. W. Scholastica, James Preston Files—1913, Baltimore City Archives. It can only be surmised that Sister Scholastica was an administrator or possibly the lead administrator of Mount Saint Agnes College at the time of her writing.

65. Letter by James Preston, James Preston Files—1913, Baltimore City Archives.

66. Staff writer, "Churchmen Will Attend Segregation Conference: Madison Avenue Representatives Will Discuss Invasion of Negroes," *Baltimore Sun*, January 21, 1924.

67. Carey A. Moore, letter to Baltimore mayor Howard Jackson on behalf of five White churches supporting racial segregation, Howard Jackson Files—1924, Baltimore City Archives. The five White churches who were represented in the letter to Mayor Jackson were (1) Babcock Memorial Presbyterian Church, (2) St. Bartholomew Protestant Episcopal Church, (3) Church of the Incarnation, Evangelical Lutheran, (4) St. John Methodist Episcopal Church South, and (5) Madison Avenue Methodist Episcopal Church.

68. Staff writer, "First Klan Church in State Dedicated in Harford County: Grand Dragon, Kleagles, Titans and Cyclopses Gather at Webster for Ceremony," *Baltimore Sun*, August 24, 1924. Emphasizing the Klan's Christian ideals, Grand Dragon Beall closed his address by dedicating the Klan church "to the battle of Christianity, the perpetuation of national honor and the chastity of American women."

69. Grant, *As Long as They Don't Move Next Door*, 36–37.

70. Staff writer, "Klan Takes Credit for New Quota Act: Imperial Wizard Tells Klanvocation East Is Stronghold of Un-Americanism," *Baltimore Sun*, September 25, 1924.

71. Andrew Holter, "Our Town: What the Rise of Nazism Looked Like in Baltimore during the 1930s," *Baltimore City Paper*, February 15, 2017, https://www.citypaper.com/news/features/bcpnews-our-town-what-the-rise-of-nazism-looked-like-in-baltimore-during-the-1930s-20170214-htmlstory.html. Decades later, Baltimore's Hampden community would retain its reputation of being unwelcoming to Black people due to perceptions of racial exclusivity. See Laura Marshallsay, 2010s. *Interpreting Druid Hill Park within the Hampden Community* (blog), 2010s, https://lmarshallsay.wordpress.com/historical-writing/interpreting-druid-hill-park-within-the-hampden-community/.

72. The Mount Royal Improvement Association (MRIA) writer, undated but would be late 1920s or early 1930s, *The MRIA*, 5.

73. William L. Marbury Sr. drafted the change to Maryland's constitution to disenfranchise Black voters in 1904, 1908, and 1910. All three attempts would fail. Ever the ardent white supremacist, Marbury had also helped to draft various versions of Baltimore's racial zoning ordinances in the 1910s. See Power, "Meade v. Dennistone," 787.

74. The Mount Royal Association pamphlet and letter are held in the library at the Maryland Historical Society.

75. Power, "Meade v. Dennistone," 793. Power argues: "White city-dwellers resisted the 'black invasion' district by district, neighborhood by neighborhood, block by block, and house by house. News accounts from the 1920s are filled with stories of angry confrontations, broken windows and other terror tactics deployed by besieged white homeowners."

76. Johns Hopkins Sheridan Libraries, Residential Security Map of Baltimore Md., 2016, https://jscholarship.library.jhu.edu/handle/1774.2/32621. The names and occupations of the people and organizations that helped create the map are (1) Mr. J. J. Requardt, Real Estate Broker; (2) Robert M. Morfort, Real Estate Broker; (3) Mr. Harry B. Wolfe, Real Estate Broker; (4) Mr. A. D. Clemens, Real Estate Broker; (5) Mr. Joseph M. Hisley, Real Estate Broker; (6)

Smith Real Estate Company, Real Estate Broker; (7) Mr. George P. Klein, Real Estate Broker; (8) Mr. Lemmon, Chief Evaluator—F.H.A.; (9) Mr. Ivan McDougal, Professor Economics and Sociology—Goucher College; (10) Piper and Hill, Real Estate Brokers; (11) Mr. H. W. Irr, Secretary, Pennsylvania Avenue F.S.L.A.; (12) Mr. F. W. Brochman, Cashier, West Baltimore Building Association; (13) Dr. Conrad, Home Owners' Loan Corporation—Towson; (14) Mr. Francis L. Smoot, State Appraiser, HOLC; (15) Mr. L. Krover, Assistant State Appraiser, HOLC; and (16) Mr. William Martein, Real Estate Operator, Baltimore.

77. See the bottom left corner of the 1937 Residential Security Map for Baltimore City. Map can be downloaded or viewed at the Johns Hopkins Sheridan Libraries, https://jscholarship.library.jhu.edu/handle/1774.2/32621. Earlier, the Baltimore City Health Department was implicated in helping create racial segregation. Now the Planning Department of Baltimore City is implicated.

78. Arnold Hirsch, "Public Policy and Residential Segregation in Baltimore, 1900–1968," Thompson v. HUD Court Files, Plaintiff's Exhibit No. 3, Case Number MJG 95-309, page 22, May 3, 2003, University of Baltimore, Langsdale Library, Special Collections.

79. Staff writer, "Housing Foes Tell Why They Oppose Homes: Crowd of 800 Boos Mayor for Favoring Colored War Homes," *Baltimore Afro-American*, July 17, 1943.

80. The White clergy included Rev. John J. Donlan (pastor of St. Dominic Catholic Church), Rev. Allen Gillis (pastor of Parkside Methodist Church), Rev. T. Vincent Fitzgerald (pastor of St. Anthony of Padua Catholic Church), and Rabbi Henry Eispruch (leader of Salem Lutheran Hebrew Center).

81. Staff writer, "Crowd of 800 Boos Mayor for Favoring Colored War Homes: Housing Foes Tell Why They Oppose Homes."

82. Staff writer, "Group to Protest Housing Proposal: To Go to Washington to Fight Plan for Negro Unit in Mount Winans," *Baltimore Sun*, 1943.

83. Hirsch, May 3, 2003, Plaintiff's Exhibit No. 3, Case Number MJG 95-309. According to Hirsch, the federal government wanted to put the public housing in Armistead Gardens "still, the mayor and HABC refused their assent, leading the FPHA [Federal Public Housing Authority] to assert its willingness to act under its own authority. . . ." However, the threat of mob violence caused the FPHA to place the public housing development on Eastern Avenue instead of Herring Run Park. Hirsch's paper quotes a federal report that apparently incorrectly switches the sites, but the essence of the threat of mob violence is what is most germane.

84. Staff writer, "Negro Housing Dispute Ends: FPHA Approves 4 Sites Recommended By HAB For Development," *Baltimore Sun*, October 26, 1943.

85. Karl Taeuber, "Public Housing and Racial Segregation in Baltimore," May 3, 2003, report generated for the Thompson v. HUD court case. The case was litigated by the Maryland ACLU. Plaintiff's Exhibit No. 2, Case Number MJG 95-309, University of Baltimore, Langsdale Library, Special Collections. The discriminatory siting of public housing was not unique to Baltimore. As historian Raymond Mohl stated with respect to public housing nationwide: "Located exclusively in black areas, these and other large public housing projects absorbed low-income black families whose housing had been demolished through urban renewal, highway construction, and code

enforcement. Essentially, these housing projects solidified black ghettoization in the postwar." Mohl, "Race and Housing in the Postwar City: An
Explosive History," *Journal of the Illinois State Historical Society* 94, no. 1
(2001): 8–30, 13.

86. This pattern is fairly apparent when one examines the racial dot map
created by Dustin Cable, formerly at the University of Virginia. I coined the
term *Black Butterfly* in 2015 after drawing the boundary of Baltimore on
Cable's map. The racial dot map is located at https://demographics.virginia
.edu/DotMap/.

87. Taeuber, May 3, 2003, Plaintiff's Exhibit No. 2, Case Number MJG 95-309.

88. Weldon Wallace, "How Mt. Washington Preserved Itself," *Baltimore Sun*,
May 21, 1973.

89. "Baltimore Neighborhoods Inc. Settles Steering Suit for $250,000," National
Fair Housing Advocate, 1992, https://fairhousing.com/news-archive
/advocate/1992/baltimore-neighborhoods-inc-settles-steering-suit-250-000.

90. See appendix D for table of repeated forced uprootings of Black people
throughout Baltimore City history.

91. Renée Gordon, "Maryland Trails: Look Back in Wonder (Part 1)," *Philadelphia
Sun*, January 18, 2013, http://www.philasun.com/travel/maryland-trails-look
-back-in-wonder-part-one/.

92. Frederick Douglass, "What to the Slave Is the Fourth of July?" (speech,
Corinthian Hall, NY, July 5, 1852).

93. As Ralph Clayton wrote: "For 45 years, thousands of families and individuals
were sent south on their final passage. For most on board, this meant a death
that came when families and loved ones were separated and 'sold South'—a
separation from which few returned. It also signified almost certain separation from one another in New Orleans; large families were rarely sold to the
same buyer." Ralph Clayton, "A Bitter Inner Harbor Legacy: The Slave
Trade," *Baltimore Sun*, July 12, 2000.

94. "The slave jails served several purposes. Slave owners leaving for a trip
could check their slaves into a jail to ensure they would not flee. Travelers
stopping in Baltimore could lock up their slaves overnight while they slept at a
nearby inn. Unwanted slaves or those considered unreliable because of
runaway attempts could be sold and housed at the jail until a ship was ready
to take them south, usually to New Orleans." Scott Shane, "The Secret
History of City Slave Trade: Blacks and Whites Alike of Modern-Day Baltimore
Have Ignored the Story of the Jails That Played a Key Role in the U.S. Slave
Trade of the 1800s," *Baltimore Sun*, July 20, 1999, https://www.baltimoresun
.com/news/bs-xpm-1999-06-20-9906220293-story.html.

95. According to Ralph Clayton: "Profits from the slave trade allowed dealers like
Woolfolk to make investments in properties throughout Baltimore and in
several Southern states. Traders like James Franklin Purvis channeled money
from 'cash for blood' into banking and brokerage businesses in the city. A
portion of that money was certainly used for loans provided for local businesses and manufacturers. In short, the blood stained money found its way
into many areas of the local economy." Ralph Clayton, *Cash for Blood: The
Baltimore to New Orleans Domestic Slave Trade* (Westminster, MD: Heritage
Books, 2007), 69. In addition, just as the *Baltimore Sun* would later assist
pro-segregationists in pushing for Baltimore Apartheid in the 1910s-1920s,

the newspaper also participated in the advertisement of slave trading between 1850 and 1860 (662).

96. Garrett Power, "Deconstructing the Slums of Baltimore," in *From Mobtown to Charm City—New Perspectives on Baltimore's Past*, ed. Jessica Elfenbein, John Breihan, and Thomas Hollowak (Baltimore: Maryland Historical Society, 2002). See also Hirsch, May 3, 2003, Plaintiff's Exhibit No. 3, Case Number MJG 95-309. For more in-depth information regarding Hopkins-related displacement in East Baltimore, read Marisela Gomez, *Race, Class, Power, and Organizing in East Baltimore: Rebuilding Abandoned Communities in America* (Lanham, MD: Lexington Books, 2013).

97. Spence Lean, "Preston Gardens: Planted on the Seeds of Racism," Baltimore City's Past, Present, and Future, http://baltimorefuture.blogspot.com /2010/12/preston-gardensplanted-on-seeds-of.html.

98. The park sits across the street from Mercy Hospital in downtown Baltimore on St. Paul Street.

99. "Need for Better Housing for Negroes Revealed in Tuberculosis Statistics," *Baltimore Municipal Journal*, August 10, 1917, bottom of first column and top of the second column.

100. "What Can Be Done to Improve the Living Conditions of Baltimore's Negro Population," third column, first full paragraph (see n. 47).

101. Donald Trump (@realDonalTrump), "Rep. Elijah Cummings has been a brutal bully," Twitter, July 27, 2019, 7:14 a.m., https://twitter.com/realDonaldTrump /status/1155073964634517505.

102. Corey Henderson, "The Reverberating Influence of Historical Trauma on the Health of African Americans in Baltimore City" (PhD diss., Morgan State University, 2017), 34.

103. Russ P. Lopez, "Public Health, the APHA, and Urban Renewal," *American Journal of Public Health* 99, no. 9 (2009): 1603-1611, 1606. Noting the role of public health departments in enforcing and implementing urban renewal, Lopez offers the following details: "In 1948, the APHA-CHH developed guidelines for inspecting housing and neighborhoods. With the passage of the 1954 Housing Act and its statutory mandate that blight be documented, these guidelines began to be used as legal justification for urban renewal areas. . . . Significantly, the standards did not condemn racial segregation in housing, only acknowledging that some evidence suggested that segregation was bad for health and that there was a need for additional study before the APHA could develop a position on the issue. . . . The public health community and the APHA were particularly involved in the necessary early step of declaring neighborhoods blighted. Blight was an ambiguous term and government officials could manipulate its meaning at will. By establishing its guidelines, the APHA supplied a scientific and seemingly impartial justification for declaring a neighborhood blighted." To be sure, many alley homes often were little more than wooden shacks without plumbing or indoor toilets. Many homes or tenements were not fit for human habitation. Those dwellings did need to be demolished. The core issue then is that during slum clearance and urban renewal, Black residents were rarely consulted in terms of how their housing could be improved and rarely allowed to stay to enjoy the newly built housing and renewed neighborhood. When housing was made available for displaced residents, their relocation needs

were often given little attention. Very little thought was given to the impact on the affected communities aside from perhaps public housing construction. But even then, not enough public housing units were built to meet the demand for housing for existing and incoming Black residents in the city.

104. Hirsch, May 3, 2003, Plaintiff's Exhibit No. 3. Case Number MJG 95-309.

105. Community Renewal Program, *Displacement and Relocation, Past and Future—Baltimore, Maryland*, March 1965, Baltimore Urban Renewal and Housing Agency, staff monograph, table 1, University of Baltimore, Langsdale Library, Special Collections. For HOPE VI displacement, see also Robin Smith, *Housing Choice for HOPE VI Relocatees* (Washington, DC: Urban Institute, April 2002).

106. Smith, *Housing Choice for HOPE VI Relocatees*, 25–36, especially the maps in the report. Since 1990, the Housing Authority of Baltimore City has demolished multiple public housing communities—Flag House, Hollander Ridge, Lexington Terrace, Murphy Homes, Lafayette Courts, Somerset Homes, Broadway, Julian, and more. Although HABC would argue that the people displaced were given Housing Choice Vouchers (formerly known as Section 8 vouchers), most residents ended up in other lower-income or redlined Black neighborhoods after HOPE VI demolition. This shows how displacement often simply results in shuffling people with lower incomes and concentrating people with lower incomes in redlined Black communities.

107. EBMC, "When Enough Is NOT Enough—beyond $100 Million," 2001, Empower Baltimore Management Corporation, PowerPoint, box 18A, folder 46, University of Baltimore, Langsdale Library, Special Collections.

108. The six Empowerment Zone areas were (1) Sandtown-Winchester, (2) Harlem Park/Lafayette Square, (3) Poppleton, (4) Pigtown/Morrill Park, (5) Middle East/Madison Park, and (6) Fells Point/Jonestown/Inner Harbor East.

109. Lawrence Brown, "Down to the Wire: Displacement and Disinvestment in Baltimore City," in *The 2015 State of Black Baltimore: Still Separate, Still Unequal* (Baltimore: Greater Baltimore Urban League, 2015).

110. Gady A. Epstein and Eric Seigel, "City, Hopkins Weigh Plan for East-Side Development," *Baltimore Sun*, January 11, 2001.

111. Baltimore Department of Housing and Community Development, *Residential Displacement: 1951–1971 Activity Analysis* (Baltimore: Department of Housing and Community Development), May 1972, Thompson v. HUD Court Files. The case was litigated by the Maryland ACLU, Plaintiff's Exhibit No. 173, Case Number MJG 95-309, page 4, table 2, University of Baltimore, Langsdale Library, Special Collections.

112. In total, Johns Hopkins Medical Institutions would displace over 2,000 Black families for its benefit, including campus expansion, student and faculty housing, and a bioscience park for Johns Hopkins Hospital. As Marisela Gomez summarized: "The Broadway Redevelopment in the 1950s and the current 2001 project are similar in their massive displacement of a historic African American community. In both redevelopment projects, approximately 800 households and businesses were displaced. They were both projects aimed at renewing the place, not the people." Gomez, *Race, Class, Power, and Organizing*, 57. See also Nancy Adess et al., *Disrupting Poverty: Coming Together to Build Financial Security for Individuals and Communities* (Seattle: The Paul G. Allen Family Foundation, March 2014), 21.

113. Department of Planning, "Residential Development Opportunities in Baltimore City" (City of Baltimore, June 2004), 5.

114. Hirsch, May 3, 2003, Plaintiff's Exhibit No. 3, Case Number MJG 95-309.

115. Hirsch, May 3, 2003, Plaintiff's Exhibit No. 3, Case Number MJG 95-309, page 69.

116. Community Renewal Program, March 1965, *Displacement and Relocation, Past and Future—Baltimore, Maryland*, table 1 (see n. 104).

117. Community Renewal Program, March 1965, *Displacement and Relocation, Past and Future—Baltimore, Maryland*, table 1.

118. Hirsch, May 3, 2003, Plaintiff's Exhibit No. 3, Case Number MJG 95-309, page 69.

119. Taeuber, May 3, 2003, Plaintiff's Exhibit No. 2, Case Number MJG 95-309, tables 4–5 on pages 103–104.

120. US District Court of Maryland lawsuit, Movement Against Destruction v. Volpe, 361 F. Supp. 1360 (D. Md. 1973). There were actually more displacements caused by highway construction in Baltimore, but the numbers were not broken out by race the way they were with urban renewal data. According to the Baltimore Department of Housing and Community Development (DHCD), there were 1,832 households displaced by highways between 1951 and 1971. So it is highly likely that 965 is an underestimate. See DHCD, "Residential Displacement, Activity Analysis, 1951–1971," DHCD, 1972, Thompson v. HUD Court Files. The case was litigated by the Maryland ACLU. Plaintiff's Exhibit No. 173, Case Number MJG 95-309. Data found in table V on page 8. University of Baltimore, Langsdale Library, Special Collections.

121. Nancy Adess et al., *Disrupting Poverty*, 21.

122. This total excludes the 100 Black families displaced by Baltimore and Ohio Railroad yard expansion, the unknown number of Black people displaced by Preston Gardens Park, and the 7,048 families displaced by equivalent private demolitions that were required by the federal government but facilitated by the private sector. For B&O Railroad yard expansion displacement, see David Terry and Eli Pousson, "Upton and Old West Baltimore," Baltimore Heritage Open Tours, November 2, 2012. Early History of South Baltimore section, https://baltimoreheritage.github.io/tours/2012/11/02/upton-old-west-baltimore/. See page 85 of National Commission on Urban Problems's *Building the American City* for a more complete explanation of equivalent private demolitions. The race of families displaced by equivalent private demolitions is not identified in the data. Therefore, the calculations here greatly underestimate the numbers of Black people displaced throughout the city's history.

123. See appendix D for a table of repeated forced uprootings of Black people throughout Baltimore City history.

124. Lean, "Preston Gardens" (see n. 97).

125. Jim Holechek, *Baltimore's Two Cross Keys Villages: One Black. One White* (New York: iUniverse, 2003), 85.

126. Gomez, *Race, Class, Power, and Organizing*, 57.

127. Alison Knezevich, "Residents of Towson Neighborhood Confront Racist Legacy of Covenants," *Baltimore Sun*, September 10, 2017, http://www.baltimoresun.com/news/maryland/baltimore-county/bs-md-co-rodgers

-forge-covenants-20170907-story.html. The racial restrictions are no longer enforceable due to the Supreme Court's 1948 decision Shelly v. Kraemer.

128. As Baltimore County states in its 2011 *Analysis of Impediments* report: "The population influx caused some developments in the County to regulate growth [and to adopt] racially restrictive covenants, development restrictions or zoning practices through which the racial composition of neighborhoods could be controlled. The number of both White residents and Black residents grew, though housing opportunities continued to be extremely restricted for Blacks. . . . Federal funding became available in the late 1930s for local housing authorities to house lower-income populations, though the initiative to develop public housing programs was left to local governments. . . . The County has maintained a deliberate decision not to build public housing in order to preserve its economic homogeneity."

129. Maryland State Advisory Committee, *The Zoning and Planning Process in Baltimore County and Its Effect on Minority Group Residents* (Maryland State Advisory Committee to the United States Commission on Civil Rights, March 1971). According to the committee: "A 1970 hearing of the U.S. Commission on Human Rights examined the use of 'discontinuous street patterns' in Baltimore County, concluding that the layout of roads had the effect of isolating Blacks from their surroundings, particularly from adjacent White residential areas. The County has also been accused of expulsive zoning practices from the 1950s to the 1980s. This refers to the rezoning of residential Black neighborhoods such as Turner Station as commercial areas, while nearby White neighborhoods are left untouched. Expulsive zoning also refers to the rezoning of areas surrounding Black neighborhoods to lower densities to create a buffer that effectively prevents expansion. As a result of zoning changes, Turner Station's population dropped from over 9,000 to 3,557 during the 1950s. Overall, arguably due to such policies and practices, the County's Black population fell from 18,026 to 17,535 between 1950 and 1960, despite the County's overall population increase during those years from 270,273 to 492,418 (82%)."

130. ACLU, "Baltimore County Signs Agreement with HUD to End Housing Discrimination," Maryland ACLU, March 15, 2016, https://www.aclu.org /news/baltimore-county-signs-agreement-hud-end-decades-housing -discrimination.

131. Ron Cassie, "A Tale of Two Cities," *Baltimore Magazine*, 2015, https://www .baltimoremagazine.com/2016/4/11/a-tale-of-two-cities-west-baltimore -before-after-freddie-gray.

132. Pamela Wood, "Baltimore County Council Rejects Housing Anti-discrimination Bill," *Baltimore Sun*, August 1, 2016, http://www .baltimoresun.com/news/maryland/baltimore-county/bs-md-co-housing -policy-vote-20160801-story.html.

133. John Lee, "Redmer Says He Will Defy Affordable Housing Agreement If Elected," WYPR, September 26, 2016, http://www.wypr.org/post/redmer -says-he-will-defy-affordable-housing-agreement-if-elected.

134. "John Olszewski Jr. Wins Baltimore County Executive, Redmer Concedes," *CBS Baltimore*, WJZ-13, November 6, 2018, https://baltimore.cbslocal.com /2018/11/06/john-olszewski-jr-wins-baltimore-county-executive/.

135. Bryna Zumer, "Opponents Criticize Plan for 'Forced Section 8' in Baltimore County," *Fox 45 News*, October 28, 2019, https://foxbaltimore.com/news /local/opponents-criticize-plan-for-forced-section-8-in-baltimore-county. See also John Lee, "Housing Voucher Bill Passes Baltimore County Council," WYPR 88.1 FM, November 4, 2019, https://www.wypr.org/post/housing -voucher-bill-passes-baltimore-county-council?fbclid=IwAR2tvUFdu _IvCTWaMkYFVFEOiqa9Wdb7lc6GIVV_hM_RguFkgLFUUKPsYxw.

136. Wilborn P. Nobles III, "Baltimore County Executive, Activist Energy Proved Decisive in Push for 'Overdue' Housing Discrimination Law," *Baltimore Sun*, November 6, 2019, https://www.baltimoresun.com/maryland /baltimore-county/bs-md-co-voucher-bill-vote-20191106 -myl64y7sgnahdlo22qipaxaooe-story.html.

137. Wilborn P. Nobles III, "County Killings Up 52% for Year," *Baltimore Sun*, November 4, 2019, https://www.baltimoresun.com/maryland/baltimore -county/bs-md-co-baltimore-county-crime-20191104 -26v4yuu4bzaaxiufhy4f25lcsq-story.html.

138. Staff correspondent, "Segregation Law in Baltimore Operates" (see n. 15).

139. Alvin Chang, "White America Is Quietly Self-Segregating," Vox, January 18, 2017, https://www.vox.com/2017/1/18/14296126/white-segregated-suburb -neighborhood-cartoon. Chang finds "data shows that as minorities move into suburbs, white families are making small and personal decisions that add velocity to the momentum of discrimination. They are increasingly choosing to self-segregate into racially isolated communities—'hunkering down,' as Lichter likes to call it—and preserving a specific kind of dream."

140. Brian Resnick, "White Fear of Demographic Change Is a Powerful Psychological Force," Vox, January 28, 2017, https://www.vox.com/science-and-health /2017/1/26/14340542/white-fear-trump-psychology-minority-majority.

Track 4. Ongoing Historical Trauma

1. Colby Itkowitz, "Trump Attacks Rep. Cummings's District, Calling It a 'Disgusting, Rat and Rodent Infested Mess,'" *Washington Post*, July 27, 2019, https://www.washingtonpost.com/politics/trump-attacks-rep -cummingss-district-calling-it-a-disgusting-rat-and-rodent-infested-mess /2019/07/27/b93c89b2-b073-11e9-bc5c-e73b603e7f38_story.html.

2. An analysis by *USA Today* reporter John Fritze found that during 64 rallies, President Trump used the language of demonization against immigrants and asylum-seekers over 500 times, including "alien"—213 times, "criminal"—189 times, "The hell out of our country"—43 times, "animal"—34 times, "killer"—32 times, "predator"—31 times, "invasion"—13 times, and "invade"—6 times. Fritze, "Trump Used Words Like 'Invasion' and 'Killer' to Discuss Immigrants at Rallies 500 Times," *USA Today*, August 8, 2019, https://www.usatoday.com/story/news/politics/elections/2019/08/08 /trump-immigrants-rhetoric-criticized-el-paso-dayton-shootings /1936742001/. As discussed in Track 3, in the first quarter of the 1900s, the language of "Negro Invasion" was deployed to repel Southern Black migrants arriving in more northern cities who were fleeing racial violence in the Deep South. In the late 2010s, the stigmatizing language of "alien," "animal," "invasion," and "predator" has been used by the Trump administration to repel Central American immigrants fleeing violence and condi-

tions caused by climate change in their countries. In both cases, the two groups of migrating people fleeing violence were dehumanized by stigmatized language and then demonized by laws.

3. According to historian Paige Glotzer, the language used by Trump—rat and rodent infestation, in particular—echoes the same language used by Baltimore's Roland Park Company to create and enforce community-wide racially restrictive covenants in the 1910s to bar Black people from owning homes in the exclusive suburban area. Paige writes: "At the turn of the 20th century, suburban development companies bought large tracts of land on the periphery of the growing city. Among the most influential was the Roland Park Company, which created some of Baltimore's first restricted communities governed by a new tool: the restrictive covenant. These documents were legal contracts that had historically been applied to single lots. The Roland Park Company had a different idea: make them community-wide. To do that, they looked to existing 'nuisance laws' that cities used to regulate property in order to prevent health hazards such as rat infestations." Glotzer, "What 'Infests' Baltimore? The Segregation History Buried in Trump's Tweets," CityLab, August 2019, https://www.citylab.com/perspective/2019/07/trump-tweets-elijah-cummings-baltimore-history-racism/594967/.

4. These include government-enforced racial segregation and uprootings, white supremacist violence, economic destruction, land confiscation, and cultural dispossession.

5. Brave Heart's conceptual framework of historical trauma can be applied to any vulnerable population that has been impacted by cataclysmic social, political, and economic disruption caused by a more powerful group of people. Brave Heart proposed her construct to explain health outcomes for Native peoples in America. Interested readers should study scholars such as Tennille Marley who explicate how historical trauma affects Native peoples' health. I have used Brave Heart's concept and Michelle Sotero's conceptual framework to explain how historical trauma applies to the descendants of Africans enslaved in the United States. See also Michelle Sotero, "The Conceptual Model of Historical Trauma: Implications for Public Health Practice and Research," *Journal of Health Disparities Research and Practice* 1, no. 1 (2006): 93–108.

6. While I focus on spatial pathways for the proliferation of historical trauma, the primary biological pathway for the intergenerational transmission of historical trauma among descendants of enslaved Africans in the United States is detailed in the academic field of epigenetics. Epigenetics can be defined as "the study of changes in organisms caused by modification of gene expression rather than alteration of the genetic code itself" (*Oxford Dictionary*). A more robust discussion of epigenetics and its impact on the bodily health of African Americans is beyond the scope of this text, however epigenetics and its health implications can be found in the following three journal articles. Darrell J. Gaskins, Alvin E. Headen, and Shelley I. White-Means, "Racial Disparities in Health and Wealth: The Effects of Slavery and Discrimination," *Review of Black Political Economy* 32, nos. 3–4 (2005): 95–110; Fatima Jackson, Latifa Jackson, and Zainab ElRadi Jackson, "Developmental Stage Epigenetic Modifications and Clinical Symptoms Associated with the Trauma and Stress of Enslavement and Institutionalized Racism," *Journal of Clinical Epigenetics* 4, no. 2 (2008): 11; Bridget J. Goosby and Chelsea Heidbrink,

"Transgenerational Consequences of Racial Discrimination for African American Health," *Social Compass* 7, no. 8 (2013): 630–643.

7. As Audrey McFarlane argues: "Racial geography shapes lives and life's opportunities; we rely on the resulting segregated racial geography to make our decisions about where to live. Racially identified places lead to distinctly different economic conditions in terms of prices, quality of schools, shopping, and other services. These differences also play a role in wealth allocations—markets for real estate are racialized and discounted or overvalued accordingly. Middle class neighborhoods will receive a racial premium or discount based on race. Schools and services will be better in and near white neighborhoods and worse in or near black neighborhoods." Audrey McFarlane, "Operatively White? Exploring the Significance of Race and Class through the Paradox of Black Middle-Classness," *Law and Contemporary Problems* 72 (2009): 176.

8. Melinda Henneberger, "A Yonkers Street: Whites, Blacks and Silence," *New York Times*, October 15, 1992, https://www.nytimes.com/1992/10/15 /nyregion/a-yonkers-street-whites-blacks-and-silence.html.

9. Ira Katznelson, *When Affirmative Action Was White: An Untold History of Racial Inequality in Twentieth-Century America* (New York: Norton, 2005).

10. Sonya Douglass Horsford, *Learning in a Burning House: Educational Inequality, Ideology, and (Dis)integration* (New York: Teachers College Press, 2011), 1.

11. Horsford, *Learning in a Burning House*, 3–6.

12. My "discovery" of the Black Butterfly was serendipitous. One day I was examining the racial dot map made by Dustin Cable, formerly with the University of Virginia. I noticed that the boundary of Baltimore needed to be prominently displayed on the map so people could immediately see how racially segregated it is today. As soon as I drew the boundary, I could see the White L pattern. Immediately afterward, I noticed something else—the pattern of a butterfly. This was in 2015, maybe a few months after Kendrick Lamar had released his masterful hip-hop album *To Pimp a Butterfly*. The title was analogous to what takes place with the city's treatment of the Black Butterfly.

13. Noliwe Rooks, *Cutting School: Privatization, Segregation, and the End of Public Segregation* (New York: New Press, 2017," 2.

14. Nick Penzenstadler and Jeff Kelly Lowenstein, "Seniors Were Sold a Risk-Free Retirement with Reverse Mortgages. Now They Face Foreclosure," *USA Today*, September 24, 2019, https://www.usatoday.com/in-depth/news/investigations /2019/06/11/seniors-face-foreclosure-retirement-after-failed-reverse -mortgage/1329043001/.

15. The complicity of White institutions and society was expressed poignantly by the National Advisory Commission on Civil Disorders (popularly known as the Kerner Commission) in their 1968 report: "Violence and destruction must be ended—in the streets of the ghetto and in the lives of people. Segregation and poverty have created in the racial ghetto a destructive environment totally unknown to most white Americans. What white Americans have never fully understood but what the Negro can never forget—is that white society is deeply implicated in the ghetto. White institutions created it, white institutions maintain it, and white society condones it." As Richard Rothstein also

argues in his book *The Color of Law*, current racial segregation is not *de facto*, it is *de jure*—or still a matter of law.

16. Karl Taeuber, "Public Housing and Racial Segregation in Baltimore, 1900–1968," Thompson v. HUD Court Files. The case was litigated by the Maryland ACLU. Plaintiff's Exhibit No. 2, Case Number MJG 95-309, May 3, 2003, University of Baltimore, Langsdale Library, Special Collections.

17. The concentration of residents with Housing Choice Vouchers in the Black Butterfly is clear when viewing maps by the Baltimore Neighborhood Indicator Alliance or when viewing the map by the Center for Budget and Policy Priorities (CBPP) and Poverty and Race Research Action Council (PPRAC)(https://www.cbpp.org/research/housing/interactive-map-where-voucher-households-live-in-the-50-largest-metropolitan-areas).

18. Alicia Mazzara and Brian Knudsen, "Where Families with Children Use Housing Vouchers: A Comparative Look at the 50 Largest Metropolitan Areas," CBPP and PPRAC, January 2, 2019, https://www.cbpp.org/research/housing/where-families-with-children-use-housing-vouchers.

19. Louis Misrendino, "Baltimore's Property Tax Privileged v. Punished," *Baltimore Sun*, July 4, 2016, http://www.baltimoresun.com/news/opinion/oped/bs-ed-property-tax-20160704-story.html. See also Louis Misrendino, "A Failed Redevelopment and Tax Policy," *Maryland Public Policy Institute*, May 22, 2015, https://www.mdpolicy.org/research/detail/a-failed-redevelopment-and-tax-policy. Lawrence Brown, "Protect Whose House? How Baltimore's Leaders Failed to Further Affordable and Fair Housing in Port Covington," *University of Baltimore Journal of Land and Development 6*, no. 2 (2018): 161–169.

20. Bradford Van Arnum, *Recreation Center Closings in Baltimore: Reconsidering Spending Priorities, Juvenile Crime, and Equity* (Baltimore: Citizens Planning and Housing Association, February 2014), 2. For school closures, see Talia Richman, "Baltimore School Board Votes to Close Five Schools," *Baltimore Sun*, January 8, 2019. This article says a total of 75 schools were closed since 2004. When adding the nine closed in 2001, this brings the total since 2000 to 84. Liz Bowie and Erika Niedowski, "City Board Acts to Close Nine Schools," *Baltimore Sun*, March 14, 2001.

21. Talia Richman, "As Baltimore Prepares to Close More Schools, Many Worry about the Communities They Anchor," *Baltimore Sun*, December 28, 2018, https://www.baltimoresun.com/maryland/baltimore-city/bs-md-ci-school-closures-20181130-story.html.

22. Sarah Yatsko, "Baltimore and the Portfolio School District Strategy," Center on Reinventing Public Education, June 2012.

23. State of Maryland and City of Baltimore, "Memorandum of Understanding for the Construction and Revitalization of Baltimore City Public Schools," Baltimore 21st Century Schools, September 16, 2013, https://baltimore21stcenturyschools.org/about/memorandum-understanding.

24. In their report *Death by a Thousand Cuts*, Journey for Justice Alliance explains the devastation that permanent closures of public schools cause already redlined Black neighborhoods: "Closing a school is one of the most traumatic things that can happen to a community; it strikes at the very core of community culture, history, and identity, and . . . produces far-reaching repercussions that negatively affect every aspect of community life. It has been

nothing short of devastating to the health and development of many of our children and youth, has put a strain on our families, has contributed to the destabilization and deterioration of our communities, has undermined many good schools and effective school improvement efforts, has destroyed relationships with quality educators, and has contributed to increased community violence." Journey for Justice Alliance, *Death by a Thousand Cuts: Racism, School Closures, and Public School Sabotage* (n.p.: Journey for Justice Alliance, May 2014).

25. Noli Brazil, "The Effects of Public Elementary School Closures on Neighborhood Housing Values in U.S. Metropolitan Areas, 2000–2010," in *Shuttered Schools: Race, Community, and School Closures in American Cities*, ed. Ebony M. Duncan-Shippy, chap. 8, 251–252 (Charlotte, NC: Information Age, 2019).

26. Richman, "Baltimore Prepares to Close More Schools."

27. Eve L. Ewing, *Ghosts in the Schoolyard: Racism and School Closings on Chicago's South Side* (Chicago: University of Chicago Press, 2018), 14, 129–130, 151–155. Consider the names of some of the schools closed by the Baltimore City Public School System since 2000: Thurgood Marshall Middle School, Dr. Lillie M. Jackson Elementary, Harriet Tubman Elementary, Thurgood Marshall High School, Paul Laurence Dunbar Middle School, Langston Hughes Elementary School, W. E. B. Du Bois High School, Malcolm X Elementary, and Martin Luther King Jr. Elementary/Middle.

28. David Armenti, "A Thorny Path: School Desegregation in Baltimore," Underbelly: The Maryland Historical Society Library, May 15, 2014, http://www.mdhs.org/underbelly/2014/05/15/a-thorny-path-school-desegregation-in-baltimore/.

29. Bettye Thomas, "Public Education and Black Protest in Baltimore 1865–1900," *Maryland Historical Society Magazine* 71, no. 3 (1976): 381–391. Thomas explains: "From 1865 through 1900 the education of black children remained the focal point of black protest in Baltimore. The establishment of public schools for blacks was viewed as a positive achievement; however, the removal of black teachers was a serious setback for the black community. Black teachers formerly employed by the Moral Improvement Association were simply dismissed. Since the school board pursued such action expecting criticism from blacks, it moved to insure the support of white teachers by stipulating that white teachers in black schools would receive salary equal to that of white teachers in white schools."

30. Lauren Camera, "Black Teachers Improve Outcomes for Black Students," *US News*, November 23, 2018, https://www.usnews.com/news/education-news/articles/2018-11-23/black-teachers-improve-outcomes-for-black-students. However, Black teachers are often burned out due to unsupportive school administrations and the extra work they do in terms of mentoring and role modeling. "The State of Teacher Diversity in American Education," The Albert Shanker Institute, September 2015, https://www.shankerinstitute.org/resource/teacherdiversity.

31. Philip Goff, Matthew C. Jackson, Brook A. Di Leone, Carmen M. Culotta, and Natalie A. DiTomasso, "The Essence of Innocence: Consequences of Dehumanizing Black Children," *Journal of Personality and Social Psychology* 106, no. 4 (2014): 526–545.

32. These data are found in Kristina Rizga's excellent article "Black Teachers Matter" in *Mother Jones* magazine. See also "The State of Teacher Diversity in American Education," 95. This is connected to the weakening of African-centered K–12 schools by charter schools as Rachel Cohen discusses in her illuminating article "The Afrocentric Education Crisis" in *American Prospect*.

33. While HABC disputes Jacobson's characterization by arguing that they provided residents with Housing Choice Vouchers (HCVs), HABC's rebuttal only confirms the point that the overwhelming majority of their residents with HCVs from public housing communities torn down by HOPE VI were displaced and dispersed throughout the city and disproportionately concentrated in Black Butterfly neighborhoods. See also Robin E. Smith, *Housing Choice for HOPE VI Relocatees* (Washington, DC: Urban Institute, 2002), particularly the maps on pages 33–36 of the report, https://www.urban.org/sites/default/files/publication/60636/410592-Housing-Choice-for-HOPE-VI-Relocatees.PDF.

34. Doug Donovan and Jean Marbella, "Dismissed: Tenants Lose, Landlords Win in Baltimore's Rent Court," *Baltimore Sun*, August 26, 2017, http://data.baltimoresun.com/news/dismissed/.

35. Melody Simmons, "Maryland Leads the U.S. in Foreclosure Filings for the Second Consecutive Month," *Baltimore Business Journal*, December 9, 2015, https://www.bizjournals.com/baltimore/blog/real-estate/2015/12/baltimores-rate-is-among-the-highest-in-the-us.html.

36. Melody Simmons, "Maryland Leads the U.S. in Foreclosure Filings." See also Donovan and Marbella, "Dismissed"; "Baltimore City Foreclosure Filings," Baltimore Neighborhood Indicator Alliance, http://www.ubalt.edu/foreclosures/index.cfm.

37. Corporation for Enterprise Development (CFED), *Racial Wealth Divide in Baltimore* (CFED, 2015); CFED is now known as Prosperity Now.

38. Melody Simmons and Joan Jacobson, "Too Big to Fail? Betting a Billion on East Baltimore," *The Daily Record*, February 1, 2011, http://thedailyrecord.com/too-big-to-fail-betting-a-billion-on-east-baltimore/.

39. Meredith Cohn, "Redevelopment of West Baltimore's Poppleton Taking Shape," *Baltimore Sun*, October 16, 2018.

40. Robbie Whelan, "BioPark Drawing Home Buyers West," *The Daily Record*, April 1, 2008, http://www.umbiopark.com/news-events/news/1034/biopark-drawing-home-buyers-west. Whelan goes on to write: "Last year, four houses in a row on the 1000 block of West Fayette Street, less than two blocks from the BioPark, sold for an average of $371,000 apiece, helping to account for a 588 percent rise in the median home sale price in the neighborhood. In 2004, the median price of a home sold in Poppleton was $59,500. Audrey Robinson, president of the Poppleton Co-Op, which is subsidized by the U.S. Department of Housing and Urban Development, said local residents are already reaping the benefits of University of Maryland's investment in the neighborhood. 'We're feeling so far so good, as long as we don't become displaced,' she said." See also Lawrence Brown, "Down to the Wire: Displacement and Disinvestment in Baltimore City," in *The 2015 State of Black Baltimore: Still Separate, Still Unequal* (Baltimore: Greater Baltimore Urban League, 2015).

41. Baltimore City's Black population in 1990 was 435,768 according to the Maryland State Data Center, http://planning.maryland.gov/MSDC/Pages/census/censusHistorical.aspx. Baltimore City's estimated Black population

in 2016 was 387,631, according to data from the US Census Bureau, *2012–2016 American Community Survey 5-Year Estimates*. This represents a population drop of 48,137.

42. Lindsay Beane, *Baltimore Blog: Populations Decline Part 1*, April 2017, http://lindsaybeane.com/2017/04/19/baltimore-blog-population-decline/. Dr. Beane arrives at her compelling thesis by showing the large population decrease in the Southern Park Heights community between 1990 and 2010. My work examining Empowerment Zones also shows a large decrease in population in the six areas just east and west of downtown in historically redlined Black communities. These are also areas that would have experienced high levels of homicide and early deaths rooted in Baltimore Apartheid.

43. Yvonne Wegner, "Housing Program Used to Break Up High-Poverty Areas in Baltimore to Stop Taking Applicants," *Baltimore Sun*, January 12, 2017, http://www.baltimoresun.com/news/maryland/baltimore-city/bs-md-ci -voucher-wait-list-20170112-story.html.

44. Johns Hopkins University Office of Worklife and Engagement, Live Near Your Work, Johns Hopkins University and Health Systems, July 1, 2018, http:// hopkinsworklife.org/housing_relocation/LNYW/index.html. See also Lawrence Brown, Ashley Bachelder, Marisela Gomez, Alicia Sherrell, and Imani Victoria Bryan, "The Rise of Anchor Institutions and the Threat to Community Health: Protecting Community Wealth, Building Community Power," *Kalfou* 3, no. 1 (2016): 79–100. See page 86 for a fuller explanation of the gentrification components of the Johns Hopkins University and Health Systems' Live Near Your Work program.

45. Melody Simmons, "Johns Hopkins Ups Ante on 'Live Near Your Work' with $36K Deal," *Baltimore Business Journal*, July 25, 2016, https://www .bizjournals.com/baltimore/blog/real-estate/2016/07/johns-hopkins-ups -the-ante-on-live-where-you-work.html.

46. Broadway Services, "Live Near Your Work Program," *On Broadway: A Newsletter for the Employees of Broadway Services*, July–September 2013, p. 6. See also *On Broadway* issues February–April 2017, p. 5, and "Live Baltimore," 2018, https://livebaltimore.com/live-near-your-work/.

47. Melody Simmons, "UM Baltimore Set to Offer 'Live Near Your Work' Grants to Employees," *Baltimore Business Journal*, January 5, 2018, https://www .bizjournals.com/baltimore/news/2018/01/05/um-baltimore-set-to-offer -live-near-your-work.html. See also University of Maryland, Baltimore, "Live Near Your Work," University of Maryland, Baltimore, 2017–2018, http:// www.umaryland.edu/live-near-your-work/.

48. Robert Reinhold, "Urbanologist Scores Baltimore: Excerpts from an AFRO interview with Dr. Homer Favor, School of Urban Affairs and Human Develop-ment, Morgan State University," *Baltimore Afro-American*, October 3, 1978, 6.

49. Jason Richardson, Bruce Mitchell, and Juan Franco, "Shifting Neighborhoods: Gentrification and Cultural Displacement in American Cities," National Community Reinvestment Coalition, March 19, 2019, https://ncrc.org /gentrification/.

50. Brandon Weigel, "Study: Baltimore Has Seen One of the Highest Rates of Gentrification in the U.S.," *Baltimore Fishbowl*, March 19, 2019, https:// baltimorefishbowl.com/stories/study-baltimore-has-seen-one-of-the-highest -rates-of-gentrification-in-the-u-s/.

51. In spite of the loss of 11.4% of its Black residents, the GRIA crowed, "Remington appears to be re-emerging as one of the great neighborhoods of Baltimore yet again." Greater Remington Improvement Association (GRIA), "Remington Neighborhood Plan," GRIA, 2017, http://www.griaonline.org/neighborhood-plan/, p. 16.

52. This is a point where the arguments of prominent urbanists such as Richard Florida, Alan Malloch, and others are fundamentally flawed. They argue that concentrated poverty is a more pressing issue than gentrification. But such an analysis can only be true if it ignores the impact of serial forced displacement in Black communities historically. Black communities have been uprooted repeatedly whether they contained concentrations of Black wealth (e.g., Black Wall Street in Tulsa or Hayti in Durham, NC) or poverty (e.g., urban renewal or demolition of public housing). From the perspective of Black communities, gentrification intensifies and deepens poverty just as all forms of forced displacement do. Gentrification increases poverty and merely shuffles people into new different areas of concentrated poverty. This is what happened previously with rural land dispossession, slum clearance, urban renewal, highway construction, mass incarceration, public housing demolition, and other forms of forced displacement.

53. Bryna Zumer, "West Balt. Residents Rally to Stop Demolition, Urge City to 'Rebuild,'" *Fox45 News*, September 6, 2018, https://foxbaltimore.com/news/local/west-balt-residents-rally-to-stop-demolition-urge-city-to-rebuild.

54. In the Oldtown community, roughly 100 families were forced to leave when Somerset Court was demolished. Pall Mall Apartments had 25 families that were forced to leave, and Park Heights Renaissance displaced 62 families. In Reservoir Hill, 186 families were relocated from Madison Park North Apartments, many willingly, but after years of deep disinvestment and apartment mismanagement. For Somerset Court demolition, see Joan Jacobson, "The Dismantling of Baltimore's Public Housing: Housing Authority Cutting 2,400 Homes for the Poor from Its Depleted Inventory," *The Abell Report*, September 2007, 2, third column. For Park Heights Renaissance displacement, see Rick Seltzer, "Baltimore Is Seeking a Developer for a Major Transformation of Park Heights," *Baltimore Business Journal*, March 9, 2016, https://www.bizjournals.com/baltimore/blog/real-estate/2016/03/baltimore-developer-park-heights.html. For Madison Park North Apartments demolition, see Yvonne Wagner and Justin Fenton, "Troubled Reservoir Hill Apartment Complex to Be Razed," *Baltimore Sun*, August 3, 2014, https://www.baltimoresun.com/news/maryland/baltimore-city/bs-md-ci-madison-park-north-20140803-story.html.

55. Andrew Zaleski, "The Great 'Innovation' Rebrand of West Baltimore," Next City, March 20, 2017, https://nextcity.org/features/view/west-baltimore-innovation-district-rebrand-tech-economy.

56. Speaking to the skepticism regarding the future direction and fair housing implications of the Perkins Somerset Oldtown Transformation Plan, Barbara Samuels (managing attorney for ACLU of Maryland's Fair Housing Project) argued: "It could go one of two ways. It's got real potential to break down what we call the 'Two Baltimores' and create an economically and racially integrated community and school there around the Perkins site. Or it could go completely the other way and become a mechanism for removing public

housing, low-income people and, specifically, low-income African-Americans who live next to this new luxury area." D. Amari Jackson, "Is the Baltimore Housing Authority a Gateway for the Gentrification of the City?," *Atlanta Black Star*, September 15, 2017, https://atlantablackstar.com/2017/09/15/baltimore-housing-authority-gateway-gentrification/. In addition, local public housing authorities are notorious for using "not in good standing" clauses to filter and screen out public housing residents and keep them from returning to the newly built mixed income community built on the site of the former public housing development. Early versions of the PSO Redevelopment plan called for demolishing one building at a time and allowing residents to remain in the Perkins Homes community while the rebuild takes place. This would certainly protect against displacement *if* the plan is implemented as promised.

57. Gregg Levine, "A History of Violence: Baltimore's 'Broken Relationship' Years in Making," *Al Jazeera America*, April 28, 2015, http://america.aljazeera.com/blogs/scrutineer/2015/4/28/a-history-of-violence-baltimores-broken-relationship-years-in-making.html. According to an *Al Jazeera* article by Gregg Levine: "In the two decades leading up to 2012, 127 citizens were killed by police in Baltimore—significantly more than other cities of similar size. Las Vegas saw 100 deaths at the hands of law enforcement, while in other like-sized cities, such as Memphis, Oklahoma City and Seattle, police killings were less than half Baltimore's number."

58. Mark Puente, "Undue Force," *Baltimore Sun*, September 28, 2014, http://data.baltimoresun.com/news/police-settlements/.

59. Doug Donavan and Mark Puente, "Freddie Gray Not the First to Come Out of Baltimore Police Van with Serious Injuries," *Baltimore Sun*, April 23, 2015, http://www.baltimoresun.com/news/maryland/baltimore-city/bs-md-gray-rough-rides-20150423-story.html.

60. Mark Puente and Meredith Cohn, "Freddie Gray among Many Suspects Who Do Not Get Medical Care from Baltimore Police," *Baltimore Sun*, May 9, 2015, http://www.baltimoresun.com/news/maryland/sun-investigates/bs-md-gray-jail-rejections-20150509-story.html. See also *Sun* reporter/analyst, "Examining Medical Rejections at Corrections Facilities," *Baltimore Sun*, May 9, 2015, http://data.baltimoresun.com/news/intake-logs/presentation-prototype-seven/.

61. Jayne Miller, "War on Drugs Contributes to Violence in Baltimore," *WBAL-TV 11 News*, October 26, 2017, https://www.wbaltv.com/article/war-on-drugs-contributes-to-violence-in-baltimore/13100359.

62. Brandon Patterson, "Black Lives Matter Organizers Labeled as 'Threat Actors' by Cybersecurity Firm," *Mother Jones*, August 3, 2015, https://www.motherjones.com/politics/2015/08/zerofox-report-baltimore-black-lives-matter/. See also Stephen Babcock, "ZeroFox under Fire for Social Media 'Threat Actors' Report during Baltimore Riots," Technical.ly, August 4, 2015, https://technical.ly/baltimore/2015/08/04/zerofox-fire-social-media-threat-actors-report-baltimore-riots/. Similar tracking on social media would be uncovered in Memphis, Tennessee, by the Memphis Police Department against Memphis Black Lives Matter activists in 2018.

63. Brandon Powers, "Eyes over Baltimore: How Police Use Military Technology to Secretly Track," *Rolling Stone*, January 6, 2017, https://www.rollingstone

.com/culture/culture-features/eyes-over-baltimore-how-police-use-military -technology-to-secretly-track-you-126885/. See also Jessica Guynn, "ACLU: Police Used Twitter, Facebook to Track Protests," *USA Today*, October 11, 2016, https://www.usatoday.com/story/tech/news/2016/10/11/aclu-police -used-twitter-facebook-data-track-protesters-baltimore-ferguson/91897034/.

64. Barbara Tasch, "An Investigation in Baltimore Has 'Opened the Floodgates' on the Use of Secretive FBI Cellphone Tracking Devices," *Business Insider*, August 28, 2015, http://www.businessinsider.com/baltimore-defense -lawyers-review-cases-where-police-used-stingrays-2015-8.

65. Monte Reel, "It's Not Spying If They're Always Watching: Uncovering Baltimore's Secret Surveillance Program," *Bloomberg Businessweek*, August 23, 2016, https://www.bloomberg.com/features/2016-baltimore-secret -surveillance/.

66. US Department of Justice, *Investigation of the Baltimore City Police Department* (Washington, DC: Civil Rights Division, US Department of Justice, August 10, 2016), 3.

67. Kevin Rector and Natalie Sherman, "Baltimore Police, Partners Create Around-the-Clock 'War Room' to Address Crime Surge," *Baltimore Sun*, July 12, 2015, http://www.baltimoresun.com/news/maryland/crime/bs-md -violence-strategy-20150712-story.html. See also Baltimore Police Commissioner Kevin Davis, "Policy 302: Rules and Regulations," Baltimore Police Department, August 26, 2017, 4–7, https://www.baltimorepolice.org/file/162 /download?token=FOK7Cfvi.

68. "The Gang Within: A Baltimore Police Scandal," *Al Jazeera*, https://www .aljazeera.com/programmes/faultlines/2018/10/gang-baltimore-police -scandal-181003055735408.html.

69. Mary Rose Madden, "How the GTTF Cops Were Caught—and Why Didn't Local Authorities Catch 'Em?," WYPR, June 6, 2018, https://www.wypr.org /post/how-gttf-cops-were-caught-and-why-didnt-local-authorities-catch-em.

70. Ava-joye Burnett, "Former BPD Sergeant Allegedly Helped GTTF Member by Planting Gun at Arrest Scene, Telling Witness to Lie," CBS Baltimore, March 6, 2019, https://baltimore.cbslocal.com/2019/03/05/former-bpd -sergeant-allegedly-helped-gttf-member-by-planting-gun-at-arrest-scene -telling-witness-to-lie/.

71. US Department of Justice, *Investigation of the Baltimore City Police Department*, 156.

72. National Advisory Commission on Civil Disorders, *Report of the National Advisory Commission on Civil Disorders* (Washington, DC: Department of Justice, 1968).

73. Regarding the central role played by President Johnson, Elizabeth Hinton wrote: "Over the five summers of Lyndon B. Johnson's presidency, the nation witnessed more than 250 incidents of urban civil disorder. . . . Unprecedented in its fury and frequency, this disorder radically reshaped the direction of Johnson's Great Society programs, resulting ultimately in a merger of antipoverty programs with anticrime programs that laid the groundwork for contemporary mass incarceration." See Hinton, "'A War within Our Own Boundaries': Lyndon Johnson's Great Society and the Rise of the Carceral State," *Journal of American History* 102, no. 1 (2015): 100–112, 100.

74. Terry v. Ohio, decided by the United States Supreme Court on June 10, 1968, Oyez, www.oyez.org/cases/1967/67.

75. Graham v. Connor, decided by the United States Supreme Court on May 15, 1989, Oyez, www.oyez.org/cases/1988/87-6571.

76. Illinois v. Wardlow, decided by the United States Supreme Court on January 12, 2000, Oyez, www.oyez.org/cases/1999/98-1036.

77. Utah v. Strieff, decided by the United States Supreme Court on June 20, 2016, Oyez, www.oyez.org/cases/2015/14-1373.

78. Shirley Li, "The Evolution of Police Militarization in Ferguson and Beyond," *The Atlantic*, August 14, 2014, https://www.theatlantic.com/national/archive/2014/08/the-evolution-of-police-militarization-in-ferguson-and-beyond/376107/.

79. Aldina Mesic, Lydia Franklin, Alev Cansever, et al., "The Relationship between Structural Racism and Black-White Disparities in Fatal Shootings at the State Level," *Journal of the National Medical Association*, 110, no. 2 (2018): 106–116. Their index comprises measuring the racial disparities in five areas—(1) residential segregation, (2) incarceration rates, (3) education attainment, (4) economic indicators, and (5) employment status.

80. Brad Smith and Malcolm Holmes, "Police Use of Excessive Force in Minority Communities: A Test of the Minority Threat, Place, and Community Accountability Hypotheses," *Social Problems* 61, no. 1 (2014): 83–104.

81. Michael Siegel, Rebecca Sherman, Cindy Li, and Anita Knopov, "The Relationship between Racial Residential Segregation and Black-White Disparities in Fatal Police Shootings at the City Level, 2013–2017," *Journal of the National Medical Association* 111, no. 6 (2019): 580–587.

82. David A. Fahrenthold, "Large Protests against Police Violence Again Fill the Streets of U.S. Cities," *Washington Post*, June 2, 2020, https://www.washingtonpost.com/politics/large-protests-against-police-violence-again-fill-streets-of-us-cities/2020/06/02/f4551a62-a51b-11ea-b473-04905b1af82b_story.html.

83. Zolan Kanno-Youngs and Katie Benner, "Trump Deploys the Full Might of Federal Law Enforcement to Crush Protests," *New York Times*, June 2, 2020, https://www.nytimes.com/2020/06/02/us/politics/trump-law-enforcement-protests.html.

84. "Read: President Trump's Call with US Governors over Protests," CNN, June 1, 2020, https://www.cnn.com/2020/06/01/politics/wh-governors-call-protests/index.html.

85. Shaila Dewan and Mike Baker, "Facing Protests over Use of Force, Police Respond with More Force," *New York Times*, https://www.nytimes.com/2020/05/31/us/police-tactics-floyd-protests.html.

86. Yamiche Alcindor, "What's in the Justice in Policing Act?," *PBS News Hour*, June 12, 2020, https://www.pbs.org/newshour/politics/whats-in-the-justice-in-policing-act.

87. Bruce Mitchell and Juan Franco, HOLC "Redlining" Maps: The Persistent Structure of Segregation and Economic Inequality (Washington, DC: National Community Reinvestment Coalition, 2018), https://ncrc.org/wp-content/uploads/dlm_uploads/2018/02/NCRC-Research-HOLC-10.pdf.

88. Sarah Mikhitarian, "Home Values Remain Low in Vast Majority of Formerly Redlined Neighborhoods," Zillow Research, 2018, https://www.zillow.com/research/home-values-redlined-areas-19674/.

89. Andre Perry, Jonathan Rothwell, and David Harshbarger, *The Devaluation of Assets in Black Neighborhoods: The Case of Residential Property* (Washington, DC: Brookings Institution Metropolitan Policy Program and Gallup, 2018).

90. National Community Reinvestment Coalition, *Home Mortgage and Small Business Lending in Baltimore and Surrounding Areas* (Washington, DC: National Community Reinvestment Coalition, November 2015), https://ncrc .org/wp-content/uploads/2015/11/ncrc_baltimore_lending_analysis_web.pdf.

91. National Community Reinvestment Coalition, *Home Mortgage Lending in St. Louis, Milwaukee, Minneapolis, and Surrounding Areas* (Washington, DC: National Community Reinvestment Coalition, 2018), https://ncrc.org/wp -content/uploads/2018/01/Home-Mortgage-Lending2.pdf. See also Mitchell and Franco, *HOLC "Redlining" Maps*, http://maps.ncrc.org/holcreport /index.html. This website contains a tremendous web tool to help communities across the nation understand how past redlining is affecting home values in their neighborhoods in urban areas today.

92. Fox and colleagues found: "Since 2010, the branch footprint in majority-black areas has shrunk 14.6%, compared to 9.7% in all other communities, with the nation's two largest banks—JPMorgan Chase & Co. and Bank of America Corp.—playing significant roles. JPMorgan had the largest disparity in net closure rates. From 2010 to 2018, it opened almost as many branches as it closed—except in majority-black communities. JPMorgan shrank its branch footprint in majority-black areas by 22.8% from 2010 to 2018, compared to a net decline of 0.2% in the rest of the U.S. Bank of America has closed more of its branches in majority-black communities, but the bank has been closing more branches nationwide, resulting in a smaller disparity. Bank of America reduced the number of branches in majority-black neighborhoods by 29.1%, compared to an 18.4% decline in non-majority-black areas." Zach Fox, Zain Tariq, Liz Thomas, and Ciaralou Palicpic, "Bank Branch Closures Take Greatest Toll on Majority-Black Areas," S&P Global Market Intelligence, July 25, 2019, https://www.spglobal.com/marketintelligence/en/news -insights/latest-news-headlines/52872925.

93. Activists for Fair Housing, *Baltimore under Siege: The Impact of Financing on The Baltimore Home Buyer (1960–1970)*, September 1971, University of Baltimore, Langsdale Library, Special Collections and in their digital collection online.

94. "Blockbusting" describes a process in real estate where agents would work to flip houses by scaring Whites with the threat of racial integration. According to Emily Lieb, blockbusting occurred when "realtors used the threat of integration to frighten whites into selling their houses, often for much less than they had paid, to be resold at enormous markup to black families desperate for decent housing." See Emily Lieb, "'Baltimore Does Not Condone Profiteering in Squalor': The Baltimore Plan and the Problem of Housing-Code Enforcement in an American City," *Planning Perspectives* 33, no. 1 (2018): 75–95, 78.

95. Aaron Glantz and Emmanuel Martinez, "Modern-Day Redlining: How Banks Block People of Color from Homeownership," *Chicago Tribune*, February 17, 2018, http://www.chicagotribune.com/business/ct-biz-modern -day-redlining-20180215-story.html#. See also Mitchell and Franco, *HOLC "Redlining" Maps*. The mechanics of subprime mortgages and the housing bubble are quite difficult often to understand, but the movie *The Big Short* does a fairly good job of breaking down what happened.

96. Jacob Rugh, Len Albright, and Douglas S. Massey, "Race, Space, and Cumulative Disadvantage: A Case Study of the Subprime Lending Collapse," *Social Problems* 62 (2015): 186–218. Rugh and colleagues show that middle-class Black homebuyers were especially targeted by Wells Fargo. "Consistent with sociological research on the black middle class, higher socioeconomic status by no means protects families from systematic discrimination, especially when they live in black neighborhoods. Indeed, higher status may even exacerbate potential losses to black income and wealth. Based on our analysis, compared with $14,904 for all African Americans, the projected cumulative cost of discrimination for blacks earning over $50,000 per year was $19,026. Our findings thus confirm those of Faber, who documents higher rates of subprime lending for higher-income blacks, and Katrin Anacker and James Carr and Debbie Bocian and colleagues, who report higher rates of foreclosure for upper-class blacks net of other factors."

97. Justin P. Steil, Len Albright, Jacob S. Rugh, and Douglas Massey, "The Social Structure of Mortgage Discrimination," *Housing Studies* 33, no. 5 (2018): 759–776, 771.

98. Marc V. Levine, "'A Third-World City in the First World': Social Exclusion, Racial Inequality, and Sustainable Development in Baltimore" in *The Social Sustainability of Cities: Diversity and the Management of Change*, ed. M. Polese and R. E. Stren, 123–156 (Toronto: University of Toronto Press, 2000). Levine discusses $2 billion in tax revenues spent along Baltimore's waterfront area. I add in more recent tax expenditures to another $1 billion invested in the White L or with predominantly White institutions: $660 million Sagamore TIF, $330 million in revenue bonds for the city hotel, $107 million Harbor Point TIF, and the $78 million EBDI TIF.

99. Lawrence Brown, "Two Baltimores: The White L vs. the Black Butterfly," *City Paper*, June 28, 2016, http://www.citypaper.com/bcpnews-two -baltimores-the-white-l-vs-the-black-butterfly-20160628-htmlstory.html.

100. HUB Staff writer, "Baltimore BLocal Partner Businesses Invest Millions in City during Program's First Year," *Johns Hopkins University HUB*, December 11, 2017, https://hub.jhu.edu/2017/12/11/blocal-progress-report -surpasses-goal/; Jacob Took, "How Do HopkinsLocal Investments Impact the City?," *The Johns Hopkins News-Letter*, February 28, 2019, https://www .jhunewsletter.com/article/2019/02/how-do-hopkinslocal-investments -impact-the-city. Many of the same corporations that are members of BLocal are members of the Greater Baltimore Committee such as Under Armour, Legg Mason, and Whiting Turner. Multiple entities of the Johns Hopkins University and hospital conglomerate are also represented on the Greater Baltimore Committee.

101. In 2019, Johns Hopkins University administrators pushed for the passage of its own private police force, giving a private entity the public authority of policing. The effort also adds more policing to a city that is under a federal consent decree for a racist pattern of policing. The Hopkins legislation was entitled the Community Safety and Strengthening Act—a dubious name given that the proposed legislation is designed to make the community safer for the benefit of Hopkins employees who are also being given public-private incentives such as Live Near Your Work to live in areas adjacent to Hopkins campuses in Central and East Baltimore. For Hopkins's attempt to block the

unionization of its nurses, see Kelly Gooch, "Johns Hopkins Stifled Unionizing Efforts, Federal Labor Board Finds," *Becker's Hospital Review*, October 31, 2018, https://www.beckershospitalreview.com/human-capital-and-risk /johns-hopkins-stifled-unionizing-efforts-federal-labor-board-finds.html.

102. Although Maryland did pass a $15 per hour minimum wage law in the 2019 legislative session, large businesses will not be required to pay workers $15 per hour until 2015. Hence, for an entire five-year period, large corporations will be able to avoid paying a living wage. Alexia Fernández-Campbell, "Maryland Just Became the Sixth State to Raise the Minimum Wage to $15 An Hour," Vox, March 28, 2019, https://www.vox.com/2019/3/28 /18285346/maryland-passes-15-minimum-wage.

103. National Nurses United, "Burdening Baltimore: How Johns Hopkins Hospital and Other Not-for-Profit Hospitals, Colleges, and Universities Fail to Pay Their Fair Share," National Nurses United, Coalition for a Humane Hopkins, and AFL-CIO, October 2019, 8. The figures for JHMI include Johns Hopkins Hospital.

104. Luke Broadwater, "University of Maryland Medical System Pays Members of Volunteer Board Hundreds of Thousands in Business Deals," *Baltimore Sun*, March 13, 2019, https://www.baltimoresun.com/news/maryland/politics /bs-md-umms-legislation-20190312-story.html.

105. Luke Broadwater, "New Audit Says Top Medical System Officials Never Read Pugh's 'Healthy Holly' Books before Paying Her $500,000," *Baltimore Sun*, December 14, 2019, https://www.baltimoresun.com/politics/bs-md-pol -umms-report-20191213-q7hoqfenczgf5kru6h4geizzb4-story.html.

106. Jeff Singer, "UMMS Self-Dealing Scandal a Product of Privatization," *Baltimore Brew*, April 1, 2019, https://baltimorebrew.com/2019/04/01 /umms-self-dealing-scandal-a-product-of-privatization/.

107. The Democracy Collaborative, "The Cleveland Model—How the Evergreen Cooperatives are Building Community Wealth," The Democracy Collaborative, 2019, https://community-wealth.org/content/cleveland -model-how-evergreen-cooperatives-are-building-community-wealth.

108. National Nurses United, "Burdening Baltimore," 8.

109. Luke Broadwater, "University of Maryland Medical System Pays Members of Volunteer Board Hundreds of Thousands in Business Deals," *Baltimore Sun*, March 13, 2019, https://www.baltimoresun.com/news/maryland/politics /bs-md-umms-legislation-20190312-story.html; David Plymyer, "Seeds for UMMS Contracting Scandal Were Sowed in Ethics-Challenged Annapolis," *Baltimore Brew*, March 22, 2019, https://baltimorebrew.com/2019/03/22 /seeds-for-umms-contracting-scandal-were-sowed-in-ethics-challenged -annapolis/; Mark Reutter, "UMMS's Bob Chrencik Built a Hospital Empire Out of Privatization," *Baltimore Brew*, March 19, 2019, https://www .baltimorebrew.com/2019/03/19/ummss-bob-chrencik-built-a-hospital -empire-out-of-privatization/.

110. McCormick Taylor and Sabra, Wang & Associates, *2015 Baltimore City Bike Master Plan* (Baltimore: Baltimore City Department of Transportation, March 2015).

111. Battelle Technology Partnership Practice, "Regional Economic and Demographic Market Analysis and Economic Impact Assessment of the Port Covington Project/Under Armour Headquarters Project" (prepared for

Sagamore Development Corporation, Baltimore, December 2015), appendixes A and B, 107–108.

112. "The Future of Baltimore's Waterfront," *Baltimore Business Journal*, May 19, 2017, https://www.bizjournals.com/baltimore/blog/real-estate /2015/04/how-real-estate-lawyer-jon-laria-became-an.html.

113. George Solis, "Mayor Pugh Vetoes $15 Minimum Wage Bill, Workers, Business Owners React," WJZ CBS Baltimore, March 24, 2017, https://baltimore .cbslocal.com/2017/03/24/mayor-pugh-vetoes-15-minimum-wage-bill/.

114. Jing Li and Richard Clinch (The Jacob France Institute), "Analysis of Patterns of Employment by Race in Baltimore City and the Baltimore Metropolitan Area," Associated Black Charities, February 2018, http:// www.abc-md.org/reports/.

115. Fern Shen, "Pugh to Veto $15 Minimum Wage Bill She Said, as a Candidate, She'd Sign," *Baltimore Brew*, March 24, 2017, https://www.baltimorebrew .com/2017/03/24/pugh-to-veto-15-minimum-wage-bill-she-said-as-a -candidate-shed-sign/.

116. Keeanga-Yamahtta Taylor, *From #BlackLivesMatter to Black Liberation* (Chicago: Haymarket Books, 2016), 80.

117. Political scientist Lester Spence argues that ignoring Black intra-racial income gaps: "causes us to gloss over the fact that neoliberal ideas and policies are not simply produced and reproduced by whites to withhold resources from blacks. . . . Black elected officials and civil rights leaders reproduce these ideas, participating in a remobilization project of sorts, one that consistently posits that the real reason black people aren't as successful as their white counterparts is because of a lack of hustle, is because they don't quite have the work ethic necessary to succeed in the modern moment." Lester Spence, *Knocking the Hustle: Against the Neoliberal Turn in Black Politics* (Brooklyn: Putnam Books, 2015), 25.

118. McFarlane, "Operatively White?," 165 (see n. 7). McFarlane goes on to argue on page 194: "What is the significance of being operatively white? The answer is not clear, but a few preliminary observations can be made. Most compelling is that the presence of the black middle class is used to excuse the disadvantage or displacement of the black poor."

119. Ben Paynter, "Nonprofit Boards Are Very Rich and Very White," Fast Company, September 6, 2017, https://www.fastcompany.com/40462347 /nonprofits-boards-are-very-rich-and-very-white.

120. Maria Sieron, "Largest Charitable Foundations in Greater Baltimore: Ranked by Total 2017 Assets," *Baltimore Business Journal*, February 21, 2018, https://www.bizjournals.com/baltimore/subscriber-only/2018/02/09 /charitable-foundations.html.

121. To Pill's elite actors category, I have added the entities such as the Greater Baltimore Committee, the Abell Foundation, and the University of Maryland Medical System. Given its roundtable structure, the Greater Baltimore Committee serves as the central hub for elite tier actors.

122. Pill also writes: "Corporate developer and major ed and med actors, particularly Johns Hopkins University and Johns Hopkins Health System, set the development agenda for specific sites and gain power to implement through resource alignment with other elites. The selective spatial engagement of high-resource actors is expressed in the city's megaprojects . . . augmented

with some state government resources, to realize elite priorities. Thus, major redevelopment overrides neighborhood revitalization, continuing the longstanding priority placed on prime waterfront sites that gain corporate interest." Madeleine Pill, "The Austerity Governance of Baltimore's Neighborhoods: 'The Conversation May Have Changed But the Systems Aren't Changing,'" *Journal of Urban Affairs* (2018): 5, doi:10.1080/07352166.2 018.1478226.

123. Pill highlights the governing arrangements that result in the maintenance of racial inequity even post-uprising: "The uprising provided an opportunity to interrogate continuity and change . . . in the context of what was constructed by all interviewed as a pivotal moment. The multitier analysis reveals little alteration despite this disruption. The political imperative to respond to the uprising did accelerate and expand top- to middle-tier interactions seeking to mitigate lower-tier marginality: "Since the unrest . . . businesses and philanthropic organizations and the institutions are really stepping forward and saying, 'We've got to do more collectively'" (Anchor 2). But though the city's governance has seen a degree of adjust-ment in style and tone, the priorities and fixes (spatial and institutional) remain the same. Small-scale changes and concessions have occurred at the granular level; for example, in terms of developers being willing to talk about local hiring and stressed neighborhood residents being targeted for anchor economic inclusion initiatives. Funding for lower-tier activities in the stressed neighborhoods was tokenistic, "because they realize if they don't, sooner or later the have-nots will be sitting on your doorstep" (Community 1); Pill, "Austerity Governance of Baltimore's Neighborhoods," 13.

124. "A Brief History," Abell Foundation, 2018, https://abell.org/brief-history.

125. Antero Pietila, *Not in My Neighborhood: How Bigotry Shaped a Great American City* (Chicago: Ivan R Dee, 2002).

126. Activists for Fair Housing, *Baltimore under Siege*, iii. See also Pietila, *Not in My Neighborhood*.

127. Monte Reel, "It's Not Spying If They're Always Watching: Uncovering Baltimore's Secret Surveillance Program," *Bloomberg Businessweek*, Au-gust 23, 2016, https://www.bloomberg.com/features/2016-baltimore-secret -surveillance/.

128. Marisela Gomez, *Race, Class, Power, and Organizing in East Baltimore: Rebuilding Abandoned Communities in America* (Lanham, MD: Lexington Books, 2013). For number of households displaced and the amount invested in EBDI, see Melody Simmons and Joan Jacobson, "Too Big to Fail: A Dream Derailed," *The Daily Record* 122, no. 82 (January 31, 2011): 11A.

129. Mark Reutter, "On a Single Day, Johns Hopkins Officials Gave Baltimore's Mayor $16,000," *Baltimore Brew*, March 4, 2019, https://www .baltimorebrew.com/2019/03/04/on-a-single-day-johns-hopkins-officials -gave-baltimores-mayor-16000/. Reutter explains: "As a private non-profit educational institution, JHU is banned from making contributions to political campaigns or to politicians. Individual citizens, however, are free to contribute to candidates of their choice, which is what Daniels and his senior staff—including five vice presidents, the university provost, and the past and current presidents of the Johns Hopkins Hospital—did on January 9. They

each contributed $1,000, $2,000 or, in the case of Daniels, $3,000 to the Committee to Elect Catherine E. Pugh. . . . A month later, on February 4, a measure to establish a private police force at Hopkins was introduced by state Senator Antonio Hayes at the 'request [of] Baltimore City Administration' or the mayor's office."

130. Mark Reutter, "UMMS's Bob Chrencik Built a Hospital Empire out of Privatization," *Baltimore Brew*, March 19, 2019, https://www.baltimorebrew .com/2019/03/19/ummss-bob-chrencik-built-a-hospital-empire-out-of -privatization/. One of the recipients of the UMMS no-bid contracts was then mayor Catherine Pugh.

131. David Plymyer, "Seeds for UMMS Contracting Scandal Were Sowed in Ethics-Challenged Annapolis," *Baltimore Brew*, March 22, 2019, https:// baltimorebrew.com/2019/03/22/seeds-for-umms-contracting-scandal-were -sowed-in-ethics-challenged-annapolis/. According to Plymyer: "When the General Assembly privatized UMMS in 1984, it took pains to free UMMS from state control, declaring that it was not a state agency and not subject to laws affecting only governmental or public entities. It did, however, provide that voting members of the board of directors were appointed by the governor. Boards appointed by the governor are rich opportunities for patronage. They tend to be top-heavy with politicians, former politicians and campaign contributors. The UMMS board was no exception."

132. Domingo Morel, *Takeover: Race, Education, and American Democracy* (New York: Oxford University Press, 2018), 11–12.

133. Morel, *Takeover*, 126.

134. John Arena, *Driven from New Orleans: How Nonprofits Betray Public Housing and Promote Privatization* (Minneapolis: University of Minnesota Press, 2012).

Track 5. Black Neighborhood Destruction

1. The scope of federally and locally funded urban renewal—authorized in the Housing Acts of 1949 and 1954—was massive. "By the time new funding for the program ended in 1974, local authorities had been awarded federal support for more than 2,100 distinct urban renewal projects with grants totaling approximately $53 billion (in 2009 dollars), as well as smaller sums for related activities." William J. Collins and Katharine L. Shester, "Slum Clearance and Urban Renewal in the United States," *American Economic Journal: Applied Economics* 5, no. 1 (2013): 239–273, 239. The same was true for highway construction which occurred at the same time urban renewal was taking place. "By the 1960s, federal highway construction was demolishing 37,000 urban housing units each year; urban renewal and redevelopment programs were destroying an equal number of mostly low-income housing units annually. . . . A large proportion of those dislocated were African Americans, and in most cities highway officials routinely routed express-ways through black neighborhoods." Mark H. Rose and Raymond A. Mohl, *Interstate: Highway Politics and Policy since 1939*, 3rd ed. (Knoxville: University of Tennessee Press, 2012), 96.

2. "A Conversation with James Baldwin," interview with James Baldwin, WGBH Media Library & Archives, June 24, 1963, http://openvault.wgbh .org/catalog/V_C03ED1927DCF46B5A8C82275DF4239F9.

3. The Maryland State Conference of the NAACP wrote a letter dated December 17, 1951, to Nathaniel S. Keith, director of the Division of Slum Clearance and Urban Redevelopment in the federal Housing and Home Finance Agency. See Thompson v. HUD files, Case MJG 95-709, Plaintiff's Exhibit No. 127, University of Baltimore, Langsdale Library, Special Collections.

4. Jessica Trounstine, *Segregation by Design: Local Politics and Inequality in American Cities* (Cambridge: Cambridge University Press, 2018), 120-131.

5. The federal government paid $600,000,000 of the cost while Baltimore City paid $300,000,000 of the cost. See League of Women Voters of Baltimore City, *Established Urban Renewal Areas*, League of Women Voters of Baltimore City, Enoch Pratt Central Library, Maryland Department, Call Number Md. XHT177 .B2L38, 1960, 27.

6. Raymond Mohl, "Urban Expressways and the Racial Restructuring of Postwar American Cities," *Economic History Yearbook*, 42, no. 2 (2001): 89-104.

7. Between 1949 and 1967, the federal government demolished 1,054,000 homes via urban renewal, highway construction/destruction, demolition on future public housing sites, and more. National Commission on Urban Problems, *Building the American City* (Washington, DC: Government Printing Office, 1968), 82–83. According to Mindy Thompson Fullilove in her book *Root Shock*: "By my estimate, 1,600 black neighborhoods were demolished by urban renewal. This massive destruction caused root shock on two levels. First, residents of each neighborhood experienced the traumatic stress of the loss of their life world. Second, because of the interconnections among all black people in the United States, the whole of Black America experienced root shock as well. Root shock, post urban renewal, disabled powerful mechanisms of community functioning, leaving the [B]lack world at an enormous disadvantage for meeting the challenges of globalization." Fullilove, *Root Shock: How Tearing Up City Neighborhoods Hurts America, and What We Can Do about It* (New York: Ballantine, 2004).

8. Thomas G. Brown, "A Brief History of the Federal War on Drugs," Independent Voter Network, May 7, 2012, https://ivn.us/2012/05/07/a-brief-history -of-the-federal-war-on-drugs/.

9. Mindy Thompson Fullilove and Rodrick Wallace, "Serial Forced Displacement in American Cities, 1916–2010," *Journal of Urban Health* 88, no. 3 (2011): 381–389. Crises included the crack cocaine epidemic, HIV/AIDS, and violence connected to the drug trade.

10. Fullilove and Wallace, "Serial Forced Displacement in American Cities," 384. According to Fullilove and Wallace, repeated forced uprootings leads to declining mutual support and increased individualism in affected communities. They explain: "A stage-state model of social disintegration was proposed to describe what happens to communities affected by such a series of policies. The stage-state model is based on the work of Alexander Leighton, who posited that communities exist in a continuum from integration to disintegration. He defined integration as internal interconnection, characterized by mutual support. He placed disintegration at the other end of the continuum of social organization and characterized it as individualism. The stage-state model hypothesized that communities that suffered from a series of negative events would exhibit partial collapse after each. In the absence of adequate mitigation, this meant that the collapse was a downhill progression

from integration towards disintegration, punctuated by changes in the state of social relationships." In her book *Root Shock*, Fullilove explains the pain of root shock: "It was the loss of a massive web of connections—a way of being—that had been destroyed by urban renewal; it was as if thousands of people, who seemed to be with me in sunlight, were at some deeper level of their being wandering lost in a dense fog, unable to find one another for the rest of their lives. It was a chorus of voices that rose in my head, with the cry, 'We have lost one another.'" Fullilove, *Root Shock: How Tearing Up City Neighborhoods Hurts America, and What We Can Do about It* (New York: Ballantine, 2004), 9–10.

11. Ntozake Shange, *If I Can Cook/You Know God Can: African American Food Memories, Meditations, and Recipes* (Boston: Beacon Press, 1999). Many thanks to Ashanté Reese for telling me about this marvelous quote!

12. Harold A. McDougall, *Black Baltimore: A New Theory of Community* (Philadelphia: Temple University Press, 1993), 54–56. McDougall highlighted the neighborhood impacts of urban renewal: "Black people were shuffled around Baltimore during the period of urban renewal, just as they were under the rubric of public housing and slum clearance. . . . The residents who were dislodged doubled up in other slums, creating a concentration of low-income, overcrowded, troubled people that no municipality could effectively serve." In effect, the Baltimore Urban Renewal and Housing Agency (BURHA) was a purveyor of concentrated poverty and helped create conditions in West Baltimore that still exist today. The City of Baltimore still does not serve Black West Baltimore effectively to this day.

13. Jonathan Wharton, "Gentrification: The New Colonialism in the Modern Era," *Forum on Public Policy: A Journal of the Oxford Roundtable*, Summer 2008. Discursive redlining also comes into play here. As Jones and Jackson write: "People who practice discursive redlining do not identify crime or violence as institutional problems or as symptoms of a city's failure to incorporate African Americans into economic and civic life in the postwar era. Instead, discursive redlining suggests that it is the people, their bodies, and behaviors that are the problem. The sorts of solutions that follow this conceptualization of the problem are obvious: patterned avoidance or systematic removal." Nikki Jones and Christina Jackson, "'You Just Don't Go Down There': Learning to Avoid the Ghetto in San Francisco," in *The Ghetto: Contemporary Global Issues and Controversies*, ed. Ray Hutchinson, chap. 4, 85–86 (n.p.: Routledge).

14. Tahira Mahdi, "White Space and Sense of Community Theory: Membership, Privilege, and Power," Medium, May 2018, https://medium.com/@Tahira-Mahdi/white-spaces-and-sense-of-community-theory-membership-privilege-and-power-b82710e26e22. In their work *Healthy Development without Displacement*, authors with the Prevention Institute write: "Displacement takes a toll on societal factors that are difficult to quantify—the social, emotional, and cultural networks that communities build up over time. Too often when there is new development in historically under-resourced areas, long-term residents are not directly involved or engaged in the planning process and instead are developed on top of, becoming marginalized or displaced from spaces that were their homes first. What outsiders may consider to be positive contributions to historically divested communities can have negative consequences, including a feeling that these changes aren't 'by

us' or 'for us' among existing residents." Part of the impact of forced displacement is the loss of control and self-determination. See Manal Aboelata, Rachel Bennett, Elva Yañez, Ana Bonilla, and Nikta Akhaven, *Healthy Development without Displacement: Realizing the Vision of Healthy Communities for All* (Oakland, CA: Prevention Institute, July 2017).

15. Martin Luther King Jr., "The Chicago Plan" (statement, Southern Christian Leadership Conference, Atlanta, GA, January 7, 1966).

16. This is effectively what has been revealed by the corruption case involving the University of Maryland Medical System in March 2019. Instead of a focus on dismantling Baltimore Apartheid, the focus of corrupt Black elected officials is often on catering to the interests of corporate campaign donors. But this dynamic of colonization and resource capture is not unique to cities such as Baltimore and Chicago. Internal colonization is a familiar strategy of powerful empires and colonizers throughout human history. To facilitate resource extraction, the more powerful group co-opts surrogate leaders from the more vulnerable group in order to broker political power and keep resources flowing out of colonized spaces and into colonizers' hands. For instance, many European nations that colonized Africa began a strategic withdrawal from sub-Saharan African nations, starting in 1957 with Ghana winning its independence from the British. Soon many other African nations would militarily overthrow their European colonial masters. However, former colonizers such as France would develop a neocolonial arrangement that would still benefit them economically. Often, many African leaders would rise to power as autocrats and serve the economic interests of their former colonial nations while presenting a veneer of political independence.

17. John Arena described this dynamic in New Orleans slightly differently. Instead of describing it as internal colonization, he describes it as a partnership by writing: "This type of regime, which governed New Orleans from the late 1970s until the late 2000s, is one that emerged in many majority black cities in the post-civil rights era. These political formations are characterized by a 'governing coalition' composed of a primarily black public wing that holds a majority of the leading positions in local government and their allied, primarily black cadre of professionals, contractors, and ministers. Assembled on the other side of the power structure is a mainly white corporate private wing that controls the most important economic institutions. These elites are, for the most part, committed to a neoliberal urban entrepreneurial development model, with their collaboration often taking the form of 'public-private' partnerships. The governing elite favors constructing policy through these private and sometimes quasi-public entities, since they are buffered from extensive citizen participation and pressure. . . . These corporate or entrepreneurial regimes facilitate and subsidize corporate-led economic development, while redistribution and welfare are jettisoned." Arena, *Driven from New Orleans: How Nonprofits Betray Public Housing and Promote Privatization* (Minneapolis: University of Minnesota Press, 2012). I argue that this dynamic is a partnership certainly (hence the complicity), but that there is an additional dynamic of internal colonization at play due to the way Black neighborhoods are treated a zones of wealth extraction via predatory taxation and subprime lending and renting.

18. Lawrence Brown, "Community Health and Baltimore Apartheid: Revisiting Development, Inequality, and Tax Policy," in *Baltimore Revisited: Stories of*

Inequality and Resistance in a U.S. City, ed. P. Nicole King, Kate Drabinski, and Joshua Clark Davis, chap. 6 (New Brunswick, NJ: Rutgers University, 2019).

19. Trounstine, *Segregation by Design*, 150–155, and all of chap. 7, "Segregation's Negative Consequences." While Trounstine shows decreased spending on police as racial segregation increases in 3,113 cities, I do not believe this is true for cities in hypersegregated metropolitan areas. Their spending may not be reflective of the results found in Trounstine's work because hypersegregated cities may be outliers compared to most other cities. For data that speak to this point, see The Center for Popular Democracy, Law for Black Lives, and Black Youth Project 100, "Freedom to Thrive: Reimagining Safety & Security in Our Communities," The Center for Popular Democracy, 2017, http://populardemocracy.org/news/publications/freedom-thrive-reimagining-safety-security-our-communities.

20. Jay Croft, "A New Report Finds Predominantly White School Districts Get $23 Billion More Than Nonwhite Ones," CNN, February 27, 2019, https://www.cnn.com/2019/02/27/us/education-funding-disparity-study-trnd/index.html. See also "$23 Billion," EdBuild, February 2019, https://edbuild.org/content/23-billion. Even though the Supreme Court's Brown v. Board of Education decision mandated a desegregation of children by race, it did not mandate a desegregation of resources.

21. Alexandra Tilsley, "Subtracting Schools from Communities," Urban Institute, March 23, 2017, https://www.urban.org/features/subtracting-schools-communities. According to Tilsley: "In urban and suburban areas, closures disproportionately affect poor or black students. Though black students are about 31 percent of the population in continually open urban schools, they make up 61 percent of the population in closed urban schools. Similarly, black students account for 14 percent of the students in suburban schools that stay open but 29 percent of students at suburban schools that close."

22. Jennifer Berkshire, "How Closing Schools Undermines Democracy," Have You Heard, October 25, 2017, https://haveyouheardblog.com/wp-content/uploads/2017/10/Have-You-Heard-28-How-Closing-Schools-Undermines-Democracy.pdf.

23. Gerald Markowitz and David Rosner, *Lead Wars: The Politics of Science and the Fate of America's Children* (Los Angeles: University of California Press, 2013).

24. Richard Rabin, "The Lead Industry and Lead Water Pipes: 'A Modest Campaign,'" *American Journal of Public Health*, 98, no. 9 (2008): 1584–1592. See also Gerald Markowitz and David Rosner, *Lead Wars: The Politics of Science and the Fate of America's Children* (Berkeley: University of California Press, 2013). Finally, see Nora Holzinger, *Toxic Traces: Historical Trauma, Slow Violence, and the Discursive Framing of Lead Exposure in Baltimore, MD* (Towson, MD: Towson University, May 2017).

25. Kim M. Cecil, Christopher J. Brubaker, Caleb M. Adler, et al., "Decreased Brain Volume in Adults with Childhood Lead Exposure," *PLoS Medicine 5*, no. 5 (2008): 741–750.

26. Jennifer L. Doleac, "New Evidence that Lead Exposure Increases Crime," Brookings Institution, June 1, 2017, https://www.brookings.edu/blog/up-front/2017/06/01/new-evidence-that-lead-exposure-increases-crime/. For a tremendous review of the literature linking crime and violence, see Kevin Drum, "Lead: America's Real Criminal Element," *Mother Jones*, February 11,

2016, https://www.motherjones.com/environment/2016/02/lead-exposure
-gasoline-crime-increase-children-health/.

27. Study authors noted: "We found that lead exposure in the first 6 years of life was positively associated with increased risk for firearm violence perpetration and victimization in early adulthood in a dose-response pattern. Findings were similar when examining the mean or peak blood lead level. Our findings are consistent with prior research reporting links between childhood lead levels and juvenile delinquency and criminal behavior." Lindsay R. Emer, Amy E. Kalkbrenner, Mallory O'Brien, Alice Yan, Ron A. Cisler, and Lance Weinhardt, "Association of Childhood Blood Lead Levels with Firearm Violence Perpetration and Victimization in Milwaukee," *Environmental Research* 180 (October 2019): 3.

28. Cecil et al., "Decreased Brain Volume in Adults with Childhood Lead Exposure." For more information on internal (hormonal) and external (epigenetic or gene-environment interactions) pathways that may explain biological sex differences in the manifestations of brain damage, see Garima Singh, Vikrant Singh, Marissa Sobolewski, Deborah A. Cory-Slechta, and Jay S. Schneider, "Sex-Dependent Effects of Developmental Lead Exposure on the Brain," *Frontiers in Genetics* 9, no. 8 (2018).

29. Michael Pell and Joshua Schneyer, "The Thousands of U.S. Locales Where Lead Poisoning Is Worse Than in Flint," Reuters, December 19, 2016, https://www.reuters.com/investigates/special-report/usa-lead-testing/.

30. Jeremy Hobson, "How Flint's Water Crisis Happened, and Why It Isn't Over," WBUR, July 10, 2018, https://www.wbur.org/hereandnow/2018/07/10/flint-water-crisis-poisoned-city; Mary Spicuzza, "State and County Investigators Have Launched Probes into Troubled Milwaukee Health Department," *Milwaukee Sentinel Journal*, October 25, 2018, https://www.jsonline.com/story/news/politics/2018/10/25/milwaukee-lead-crisis-state-county-investigators-probe-health-agency/1755577002/; John Byrne and Michael Hawthorne, "City Tests Confirm Some Chicago Homes with Water Meters Have Lead in Tap Water," *Chicago Tribune*, November 2, 2018, https://www.chicagotribune.com/news/local/politics/ct-met-rahm-emanuel-lead-pipe-replacement-study-20181101-story.html; Nicole Hudson, "Seeing Inequity: A St. Louis Lead Crisis," Medium, November 29, 2016, https://medium.com/forward-through-ferguson/seeing-inequity-a-st-louis-lead-crisis-1c55dd24d1e1; Rachel Dissell and Brie Zeltner, "Cleveland Lead Poisoning, 2 Year Progress Report: Toxic Neglect," *Cleveland.com*, October 22, 2018, https://www.cleveland.com/healthfit/2017/10/cleveland_lead_poisoning_2_yea.html; Karen Bouffard and Christine MacDonald, "Detroit Kids' Lead Poisoning Rate Higher Than Flint," *Detroit News*, November 14, 2017, https://www.detroitnews.com/story/news/local/detroit-city/2017/11/14/lead-poisoning-children-detroit/107683688/; Lawrence Brown, "Baltimore's Ongoing Lead Poisoning Crisis & the Link to Violent Crime," Medium, September 10, 2018, https://medium.com/@BmoreDoc/baltimores-ongoing-lead-poisoning-crisis-b53870c4a142.

31. Robert J. Simpson and Alix S. Winter, "The Racial Ecology of Lead Poisoning: Toxic Inequality in Chicago Neighborhoods, 1995-2013," *Du Bois Review* (2016): 1-23. As Simpson and Winter concluded: "Lead toxicity is a source of ecological inequity by race and a pathway through which racial inequality literally gets into the body."

32. Trounstine, *Segregation by Design*, 150–155.
33. Emily Benfer, "Contaminated Childhood: The Chronic Lead Poisoning of Low-Income Children and Communities of Color in the United States," *Health Affairs*, August 8, 2017, https://www.healthaffairs.org/do/10.1377/hblog20170808.061398/full/.
34. American Academy of Pediatrics Council on Environmental Health, "Prevention of Childhood Lead Toxicity," *Pediatrics* 138, no. 1 (2016), http://pediatrics.aappublications.org/content/early/2016/06/16/peds.2016-1493.
35. "Strategic Plan to End Childhood Lead Poisoning: A Blueprint for Action," Green & Healthy Homes Initiative, October 2016, http://www.greenandhealthyhomes.org/get-help/lead-action-plans.
36. For discriminatory renting by race, see Leah Binkovitz, "Study: Black Renter Households Pay a Rent Premium," Rice Kinder Institute for Urban Research, September 17, 2018, https://kinder.rice.edu/2018/09/14/study-black-renter-households-pay-rent-premium. For predatory mortgage lending by race, see Ira Goldstein and Dan Urevick-Ackelsberg, *Subprime Lending, Mortgage Foreclosures and Race: How Far Have We Come and How Far Have We to Go?* (n.p.: The Reinvestment Fund, 2007).
37. Unknown Baltimore City employee, "Baltimore, Seventh in Population, Is the Sixteenth City in Point of Land Area," *Baltimore Municipal Journal*, September 14, 1917. In the article, the data showed that Baltimore had a higher density of population per acre than New York, Chicago, Philadelphia, St. Louis, Boston, and all other cities listed. This means that the areas where Black people lived were likely the most densely populated and overcrowded in the nation. See also Emily Lieb, "'Baltimore Does Not Condone Profiteering in Squalor': The Baltimore Plan and the Problem of Housing-Code Enforcement in an American City," *Planning Perspectives* 33, no. 1 (2018): 75–95. On page 82, Lieb writes: "To the Urban League, the main problem was that 20% of the city's population lived in 2% of its housing." This was in 1935–1936. Hence, Black neighborhoods were still disproportionately concentrated in a very small area and in a very small percentage of the city's housing stock. Overcrowding would have been an issue during this time period as well.
38. Eve L. Ewing, *Ghosts in the Schoolyard: Racism and School Closings on Chicago's South Side* (Chicago: University of Chicago Press, 2018), 66–67.
39. Edward Goetz, *New Deal Ruins: Race, Economic Justice, and Public Housing Policy* (Ithaca, NY: Cornell University Press, 2013).
40. Lawrence Brown et al., "The Rise of Anchor Institutions and the Threat to Community Health: Protecting Community Wealth, Building Community Power," *Kalfou* 3, no. 1 (2016): 79–100, 80–81.
41. The Water Taxpayer Protection Act passed the Maryland General Assembly in 2019, making the dispossession of homes over water bills illegal.
42. James Baldwin, "A Report from Occupied Territory," *The Nation*, July 11, 1966.
43. Mark Moran, "Study Exposes Mental Health Effects of Police Shootings on Black Communities," *Psychiatric News*, July 2018, https://psychnews.psychiatryonline.org/doi/full/10.1176/appi.pn.2018.7b3. See also Jacob Bor, Atheendar S. Venkataramani, David R. Williams, and Alexander C. Tsai, "Police Killings and Their Spillover Effects on the Mental Health of Black Americans: A Population-Based, Quasi-Experimental Study," *The Lancet* 392, no. (2018): 302–310.

44. Jenna Wortham, "On Racial Violence: Racism's Psychological Toll," *New York Times Magazine*, June 24, 2015. Interview with Dr. Monnica Williams, psychologist and director of the University of Louisville's Center for Mental Health Disparities.

45. Young Moose and Martina Lynch, "No SunShine," May 19, 2015, YouTube video, 3:09, https://m.youtube.com/watch?v=ggU4toZFVbA.

46. With respect to the impact of exposure to racism on social media, Morgan Maxwell highlights how social media plays a role in exacerbating race-based traumatic stress: "Extensive social media use and increased perceptions of racism among young African American adults may put their psychological and physical health at risk. Moreover, as young African American adults will likely continue to use Facebook and Twitter for years to come, their accumulated perceptions of racism may become riskier for their health as they age. . . . Insofar as both forms of social media, by way of perceived racism, predicted anger expression, results from this study suggest extensive social media use may undermine the cardiovascular health of African Americans adults. Taken together, findings from this study suggest Facebook and Twitter use (via perceptions of racism and associated stress and anticipatory bodily alarm responses) may compromise the health of young African American adults." See Morgan L. Maxwell, "Rage and Social Media Use: The Effect of Social Media on Perceptions of Racism, Stress Appraisal, and Anger Expression among Young African American Adults" (PhD diss., Virginia Commonwealth University, 2016), 117.

47. Brad Smith and Malcolm Holmes, "Police Use of Excessive Force in Minority Communities: A Test of the Minority Threat, Place, and Community Accountability Hypotheses," *Social Problems* 61, no. 1 (2014): 83–104.

48. Michelle Jacobs, "The Violent State: Black Women's Invisible Struggle against Police Violence," *William and Mary Journal of Women and the Law* 24, no. 39 (2017): 39–100.

49. Harper Jean Tobin, Raffi Freedman-Gurspan, and Lisa Mottet, *A Blueprint for Equality: A Federal Agenda for Transgender People* (Washington, DC: National Center for Transgender Equality, June 2015), 25. "Unfortunately, law enforcement is as often a part of the problem as it is part of the solution. Half of transgender people report they are uncomfortable seeking police assistance. More than one-fifth (22%) of transgender people who had interacted with police reported police harassment, and 6% of transgender individuals reported that they experienced bias-motivated assault by officers. Black transgender people reported much higher rates of biased harassment and assault (38% and 15%)."

50. Marisela Gomez, "Policing, Community Fragmentation, and Public Health: Observations from Baltimore," *Journal of Urban Health* 93, no. Suppl 1 (April 2016): 154–167.

51. Nancy Krieger, Jarvis Chen, Pamela Waterman, Mathew Kiang, and Justin Feldman, "Police Killings and Police Deaths Are Public Health Data and Can Be Counted," *PLoS Medicine* 12, no. 12 (2015): e1001915.

52. Tanya Sharpe argues: "Grieving African American survivors of homicide victims, community violence and state sanctioned police violence often find themselves taking bold risks in their efforts to cope with such tragedies. In this context, the audacity to grieve is often actualized in the form of political

protests, anger and disillusionment in systems responsible for the provision of legal, mental and medical care services. The tragic irony is that for African Americans, the audacity to be fearless as one grieves, courageous as one grieves, and yes, angry as one grieves is not often met with the same level of support and understanding as we have seen displayed for other populations." Sharpe, "The Audacity to Grieve: African American Experiences of Coping with Violence," Exit-Wounds, May 2, 2018, https://exit-wounds-tsharpe .weebly.com/exit-wounds/may-02nd-2018.

53. Rob Nixon, *Slow Violence and the Environmentalism of the Poor* (Cambridge, MA: Harvard University Press, 2013).

54. Dana E. Goin, Kara Rudolph, and Jennifer Ahern, "Predictors of Firearm Violence in Urban Communities: A Machine-Learning Approach," *Health and Place* 51 (2018): 61–67.

55. Gregor Aisch, Eric Buth, Matthew Bloch, Amanda Cox, and Kevin Quealy, "The Best and Worst Places to Grow Up: How Your Area Compares," *New York Times*, May 4, 2015, https://www.nytimes.com/interactive/2015/05/03 /upshot/the-best-and-worst-places-to-grow-up-how-your-area-compares .html. See also Zenthia Prince, "Baltimore Ranks Lowest in Upward Mobility for Poor Boys," *The Afro-American*, August 29, 2016, https://www.afro.com /baltimore-ranks-lowest-in-upward-mobility-for-poor-boys/.

56. The Economist Data Team, "Murder Rates in 50 American Cities," *The Economist*, February 7, 2017, https://www.economist.com/graphic-detail /2017/02/07/murder-rates-in-50-american-cities.

57. Douglass Massey and Jonathan Tannen, "A Research Note on Trends in Black Hypersegregation," *Demography* 52, no. 3 (2015): 1025–1034.

58. David McFadden, "FBI: Baltimore Homicide Rate Topped US Big Cities in 2017," Associated Press News, September 25, 2018, https://www.apnews .com/4ddfc91a71ce4a3099083a8d3c2158ad.

59. Samuel Sinyangwe, DeRay Mckesson, and Brittany Packyetti, "Mapping Police Violence," Campaign Zero, 2018, https://mappingpoliceviolence.org /cities.

60. Regarding their research, Siegel et al. write: "Our finding that racial segrega- tion is a strong predictor of the Black-White disparity in fatal police shootings is consistent with the minority threat hypothesis, which holds that police officers view neighborhoods that are highly segregated—that is predomi- nantly occupied by Black residents—as being inherently more threaten- ing. . . . The problem of fatal police shootings has typically been viewed at the individual level; interventions such as inherent bias training aim to alter the way police officers interact with Black individuals. Our research suggests that what is needed is training that changes the way police interact with Black neighborhoods." Michael Siegel, Rebecca Sherman, Cindy Li, and Anita Knopov, "The Relationship between Racial Residential Segregation and Black-White Disparities in Fatal Police Shootings at the City Level, 2013–2017," *Journal of the National Medical Association* 111, no. 6 (2019): 580–587, 6.

61. Young Moose and Lynch, "No SunShine." With respect to the use of n—s by Martina Lynch in "No SunShine," scholar Robin D. G. Kelley argues that "above all, 'Nigga' speaks to a collective identity shaped by class conscious- ness, the character of inner-city space, police repression, poverty, and the constant threat of intracranial violence fed by a dying economy. . . . In fact,

'Nigga' is frequently employed to distinguish urban black working-class males from the black bourgeoisie and African Americans in positions of institutional authority." See Robin D. G. Kelley, "Kickin' Reality, Kickin' Ballistics: Gangsta Rap and Postindustrial Los Angeles," in *Droppin' Science: Critical Essays on Rap Music and Hip Hop Culture*, ed. William Eric Perkins (Philadelphia: Temple University Press, 1996).

62. Peter Levy, *The Great Uprising: Race Riots in Urban America during the 1960s* (Cambridge: Cambridge University Press, 2017), 9.

63. Walter Rucker and James Nathaniel Upton, *Encyclopedia of American Race Riots* (Westport, CT: Greenwood Press, 2007). Rucker and Upton go on to argue: "For the most part, rioters from the 1960s onward struck police and property without taking life or destroying public service buildings. They revealed a commonality of purpose: rejecting the system's legitimacy without endeavoring to overthrow its government. Spontaneous and largely unorganized, black rioters considered their actions justifiable challenge to white racial views and official policies. They spoke for themselves and stimulated federal programs, serving as momentary change agents and extensions of the civil rights struggle."

64. Levy, *The Great Uprising*, 11.

65. In his dissertation, Corey Henderson interviewed Black elders in Baltimore who discussed their experiences during segregation. Some themes that emerged were "making do" (with few resources), sticking together, and ample presence of mentors modeling positive behaviors, particularly around work habits and obtaining an education. There was a sense of ascendancy—that the community was "moving on up." But between 1950 and 2000, Baltimore would lose 100,000 manufacturing jobs. This would lead to the decimation of well-paying jobs especially for folks with lower levels of education. The rise of manufacturing companies going out of business or moving out of the city (to the suburbs or overseas) meant that Black neighborhoods would be left without the types of economic opportunity that existed at the time. This hit Black men especially hard as many manufacturing jobs were worked by men at the time. Therefore, the severance of communal bonds was exacerbated by the increased inability to "make do" (with jobs leaving the city), the increased difficulty to stick together (in the face of rapid and repeated uprootings), and a decline in work modeling as labor prospects disappear. Repeated uprootings accelerated while economic opportunity was drying up during 1950s–2000s and this contributed to the destruction of Black neighborhoods. His model of historical trauma also postulates that there is decreased transmission of history and memory that happens alongside increased lost connections with so much migration, displacement, and diffusion. Henderson, "The Reverberating Influence of Historical Trauma on the Health of African Americans in Baltimore City" (PhD diss., Morgan State University, 2017), 114. Sonya Douglass Horsford made similar comments with respect to Black public schools before desegregation. She writes: "There was 'shared participation' among educators, parents, and community members, and the school was embedded within and interdependent with the Black community. These bonds existed between the schools and their communities as well as among the schools' students, teachers, and principals. In fact, much of the research literature on all-Black schools captures the communal bonds,

collective work, and caring that characterize the type of safe, supportive, learning environment that many Negro students enjoyed pre-*Brown*." Horsford, *Learning in a Burning House: Educational Inequality, Ideology, and (Dis)integration* (New York: Teachers College Press, 2011), 37.

66. Gady A. Epstein and Eric Siegal, "City, Hopkins Weigh Plan for East-Side Development," *Baltimore Sun*, January 11, 2001. The article discusses several community leaders stating that they were not informed about the City-Hopkins planned redevelopment initiative and quotes Lucille Gorham who was by this time the president of the Middle East Community Organization. Glenn Ross, head of the McElderry Park Community Association told the *Sun*: "We were really upset that a lot of us didn't know about it and had no idea what was going on. Here's a big plan coming down and the people don't have a clue what's going on." See also Melody Simmons and Joan Jacobson, "Too Big to Fail: A Dream Derailed," *The Daily Record* 122, no. 82 (2011): 11A.

67. Epstein and Siegal, "City, Hopkins Weigh Plan."

68. Jacques Kelly, "Lucille Gorham, Neighborhood Activist," *Baltimore Sun*, November 7, 2012.

69. Kelly, "Lucille Gorham."

70. The Claim for Replacement Housing document was signed by Lucille Gorham and by EBDI's Arlene Conn.

71. Melody Simmons, "Activist's Children Fear Foreclosure of Her Home," *Maryland Daily Record*, 2013, https://thedailyrecord.com/2013/04/29/activists-children-fear-foreclosure-of-her-home/.

Track 6. Make Black Neighborhoods Matter

1. As Jason Harris argues: "We find many of our communities in this state now, school under-funded and understaffed, infrastructure for neighborhoods (roads, waste and water lines, electrical lines) in disrepair or in peril at the slightest storm. A neighborhood that can only count on a gas station for grocery staples exists in an exigent state. A school where students and staff cannot use the water fountains because the plumbing supplying the water is in an exigent state. While the corporate community has plans such as the 'Vision 2030' plan, they do not take into account the day to day issues facing our communities." Harris, *Redlines: Baltimore 2028—an Anthology of Speculative Fiction* (Baltimore: Redlines Publishing, 2012), v.

2. Wangari Maathai, *The Challenge for Africa* (New York: Anchor Books, 2010), 133–139. For neighborhood-based decision making, I draw inspiration from Maathai's model practiced in Kenya as described in her book. She describes neighborhood councils of 15 people that are elected by a community to make decisions for the area in question.

3. In a ROAR article entitled "Municipalism and the Feminization of Politics," Laura Roth and Kate Shea Baird describe a political organizing methodology called municipalism. Roth and Baird describe what I see as essential components of deeply democratic decision-making structures in communities: "Municipalism, as we understand it, is defined by a set of related characteristics. First, by the construction of a distinctive political organization that reflects the diversity of the local political landscape and responds to local issues and circumstances. Second, by open and participatory decision-making processes that harness the collective intelligence of the

community. Third, by an organizational structure that is relatively horizontal (for example, based on neighborhood assemblies) and that guides the work of elected representatives. Fourth, by a creative tension between those inside and outside of local institutions: municipalism understands that the capacity for institutional action depends on strong, organized movements in the streets that push elected leaders. For this reason, the movement welcomes pressure from outside the institutions and seeks to open up genuinely democratic decision-making mechanisms within them." Their first and second components can be achieved through Maathai's neighborhood council approach. The neighborhood council could hold neighborhood assemblies to broaden the conversations and increase community participation in community development. Neighborhood assemblies should be held frequently—perhaps bimonthly or quarterly—to ensure residents are included at every step of decision making. The fourth component depends on government officials also including advocates for social justice and racial equity in policy discussions, formulation, and implementation. I call this hybrid model the Maathian feminist municipalist approach to community empowerment and community economic development. See Roth and Baird, "Municipalism and the Feminization of Politics," *ROAR*, no. 6 (September 2017). Web link: https://roarmag.org /magazine/municipalism-feminization-urban-politics/.

4. Baltimore City Public Schools, "Restorative Practices," Baltimore City Public School System, 2018, http://www.baltimorecityschools.org /restorativepractices. See also Baltimore City Public Schools, *Financial Recovery Plan*, August 1, 2017, Baltimore City Public School System, Appendix A (Board Approved School Closures, 2004-2005 to 2017-2018). Finally, see Liz Bowie and Erika Niedowski, "City Board Acts to Shut Nine Schools," *Baltimore Sun*, March 14, 2001, http://articles.baltimoresun.com/2001-03 -14/news/0103140291_1_school-board-lafayette-elementary-school-year.

5. Teachers' Democracy Project, "The Decline in Black Teachers," 2016, http://www.tdpbaltimore.org/teachers/.

6. Luke Broadwater, "Baltimore's Quick Economic Growth Contributes to Loss in State Aid to Schools," *Baltimore Sun*, February 2, 2016, http://www .baltimoresun.com/news/maryland/baltimore-city/bs-md-ci-school-funds -20160208-story.html.

7. This loophole was not closed until 2018 due to legislation signed by Governor Larry Hogan. However, legislation by then Delegate Mary Washington's bill would have resulted in an immediate fix, whereas Hogan's legislation requires a delay of four years until the additional funds are fully allocated to public schools. This does not even cover the fact that gambling disproportionately results in money from lower-income populations being used to fund education as opposed to using more money from wealthier entities and individuals.

8. "City Schools' Deep Freeze," editorial, *Baltimore Sun*, January 4, 2018, http://www.baltimoresun.com/news/opinion/editorial/bs-ed-0105-city -schools-20180104-story.html.

9. Tyler Tynes, "Baltimore Schools Have Returned Millions in State Funds for Heating Repairs," *Baltimore Sun*, January 4, 2018, http://www.baltimoresun .com/news/maryland/education/bs-md-ci-schools-money-returned -20180104-story.html. According to Tynes: "Since 2009, Baltimore city

schools have lost around $66 million in state funding for repairs, according to the *Baltimore Sun*. Approved projects were more expensive than assumed. Repairs took too long. And any money allocated for new heating systems vanished overnight. The Maryland Public School Construction Program listed Baltimore City as only having 17 percent of its schools in 'good' condition. A 2012 Jacobs Report revealed that only 3 percent of the district's 18.5 million square footage was built within the last 25 years, 74 percent . . . was built between 1946 and 1985."

10. In terms of school choice, specialized programs that boost access to the city's elite high schools are mostly found in White L communities, giving rise to an increased opportunity for White students to be admitted into the elite schools. See Melissa Schober, "The Dirty Secret in the Data: Equity in Baltimore Schools Is a Long Way Off," *Baltimore Brew*, March 3, 2019, https://www.baltimorebrew.com/2019/03/27/the-dirty-secret-in-the-data-equity-in-baltimore-schools-is-a-long-way-off/.

11. American Civil Liberties Union (ACLU), "ACLU of Maryland Applauds Education Funding Increase; Calls It Important Step toward Educational Adequacy for Schoolchildren," ACLU, May 6, 2002, https://www.aclu.org/news/aclu-maryland-applauds-education-funding-increase-calls-it-important-step-toward-educational.

12. Molly Rath, "100 Years: The State Takes Over City Schools," *Baltimore Magazine*, 2007, http://www.baltimoremagazine.net/old-site/features/2007/08/100-years-the-state-takes-over-city-schools.

13. Maryland ACLU and NAACP Legal Defense Fund (LDF), "Letter to Governor Hogan Regarding *Bradford v. Maryland State Board of Education* Lawsuit," Maryland ACLU and NAACP LDF, January 22, 2019.

14. This study was led by Stephanie Smith. See Oscar Perry Abello, "Baltimore Reckons with Its Legacy of Redlining," Next City, November 22, 2017, https://nextcity.org/daily/entry/baltimore-reckons-legacy-redlining.

15. Sonya Douglass Horsford, *Learning in a Burning House: Educational Inequality, Ideology, and (Dis)integration* (New York: Teachers College Press, 2011), 6.

16. Racial Equity Block Grants (REBGs) should be based on an algorithm with following criteria:

- school hypersegregation status—extra funding at 70%, 80%, 90%, 95%, and 99% Black student population
- percentage of children poisoned by toxic lead and rate of lead paint violations in neighborhood where the school is located
- violent crime rate in the community statistical area (as an indicator for the amount of trauma or PTSD that is likely to affect children in the school)
- neighborhood bank redlining (as measured by 1937 Residential Security Map) and recent redlining (measured by NCRC data)
- number of permanent school closures in the community statistical area or neighborhood
- median annual household income below $35,000 among families of students attending the school
- the percentage of students, teachers, and administrators enrolled in the school that have experienced a school closure (schools with higher percentages should receive more funding)

17. This should include funding to completely replace lead pipes or other infrastructure that exposes children to toxic lead in city schools.

18. Bettina Love cuts to the heart of the matter regarding curriculum, testing, and teaching strategies: "Education is crowded with studies that acknowledge dark children's pain but never the source of their pain, the legacy that pain has left, or how that pain can be healed. I have seen professional development sessions titled 'The Crisis in Black Education,' 'The Problem with Black Boys,' and 'Addressing a Poverty Mindset.' These types of workshops White-Splain Black folx' challenges to White folx but rarely discuss the topics of redlining, housing discrimination, White flight, gentrification, police brutality, racial health disparities, and high employment. . . . Teaching strategies and education reform models must offer more than educational survival tactics to dark children—test-taking skills, acronyms, character education, No Child Left Behind, Race to the Top, charter schools, school choice. They need to be rooted in an abolitionist praxis that, with urgency, embraces what seems impossible: education for collective dignity and human power for justice." Love, *We Want to Do More Than Survive: Abolitionist Teaching and the Pursuit of Educational Freedom* (Boston: Beacon Press, 2019), 13.

19. Baltimore City Public Schools, "Members of the Board. Baltimore City Public Schools," 2018, http://www.baltimorecityschools.org//site/Default .aspx?PageID=24788. See also Talia Richman, "Mayor Pugh Appoints Two to Baltimore School Board," *Baltimore Sun*, January 11, 2018, http://www .baltimoresun.com/news/maryland/education/k-12/bs-md-ci-school-board -appointments-20180109-story.html. From 1997 to 2017, all Baltimore City Public Schools board members or commissioners were jointly selected by the mayor of Baltimore and the governor of Maryland. In 2018, Mayor Pugh solely appointed two new board commissioners. Starting in 2022, two board members will be elected. But seven commissioner seats will still be filled by appointees. In other words, until 2022, Baltimore City voters do not have a direct democratic vote on who serves as board commissioners for Baltimore City Public Schools.

20. See appendix E for BMORE Caucus's statement regarding how Baltimore City Public Schools can institute racial equity.

21. "Through this policy, City Schools owns its role in creating and implement- ing policies and practices that result in predictably lower academic and graduation outcomes and disproportionate action, for students of color than for their white peers. . . . Rather than continuing to perpetuate and contribute to institutional racism, Baltimore City Schools must move to disrupt and dismantle it in every area of our work. Our Board, school-based staff, and office-based staff will work together to aggressively and efficiently eliminate inequitable practices, systems, and structures that create advantages for some students and families while disadvantaging others. We will allocate resources to replace those inequitable practices, systems, and structures with new ones to ensure that we provide racially equitable education and environments to children and families of color." Baltimore City Public Schools System, "Equity," draft, Baltimore City Board of School Commissioners, April 16, 2019, 1.

22. Baltimore Urban Renewal and Housing Agency (BURHA), "It's Happening in Baltimore!," 1955, BURHA, Maryland Department, Enoch Pratt Central

Library. According to BURHA, the following agencies were combined: "The Housing Authority of Baltimore City (HABC), the Baltimore Redevelopment Commission, the Housing Bureau of the Health Department, the Neighborhood Planning unit of the Department of Planning, and the Area Projects formerly attached to the Department of Public Welfare" (3).

23. The Baltimore Department of Housing and Community Development, "Residential Displacement: 1951–1971 Activity Analysis," Planning Division of the Department of Housing and Community Development, 1972. Located in the Thompson v. HUD Files, Exhibit Number 173, Case Number MJG 95-309, University of Baltimore, Langsdale Library, Special Collections. Both DHCD and HABC were under one commissioner until 2017 when Mayor Catherine Pugh decoupled the two agencies. Additionally, displacement due to urban renewal, new public housing, new public improvements (schools and libraries), and highway construction were counted in the BURHA/DHCD report. Of the 1.9-mile stretch of highway built in West Baltimore through Harlem Park, historian Raymond Mohl noted: "It sent an inner-city Black community into rapid decline and still serves as a reminder of the huge social costs of the Interstate era." See Raymond Mohl, *Interstate: Highway Politics and Policy since 1939*, 3rd ed. (Knoxville: University of Tennessee Press, 2012), 132.

24. Luke Broadwater, "Baltimore Mayor Pugh to Launch New Neighborhood Investment Fund with $55M from Garage Leases," *Baltimore Sun*, May 2, 2018, https://www.baltimoresun.com/news/maryland/politics/bs-md-ci-neighborhood-impact-fund-20180501-story.html. See also Jayne Miller (@jemillerwbal), "@MayorPugh Announces $55 Mil Neighborhood Impact Investment Fund" Twitter, May 2, 2018, 7:05 a.m.

25. Luke Broadwater, "Baltimore Mayor Pugh to Launch New Neighborhood Investment Fund with $55M from Garage Leases," *Baltimore Sun*, May 2, 2018, https:///www.baltimoresun.com/news/maryland/politics/bs-md-ci-neighborhood-impact-fund-20180501-story,amp.html. As Broadwater writes: "The nonprofit's goals would be to invest in a variety of real estate projects, including those offering affordable housing, market-rate housing and smaller commercial developments. Investments located within new federally approved Opportunity Zones also could flow through the nonprofit, city officials said." In terms of outsiders benefiting, Opportunity Zones are designed to attract investors from across the nation to "invest" in lower-income urban areas.

26. Community enterprises can include community land trusts (for deeply affordable housing and community gardens), cooperatives (for collective economic development and addresses community needs), community investment trusts, public banks, universal municipal health care, or other type of structures designed democratize decision making and boost community wealth.

27. Notable Project CORE awardees include EBDI for a townhomes preparation project in "Eager Park" (the name of the community named by Lucille Gorham as Middle East was changed to Eager Park), Mount Royal CDC for the $100 million Innovation Village project in Reservoir Hill, and TRF Development Partners (now renamed) for development and vacant rehabilitation work in Oliver. Each of these projects benefits corporate developers and helps facilitate the influx of a wealthier and whiter demographic to move in.

As discussed previously, gentrification is not the private market operating randomly; it is often subsidized by public dollars.

28. Enterprise Zone information found in the TIF applications for both developments: Harbor Point TIF application (page 11) and Port Covington TIF application (page 32).

29. Mark Reutter, "Citizens Are Starting to Question Harbor Point TIF Subsidies," *Baltimore Brew*, August 3, 2013, https://www.baltimorebrew.com/2013/08/03/citizens-are-starting-to-question-harbor-point-tif-subsidies/; Natalie Sherman, "17 Things to Know about the Port Covington TIF," *Baltimore Sun*, April 29, 2016, https://www.baltimoresun.com/business/bs-bz-things-to-know-about-port-covington-20160429-story.html.

30. Robert Rehrmann, Matthew Bennett, Benjamin Blank, Mya Coover, Mindy McConville, Heather Ruby, and Michael Sanelli, *Evaluation of the Enterprise Zone Tax Credit* (Annapolis: Maryland Department of Legislative Services, Office of Policy Analysis, August 2014). According to the Department of Legislative Services, "While Enterprise Zone tax credits may incentivize some businesses to create additional jobs within enterprise zones, the tax credit is not effective in providing employment to zone residents that are chronically unemployed and/or live in poverty. A number of factors contribute to this problem, including skills mismatches for new jobs created, lower than average educational attainment levels of zone residents, and labor mobility. As such, improved educational opportunities and/or additional job training programs for residents may be more effective in enabling those residents to better compete for jobs created in enterprise zones" (vii).

31. Timothy Weaver, "The Problem with Opportunity Zones," CityLab, May 16, 2018, https://www.citylab.com/equity/2018/05/the-problem-with-opportunity-zones/560510/. Weaver writes: "Sadly, these policies almost inevitably result in tax giveaways for investment that would have occurred anyway, as we're beginning to see with opportunity zones. Under such circumstances, displacement from gentrification and rising profits for corporate developers are the likely result." See also Samuel Stein, *Capital City: Gentrification and the Real Estate State* (London: Verso, 2019), 154. Especially enchanting is Stein's discussion of Donald Trump as "The Developer President" in chapter 4, pages 116–155.

32. Jeff Ernsthausen and Justin Elliott, "One Trump Tax Cut Was Meant to Help the Poor. A Billionaire Ended Up Winning Big," ProPublica, June 19, 2019, https://www.propublica.org/article/trump-inc-podcast-one-trump-tax-cut-meant-to-help-the-poor-a-billionaire-ended-up-winning-big.

33. "Instead, billions of untaxed investment profits are beginning to pour into high-end apartment buildings and hotels, storage facilities that employ only a handful of workers, and student housing in bustling college towns, among other projects. Many of the projects that will enjoy special tax status were underway long before the opportunity-zone provision was enacted. Financial institutions are boasting about the tax savings that await those who invest in real estate in affluent neighborhoods." Jesse Drucker and Eric Lipton, "How a Trump Tax Break to Help Poor Communities Became a Windfall for the Rich," *New York Times*, August 31, 2019, https://www.nytimes.com/2019/08/31/business/the-trump-associates-benefiting-from-a-tax-break-for-poor-communities.html. See also David Yaffe-Bellany, "The Trump Associates

Benefiting from a Tax Break for Poor Communities," *New York Times*, August 31, 2019, https://www.nytimes.com/2019/08/31/business/the-trump -associates-benefiting-from-a-tax-break-for-poor-communities.html.

34. Marjorie Kelly and Sarah McKinley, *Cities Building Community Wealth* (Democracy Collaborative, November 2015). See also Democracy Collabora- tive, "Elements of the Democratic Economy," Democracy Collaborative, August 18, 2018, https://thenextsystem.org/elements.

35. Jessica Gordon Nembhard, *Collective Courage: A History of African American Cooperative Economic Thought and Practice* (University Park: Pennsylvania State University Press, 2014). Nembhard detailed the myriad ways that Black people have used collective economic approaches in her book.

36. Baltimore Black Worker Center, *The State of Black Workers in Baltimore* (Baltimore: Baltimore Black Worker Center, 2018), https:// bmoreblackworkercenter.org/our-report/. The worker center argues: "Black communities are facing a dual job crisis of unemployment and lack of quality jobs. Equity and justice require addressing various forms of oppres- sions and how they affect Black workers. Real change for Black workers will only come from Black workers building power together through organizing, demanding justice, and transforming the current racist, capitalist, and patriarchal systems that govern our world." Their nine strategies are (1) make Black neighborhoods matter in city economic development policy, (2) place Black health and well-being at the center of policy decisions, (3) invest in public sector jobs—resist attempts to privatize existing public sector jobs, (4) expand opportunities for Black workers at large private institutions and businesses, (5) support unionization—provide a boost to wages and benefits for Black workers, (6) invest in transit equity to connect Black workers to city and regional jobs, (7) capitalize businesses that hire Black workers, especially in Black neighborhoods, (8) increase economic democracy and Black-owned community enterprises, and (9) eliminate discrimination in all forms of enforcing civil and human rights of Black workers.

37. These tools and strategies include TIFs, PILOTs, NIIF, Opportunity Zones, GO bonds, and general tax breaks.

38. Just two examples of community gardens in South Baltimore are the Filbert Street Community Garden in Curtis Bay and the Black Yield Institute in Cherry Hill.

39. National Community Reinvestment Coalition (NCRC), *Home Mortgage and Small Business Lending in Baltimore and Surrounding Areas* (Washington, DC: NCRC, November 2015), https://ncrc.org/wp-content/uploads/2015/11 /ncrc_baltimore_lending_analysis_web.pdf.

40. Democracy Collaborative, "The Cleveland Model—How the Evergreen Cooperatives are Building Community Wealth," Democracy Collaborative 2018, https://community-wealth.org/content/cleveland-model-how -evergreen-cooperatives-are-building-community-wealth/.

41. Evergreen Cooperative Corporation, "We Couldn't Do It without Our Anchor Partners," Evergreen Cooperatives, 2016, http://www.evgoh.com.

42. Mercy Corps Northwest, "Community Investment Trust," Mercy Corps Northwest, 2018, https://www.mercycorpsnw.org/community/investment -trust/. See also Kevin Johnson, "REITs for Good: Nonprofit Turns High- Dollar Investment Tool Upside-Down," *Nonprofit Quarterly*, June 6, 2017,

https://nonprofitquarterly.org/2017/06/06/reits-good-nonprofit-turns-high-dollar-investment-tool-upside/.

43. This number is derived from the roughly 6,000–7,000 rental evictions per year and the roughly 3,000–4,000 mortgage foreclosures per year. Melody Simmons, "Maryland Leads the U.S. in Foreclosure Filings for the Second Consecutive Month," *Baltimore Business Journal*, December 9, 2015." See also Doug Donovan and Jean Marbella, "Dismissed: Tenants Lose, Landlords Win in Baltimore's Rent Court," *Baltimore Sun*, August 26, 2017; Baltimore Neighborhood Indicator Alliance (BNIA), "Baltimore City Foreclosure Filings," BNIA, 2011, http://www.ubalt.edu/foreclosures/index.cfm.

44. Dawn Phillips, Robbie Clark, Tammy Lee, and Alexandra Desautels, *Rebuilding Neighborhoods, Restoring Health: A Report on the Impacts of Foreclosures on Public Health* (Oakland, CA: Causa Just :: Just Causa and the Alameda County Public Health Department, 2010), http://www.acphd.org/media/53643/foreclose2.pdf.

45. Matt Hill, "Our Budget Our Values, Part 1: Spending Priorities and 20/20," Baltimore Housing Roundtable, November 8, 2017, https://www.baltimorehousingroundtable.org/publications. The Baltimore Housing Roundtable would later change its name to the Fair Development Roundtable.

46. Baynard Woods, "Battle for Tubman House: Baltimore Residents Rally for Community Center," *The Guardian*, April 23, 2016, https://www.theguardian.com/us-news/2016/apr/23/freddie-gray-baltimore-harriet-tubman-house-community.

47. Marjoleine Kars, "Maroons and Marronage," *Oxford Bibliographies*, May 2016, http://www.oxfordbibliographies.com/view/document/obo-9780199730414/obo-9780199730414-0229.xml.

48. Michael Yockel, "Small Wonder," *Baltimore Style*, March 23, 2017, https://civicworks.com/small-wonder/. See also Haniya Rae, "Tiny Homes Are Baby Steps toward Reversing the Housing Crisis," CityLab, July 14, 2017, https://www.citylab.com/equity/2017/07/tiny-houses-are-baby-steps-toward-reducing-blight/533736/.

49. Smalltimore Homes, "An Affordable Housing Initiative: Smalltimore Homes," Smalltimore Homes.org, 2018, https://www.smalltimorehomes.org/.

50. Jing Li and Richard Clinch, "Analysis of Patterns of Employment by Race in Baltimore City and the Baltimore Metropolitan Area," Associated Black Charities, February 2018, http://www.abc-md.org/reports/.

51. Doug Donovan and Jean Marbella, "Dismissed: Tenants Lose, Landlords Win in Baltimore's Rent Court," *Baltimore Sun*, August 26, 2017.

52. Lawrence Lanahan, *The Lines between Us: Two Families and a Quest to Cross Baltimore's Racial Divide* (New York: New Press, 2019), 288. See quote by Lawrence Brown.

53. Samuel Roberts, *Infectious Fear: Politics, Disease, and the Health Effects of Segregation* (Chapel Hill: University of North Carolina Press, 2009), 170.

54. Staff writer, "To Aid 90,000 Negroes Mayor Is Authorized to Name Housing Committee—Suburban Colony Proposed," *Baltimore Sun*, February 24, 1917.

55. Staff writer, "New Segregation Plan: Mayor Begins Work of Securing a Special Ordinance," *Baltimore Sun*, July 2, 1918. Commissioner Black is shown offering at least tepid opposition to Mayor Preston in the article, but not based on the issue of the fairness of Mayor Preston's plan. Instead he opposed it

based on its perceived ability to be effective. Assistant Commissioner Howard, on the other hand, usually worked in tandem with Mayor Preston. See Special correspondent, "Races Confer in Baltimore: Mayor and Prominent White Citizens Meet Representative Colored Men," *New York Age*, March 30, 1918.

56. Staff writer, "Site for City Hospital Tentatively Selected," *Baltimore Sun*, March 18, 1921.

57. Corey Henderson, "The Reverberating Influence of Historical Trauma on the Health of African Americans in Baltimore City" (PhD diss., Morgan State University, 2017), 34.

58. Luke Broadwater, "Advocates Say Lead Paint Industry Should Be Held Liable in Poisoning of Baltimore Children," *Baltimore Sun*, February 27, 2016.

59. Baltimore City Department of Health, *One Hundred and Forty-Ninth Annual Report of the Department of Health, 1963* (City of Baltimore, 1964), 17.

60. Anne Barry-Jester, "Baltimore's Toxic Legacy of Lead Paint," FiveThirtyEight, May 7, 2015, https://fivethirtyeight.com/features/baltimores-toxic-legacy-of-lead-paint/.

61. Lawrence Brown, "Baltimore's Ongoing Lead Poisoning Crisis & the Link to Violent Crime," Medium, September 18, 2018, https://link.medium.com/QDSwzxaq60.

62. As Malcolm Rio argued: "Baltimore's streetcars also helped marginalized communities better connect to their spaces of labor. The commitment to public transit infrastructure that enabled more egalitarian mobility began to erode in 1948 when the automotive cartel, National City Lines (NCL), purchased Baltimore's streetcar system. Stoerkel and Tamminen point out that under the governance of General Motors, Firestone Tires, Standard Oil, and other automotive corporations, NCL swiftly uprooted the city's streetcar infrastructure in a deliberate attempt to monopolize the sale of buses. The turn away from integrated mass transit intensified with the Great Migration of African-Americans from the South, which further spurred white flight, suburbanization, and automobile dependence." Rio, "Black Mobility Matters: An Exploratory Study of Uber, Hacking, and the Commons in Baltimore," *Architecture, Media, Politics, Society*, 10, no. 4 (2016): 6.

63. Mallory Sofastaii, "Twenty Bike Share Stations in Baltimore to Open on Oct. 28," WMAR Baltimore, October 27, 2016, https://www.wmar2news.com/news/region/baltimore-city/twenty-bike-share-stations-in-baltimore-to-open-on-october-28. See also David Dudley, "Enlisting Bikes in the Fight against Inequality," CityLab, December 2016, https://www.citylab.com/transportation/2016/12/enlisting-bikes-in-the-fight-against-inequality/511088/.

64. Andrew Zaleski, "A $9 Billion Highway That Promises to Pay for Itself," CityLab, September 26, 2017, https://www.citylab.com/transportation/2017/09/a-9-billion-highway-that-promises-to-pay-for-itself/541119/.

65. Rob Thubron, "China Unveils Electric Road Train That Runs on Painted 'Tracks,'" Techspot, June 6, 2017, https://www.techspot.com/news/69593-china-unveils-electric-road-train-runs-painted-tracks.html.

66. Oscar Perry Abello, "Baltimore Reckons with Its Legacy of Redlining," Next City, November 22, 2017, https://nextcity.org/daily/entry/baltimore-reckons-legacy-redlining.

67. Ian Duncan, "Study Finds Deep Racial Disparities in Way Baltimore Allocates Public Construction Dollars," *Baltimore Sun*, December 12, 2017,

http://www.baltimoresun.com/news/maryland/baltimore-city/bs-md-ci
-capital-budget-race-inequality-20171211-story.html.

68. In fact, Jessica Trounstine cogently argues in *Segregation by Design* that racial-spatial inequity in municipal funding for public goods is one of the great harms of racial segregation. During the early and mid-1900s, disproportion- ately more public dollars from capital budgets were allocated to wealthier White neighborhoods while Black neighborhoods were denied critical municipal funds. Trounstine, *Segregation by Design: Local Politics and Inequality in American Cities* (Cambridge: Cambridge University Press, 2018), 1–3, 23–40.

69. Jayne Miller, "I-Team Raises New Questions about Accuracy, Reliability of Baltimore Water Bills," WBAL-TV, October 22, 2019, https://www.wbaltv.com /article/i-team-questions-accuracy-reliability-baltimore-water-bills/29550555.

70. Mark Reutter, "Special 'Garbage Day' at Cross Keys Costs the City $100,000," *Baltimore Brew*, November 26, 2019, https://www .baltimorebrew.com/2019/11/26/special-garbage-day-at-cross-keys-cost-the -city-100000/.

71. "For instance, residents of Patterson Park in the southeastern section made 580 requests for a cleanup in the period analyzed by *The Sun*. All were completed on time, according to the database. This section of the city is home to several predominantly white, wealthier neighborhoods like Fells Point and Canton, though there are large swaths of the quadrant that are more racially and economically diverse, including areas of deep poverty. Residents of Carrollton Ridge, a much poorer community dotted with vacant houses, made 320 calls in the first 10 months of the year. Just 5% were answered on time. The southwest- ern section includes many predominantly black neighborhoods, including Harlem Park and Cherry Hill." Talia Richman and Christine Zhang, "Call 311 for a Dirty Alley in Baltimore? City's Response Depends on Where You Live," *Baltimore Sun*, December 11, 2019, https://www.baltimoresun.com/politics/bs -md-pol-311-response-20191211-ogy5qp5vkbdox04cmz73zvpvvi-story.html.

72. These aforementioned instances of structural advantage for White L communi- ties shed light on how benefits accrue in wealthier and demographically whiter neighborhoods. Interestingly, in each of the three instances above, no culprit is named or identified by media outlets as the source for the inequity. No one will be punished or sent to jail due to these infractions. Structurally advantaging wealthy communities is rarely viewed as a criminal offense although such actions are tantamount to robbing redlined Black neighborhoods of crucial resources. But in each instance, it is likely that someone in White L communi- ties relied on personal connections with people they know in DPW or someone in DPW made arrangements to not bill Ritz Carlton condominium owners for nearly 10 years (and no one double checked to catch the error).

73. Lawrence Brown, "Community Health and Baltimore Apartheid: Revisiting Development, Inequality, and Tax Policy," in *Baltimore Revisited: Stories of Inequality and Resistance in a U.S. City*, ed. P. Nicole King, Kate Drabinski, and Joshua Clark Davis, chap. 6 (New Brunswick, NJ: Rutgers University Press, 2019).

74. Faith Tandoc, "The Great Debate: Financing Harbor Point," Citizens Planning and Housing Association, July 16, 2013, http://www.cphabaltimore .org/2013/07/the-great-debate-financing-harbor-point/. See also Mark Reutter, "Council Panel Approves Harbor Point TIF as Chairman Storms

Out," *Baltimore Brew*, August 8, 2013, https://baltimorebrew.com/2013/08
/08/council-panel-approves-harbor-point-tif-as-chairman-storms-out/.

75. Lawrence Brown, "Protect Whose House? How Baltimore's Leaders Failed to
Further Affordable and Fair Housing in Port Covington," *University of
Baltimore Journal of Land and Development* 6, no. 2 (2018): 161–169, 168.

76. Lawrence Lanahan, *The Lines between Us: Two Families and a Quest to Cross
Baltimore's Racial Divide* (New York: New Press, 2019), 257–266. Housing
advocates who testified included Barbara Samuels (Maryland ACLU),
Anthony Williams (Housing Our Neighbors), Adam Schneider (Healthcare for
the Homeless), and Lawrence Brown (Morgan State University).

77. Peter Sicher, "Hopkins and Other Institutions Pay Baltimore $20.4 Million to
Avoid Tax Increases," *Johns Hopkins News-Letter*, July 15, 2010, https://
nlonthedl.wordpress.com/2010/07/15/hopkins-and-other-institutions-pay
-baltimore-20-4-million-to-avoid-tax-increases/. See also Rollin Hu,
"Hopkins Avoiding Taxes Is Civic Disengagement," *Johns Hopkins News-
Letter*, November 8, 2018, https://www.jhunewsletter.com/article/2018/11
/hopkins-avoiding-taxes-is-civic-disengagement.

78. Daphne A. Kenyon and Adam H. Langley, "Payments in Lieu of Taxes by
Nonprofits: Case Studies," Tax Analysts, *State Tax Notes,* July 18, 2011, 177.

79. According to Wagner: "Hospitals included in the agreement are Bon Secours,
Johns Hopkins Hospital & Johns Hopkins Bayview Medical Center, MedStar
Good Samaritan, MedStar Union Memorial, Mercy Medical Center, Sinai
LifeBridge, St. Agnes Healthcare, University of Maryland Medical Center and
University of Maryland Medical Center Midtown Campus. Participating
colleges and universities are Johns Hopkins University, Loyola University
Maryland, Maryland Institute College of Art and Notre Dame of Maryland
University." Yvonne Wagner, "City Enters $60 Million, 10-Year Agreement
with Baltimore Institutions to Help Fund Public Services," *Baltimore Sun*,
May 31, 2016, https://www.baltimoresun.com/maryland/baltimore-city/bs
-md-ci-mou-20160531-story.html.

80. Consider that at the University of Maryland Medical System—the same
hospital at the center of the Healthy Holly corruption scandal—11 administrators made more than $588,000 a year in salaries. In other words, 11 people
were paid more in salaries than the city was paid in taxes by the private
University of Maryland Medical System. As I wrote in Track 4, if administrators' salaries were cut in half, it would amount to $3.23 million that could have
been used to pay its non-administrative workers a higher salary or fund
cooperative enterprises that would increase community wealth building.
Baltimore City is likely losing tens of millions of dollars by signing PILOT
agreements instead of ensuring the 11 institutions are paying an equitable tax
rate. To wit, the Coalition for a Humane Hopkins wrote in a letter to Mayor
Jack Young: "Combined, if the three Johns Hopkins institutions were
for-profits, they would pay $65.4 million in annual property taxes to the City
of Baltimore." In other words, just the affiliated three Hopkins institutions
alone could generate an additional roughly $60 million compared to the $6
million being collected now by the city from the allied universities and
hospital nonprofits.

81. National Nurses United, *Burdening Baltimore: How Johns Hopkins Hospital and
Other Not-for-Profit Hospitals, Colleges, and Universities Fail to Pay Their Fair*

Share (Baltimore: National Nurses United, Coalition for a Humane Hopkins, and AFL-CIO, October 2019), 4.

82. National Nurses United, *Burdening Baltimore*, 3.

83. Louis Misrendino, "Baltimore's Property Tax Privileged v. Punished," *Baltimore Sun*, July 4, 2016, http://www.baltimoresun.com/news/opinion /oped/bs-ed-property-tax-20160704-story.html. See also Louis Misrendino, "A Failed Redevelopment and Tax Policy," Maryland Public Policy Institute, May 22, 2015, https://www.mdpolicy.org/research/detail/a-failed -redevelopment-and-tax-policy. Finally see Lawrence Brown, "Two Balti- mores: The White L vs. the Black Butterfly," *Baltimore City Paper*, June 28, 2016, http://www.citypaper.com/bcpnews-two-baltimores-the-white-l-vs -the-black-butterfly-20160628-htmlstory.html.

84. Robert Cenname, City Council Bill 19-0414, City of Baltimore Memo, July 24, 2019, https://baltimore.legistar.com/View.ashx?M=F&ID =7553327&GUID=2290D5D9-0CF4-4398-B3B8-C209FFF3E953. Special thanks to Melissa Schober for bringing this bill to my attention.

85. The Baltimore Black Worker Center has a tremendous analysis of the lack of racial equity in the field of labor and workforce development in a report entitled *The State of Black Workers in Baltimore*, which adds more to the picture of the *Dashboard Report: Analysis and Metrics of Baltimore City's African American Middle Class* report produced by Associated Black Charities. Equity Matters collaborated on a report entitled *Place Matters for Health in Baltimore: Ensuring Opportunities for Good Health for All*. The report exam- ines health equity in the city. The National Community Reinvestment Coalition has a report on racial inequity in redlining in bank lending entitled *Home Mortgage and Small Business Lending in Baltimore and Surrounding Areas*. Racial inequity in subprime lending by Wells Fargo is explored by Jacob Rugh and colleagues in their academic paper entitled *Race, Space, and Cumulative Disadvantage: A Case Study of the Subprime Lending Collapse*. The Justice Policy Institute and Prison Policy Initiative wrote a report examining the cost of corrections by neighborhood in their report entitled *The Right Investment? Corrections Spending in Baltimore City*. The city allocation of parks is examined in a journal article entitled "Parks and People: An Environmen- tal Justice Inquiry in Baltimore, Maryland." City recreation centers were analyzed in a report entitled *Recreation Center Closings in Baltimore: Reconsid- ering Spending Priorities, Juvenile Crime, and Equity* by the Citizens Planning and Housing Association. Alec MacGillis explores Baltimore's transit system in his article *The Third Rail* in the journal *Places*.

Track 7. Healing the Black Butterfly

1. This, in part, is written specifically to contest the notion argued for by Alan Mallach in *The Divided City* who argues for slow and incremental solutions to radical problems. Mallach presents readers with a spectrum of government action, ranging from incrementalism on one end and utopianism on the other. He presents utopianism as a radical strategy and presents dismantling racism and radical change as a "distant prospect" (256). His disdain regarding radical change to dismantle urban apartheid amounts to a liberal fatalism and settling for incremental and "pragmatic" changes that will leave urban

apartheid intact. If radical change to impose urban apartheid can take place with intention (as it has for the past 110 years), then so too can radical change to dismantle urban apartheid take place with intention today. See Mallach, *The Divided City: Poverty and Prosperity in Urban America* (Washington, DC: Island Press, 2018), 255–257.

2. Jaisal Noor, "Privatization and Kickbacks: Why the Healthy Holly Scandal Is Bigger Than Baltimore's Mayor," *The Real News*, April 3, 2019, https:// therealnews.com/stories/privatization-and-kickbacks-why-the-healthy-holly -scandal-is-bigger-than-baltimores-mayor.

3. According to Goldman Sachs, a social impact bond is an "innovative and emerging financial instrument that leverages private investment to support high-impact social programs." Goldman Sachs, "Social Impact Bonds," Goldman Sachs, October 2, 2014, https://www.goldmansachs.com/insights /pages/social-impact-bonds.html.

4. Jennifer Brown, "Denver Sold Bonds to Reduce the Human and Financial Costs of Homelessness. The Results So Far Are Promising," *Denver Post*, March 19, 2018, https://www.denverpost.com/2018/03/19/denver -homeless-bonds/. Undoubtedly, cities employing this strategy will need technical assistance in terms of how to set up such a bond. Maria Hernandez runs Impact4Health, a consulting firm that provides technical assistance on social impact bonds. Jeffrey Liebman also started the Harvard Social Impact Bond Technical Assistance Lab to provide similar assistance. While experts such as Hernandez and Liebman can provide technical assistance, the vision and execution of the Racial Equity Social Impact Bond should be driven by the residents of the city utilizing an authentic racial equity approach. See Impact4Health, "Innovations to Advance Health Equity," Impact4Health LLC, 2018, http://www.impact4health.com. See also Ashley Pettus, "Social Impact Bonds," *Harvard Magazine*, July–August 2013, https:// harvardmagazine.com/2013/07/social-impact-bonds.

5. Maria Sieron, "Largest Charitable Foundations in Greater Baltimore: Ranked by Total 2017 Assets," *Baltimore Business Journal*, 2018, https:// www.bizjournals.com/baltimore/subscriber-only/2018/02/09/charitable -foundations.html.

6. Jeffrey C. Walker, "Solving the World's Biggest Problems: Better Philan- thropy through Systems Change," *Stanford Social Innovation Review*, April 5, 2017, https://ssir.org/articles/entry/better_philanthropy_through_systems _change#.

7. Mark Reutter, "Closing Rec Centers and Slashing Youth Programs Were Root Causes of Riot, Councilman Asserts," *Baltimore Brew*, May 4, 2015, https:// www.baltimorebrew.com/2015/05/04/closing-rec-centers-and-slashing -youth-programs-were-root-causes-of-riot-councilman-asserts/.

8. In other words, since 95.59% of the $493.74 million allocated for the Balti- more Police Department is paid using city dollars (from the city's General Fund), the remaining 4.41% of the police budget is paid for with state, federal, or private dollars. Therefore, most of the Baltimore Police Department's budget is paid for by the City of Baltimore, whereas most of the budget for the Baltimore City Health Department is paid with dollars from state, federal, and private dollars.

9. "Baltimore City Bureau of the Budget and Management Research," Open Budget Baltimore, 2018, http://openbudget.baltimorecity.gov/. In Baltimore's strong mayor system, the budgets are determined by the mayor.

10. "Baltimore City Bureau of the Budget and Management Research."

11. The Center for Popular Democracy, Law for Black Lives, and Black Youth Project 100, *Freedom to Thrive: Reimagining Safety & Security in Our Communities*, The Center for Popular Democracy, 2017, https://populardemocracy.app.box.com/v/FreedomtoThrive.

12. Open Society Institute—Baltimore, *Blueprint for Baltimore: 2020 and Beyond*, January 2020, https://www.osibaltimore.org/blueprint/. After filtering, there were 4,836 valid survey responses.

13. Evan Serpick, "Baltimore Residents' Priorities Sharply at Odds With Proposed City Budget," Open Society Institute—Baltimore, June 18, 2020, https://www.osibaltimore.org/2020/06/baltimore-residents-priorities -sharply-at-odds-with-proposed-city-budget/.

14. "I argue that individual and collective historical trauma and the ways in which it manifests in the present, are largely ignored in conceptions and definitions of peacebuilding. Because of the masked ways in which it manifests, and the discrete responses to these manifestations (which includes positive resilience), peacebuilders do not ordinarily view historical trauma, nor lifespan trauma as part of their sphere of activity." Sarah Malotane, "Restorative Justice as a Tool for Peacebuilding: A South African Case Study" (PhD diss., University of KwaZulu-Natal, 2012), 63, https://www .academia.edu/22228614/Restorative_Justice_as_a_tool_for_peacebuilding _A_South_African_case_study.

15. Malotane, "Restorative Justice as a Tool for Peacebuilding."

16. Malotane's Invisible/Visible Structure of Violence model powerfully illustrates the context in which violence takes place. Her model along with her work discussed in *Open Guide to a Deeper, Wider, and Longer Analysis of Violence* (doi:10.13140/RG.2.2.34209.20321) clearly describes how invisible violence manifests and helps to create visible violence that wreaks havoc in too many of our redlined Black communities. Given her deep expertise on the subject of peacebuilding, Sarah Malotane could serve as a consultant for how this work can be done in cities that are interested in dismantling police forces and building peacebuilding authorities.

17. Jayne Miller, "Oliver Community Bucks Baltimore's Trend of Violence with Turnaround," WBAL-TV, February 2, 2017, http://www.wbaltv.com/article /oliver-community-bucks-baltimores-trend-of-violence-with-turnaround /8668220.

18. Sarah Holder, "What Happened to Crime in Camden?," CityLab, January 10, 2018, https://www.citylab.com/equity/2018/01/what-happened-to-crime-in -camden/549542/. The example of Camden does not mean that the city is now a shining beacon of policing. Rather, it shows that the sky does not start falling simply because a police force is disbanded.

19. Jessica Trounstine, *Segregation by Design: Local Politics and Inequality in American Cities* (Cambridge: Cambridge University Press, 2018), 150–155. See also Alberto Alesina, Reza Baqir, and William Easterly, "Public Goods and Ethnic Fractionalization," *Quarterly Journal of Economics*, November 1999, 1243. Alesina and colleagues' findings precede Trounstine's similar

results. They write in their paper: "Results show that the shares of spending on productive public goods—education, roads, sewers and trash pickup—in U.S. cities (metro areas/urban counties) are inversely related to the city's (metro area's/county's) ethnic fragmentation, even after controlling for other socioeconomic and demographic determinants."

20. Vickie Connor, "Maryland Looks to End Income-Based Housing Discrimination," Capital News Service, December 15, 2016, https://cnsmaryland.org /2016/12/15/maryland-looks-to-end-income-based-housing-discrimination/.

21. Edward G. Goetz, *The One Way Street of Integration: Fair Housing and the Pursuit of Racial Justice in American Cities* (Ithaca, NY: Cornell University Press, 2018), 114–118. Goetz also criticizes housing mobility strategies along the lines of acquiescing to the tolerance levels of White residents and ignoring the burdens imposed on Black people to do the integrating. He argues: "The difficulty of the fair housing integration argument is not so much its ends as its means. That is, the key problem is not so much *integration* as it is the *integrating*, especially when such efforts burden disadvantaged groups. The pursuit of residential integration, as a rule, either assumes or subordinates the residential preferences of people of color. Integration, it is understood, will not work without white acquiescence, and thus the terms of integration must be those that whites accept. Such a bind requires that the interests of communities of color be subsidiary to those of whites during the process of integrating. In addition, as a result of existing inequities of power, integration almost exclusively involves managing the settlement decisions of people of color and certainly not those of whites" (31–32). This argument echoes Sonya Douglass Horsford, namely that integration is often focused on mixing bodies, but not ensuring equitable resource allocation. After the litigation struggle to implement Brown v. Board of Education, she writes: "Attention to racial balance, however, quickly took precedence over the principal fight for equal resources" (20). Horsford, *Learning in a Burning House: Educational Inequality, Ideology, and (Dis)Integration* (New York: Teachers College Press, 2011).

22. Sarah Malotane, "Invisible Violence, Invisible Wounding: Effects of Internalised Racism in South Africa," Spring 2018. https://www.academia.edu /7323264/Invisible_Violence_Invisible_Wounding_Effects_of_internalised _racism. See also Sarah Malotane, *Disrupting Denial: Analysing Narratives of Invisible/Visible Violence & Trauma* (n.p.: New Adventure Publishing, 2018).

23. Terry Keleher, Racial Equity Impact Assessment Toolkit. *Applied Research Center* (now *Race Forward: The Center for Racial Justice Innovation*), 2009, https://www.raceforward.org/practice/tools/racial-equity-impact -assessment-toolkit.

24. Sage Howard, "How Black Co-ops Can Fight Institutional Racism," Vice, August 9, 2016, https://www.vice.com/en_us/article/jmk8qk/how-black-co -ops-can-fight-institutional-racism. Jessica Gordon Nembhard explains: "Businesses that practice cooperative economics are owned by a collective of people. The important part is that the people are not owning it for the purpose of making a profit, but for the purpose of satisfying a need or addressing a problem. Another unique piece is the democratic governing structure. Everybody who owns it has one vote regardless of how much money they put into it. If you choose to put more money into that enterprise, that's

your choice, and you can get a return. But your ability to make the decisions for the enterprise are equal to anyone else's. It's a way to democratize and make more grassroots ownership possible."

25. Agatha So, "OSI Baltimore," Open Society Institute—Baltimore, 2014, https://www.osibaltimore.org/fellow/agatha-so/. See also Agatha So, "Pathways to Homeownership," PowerPoint, May 18, 2016.

26. Potomac Association of Housing Cooperatives (PAHC), "Non-profit Housing & Public Service in Baltimore, Maryland," PAHC, 2018, https://www .potomacassoc.org.

27. Jared Ball, "Pitfalls of (Black) Capitalism and Banking," iMIXWHATi-LIKE!, November 4, 2017, https://imixwhatilike.org/2017/11/04/pitfalls -black-capitalism-banking/.

28. Mehrsa Baradaran, *The Color of Money: Black Banks and the Racial Wealth Gap* (Cambridge, MA: Harvard University Press, 2017).

29. "About Us," OneUnited Bank, 2018, https://www.oneunited.com/about-us/.

30. "Community Land Trust Home Loan," 2018, OneUnited Bank, 2018, https://www.oneunited.com/loans/home-loans/community-land-trust -home-loan/. See also Oscar Perry Abello, "A Movement to Put Money into Black-Owned Banks," Next City, August 4, 2016, https://nextcity.org/daily /entry/bankblack-movement-black-owned-banks-justin-moore.

31. Evergreen Cooperative Corporation, "About Us," 2016, http://www.evgoh.com /about-us/.

32. Jacob Took, "How Do HopkinsLocal Investments Impact the City?," *Johns Hopkins News-Letter*, February 28, 2019, https://www.jhunewsletter.com /article/2019/02/how-do-hopkinslocal-investments-impact-the-city.

33. The reason one can say they did not work is simple—redlined Black communi-ties still exist all across the nation. In the case of President Trump's Opportu-nity Zones, it will also fail to improve Black neighborhoods and work for the benefit of existing Black residents.

34. Bruce Mitchell and Juan Franco, "HOLC 'Redlining' Maps: The Persistent Structure of Segregation and Economic Inequality," *National Community Reinvestment Coalition*, 2018, https://ncrc.org/wp-content/uploads/dlm _uploads/2018/02/NCRC-Research-HOLC-10.pdf; Sarah Mikhitarian, "Home Values Remain Low in Vast Majority of Formerly Redlined Neighbor-hoods," Zillow Research, 2018, https://www.zillow.com/research/home -values-redlined-areas-19674/; Andre Perry, Jonathan Rothwell, and David Harshbarger, *The Devaluation of Assets in Black Neighborhoods: The Case of Residential Property* (Washington, DC: Brookings Institution, 2018), https:// www.brookings.edu/research/devaluation-of-assets-in-black-neighborhoods /; Jacob Rugh, Len Albright, and Douglas S. Massey, "Race, Space, and Cumulative Disadvantage: A Case Study of the Subprime Lending Collapse," *Social Problems* 62 (2015): 186–218. Rugh and colleagues show that middle-class Black homebuyers were especially targeted by Wells Fargo. "Consistent with sociological research on the black middle class, higher socioeconomic status by no means protects families from systematic discrimination, especially when they live in black neighborhoods. Indeed, higher status may even exacerbate potential losses to black income and wealth. Based on our analysis, compared with $14,904 for all African Americans, the projected cumulative cost of discrimination for blacks earning over $50,000 per year

was $19,026. Our findings thus confirm those of Faber, who documents higher rates of subprime lending for higher income blacks, and Katrin Anacker and James Carr and Debbie Bocian and colleagues, who report higher rates of foreclosure for upper-class blacks net of other factors."

35. There are instances where a community was color-coded green in 1937 by HOLC, but became a redlined community (i.e., east of York Road in north-central Baltimore). In those instances, such communities should also be included as a recipient of CRA dollars.

36. Sarah Kliff, "An Exclusive Look at Cory Booker's Plan to Fight Wealth Inequality: Give Poor Kids Money," Vox, October 22, 2018, https://www.vox .com/policy-and-politics/2018/10/22/17999558/cory-booker-baby-bonds.

37. Anna Wolfe, "Fifteen Black Moms to Receive $1,000 Monthly in Basic Income Experiment," *Mississippi Today*, September 13, 2018, https://mississippitoday .org/2018/09/13/fifteen-black-moms-to-receive-1000-monthly-in-basic -income-experiment/.

38. Alexandra Roon-Hendricks, "Will 'Basic Income' Become the California Norm? Stockton Starts $500 No-Strings Payments," *Sacramento Bee*, February 16, 2019, https://www.sacbee.com/news/local/article226280230 .html.

39. National League of Cities (NLC), "Universal Basic Income: Who's Piloting It?," NLC, 2019, https://www.nlc.org/universal-basic-income-whos-piloting-it.

40. Amy Goldstein, "New York City Mayor Vows Health Care for All—Including Undocumented Immigrants," *Washington Post*, January 8, 2019, https://www .washingtonpost.com/national/health-science/new-yorks-mayor-de-blasio -vows-health-care-for-all--including-undocumented-immigrants/2019/01/08/.

41. Mindy Thompson Fullilove, *Urban Alchemy: Restoring Joy in America's Sorted-Out Cities* (New York: New Village Press, 2013).

42. In a stunning collection of short academic journal articles edited by Lisa K. Bates and colleagues collectively entitled *Race and Spatial Imaginary: Planning Otherwise*, a variety of authors offer important insights for a Black or Afrofuturistic urban planning approach. In her essay, Anna Livia Brand argues: "We have to name and name again, search and search again for what is tacitly hidden in our landscapes and for the voices whose claims on the future are silenced by the hegemony of the white/spatial/racial/colonial/ post-colonial imagination. . . . Plan making is imagining. It is envisioning a future that details—both through words and images—who will inhabit where. It is a pronouncement of inclusion and exclusion—both of bodies, but also of racialized landscapes. For planning futures to be different, they have to be full to the rafters with non-white, non-supremacist imaginations." Brand, "Say Its Name—Planning Is the White Spatial Imaginary, or Reading McKittrick and Woods as Planning Text," *Planning Theory and Practice* 19, no. (2018): 269–272.

In the essay "Wakanda! Take the Wheel! Visions of a Black Green City," C. N. E. Corbin argues that the film *Black Panther* provides a glimpse of what could be imagined through an Afrofuturistic urban planning approach: "Birnin Zana, Wakanda's capital city, also known as the Golden City, gives us a glimpse of a non-white, urban, environmentally just future grounded in an African aesthetic. In so doing it also grants us a vision of a Black green city in the now and present. . . . The Golden City demonstrates that these are urban creations of a different ideology for a different land and for a different culture. The concept art depicts a new Black green urban aesthetic grounded in understandings of African cultural productions; shapes, colors, designs, and functions." Corbin, "Wakanda! Take the Wheel! Visions of a Black Green City," *Planning Theory and Practice* 19, no. 2 (2018): 273–276.

In her essay, Andrea R. Roberts argues for the utilization of what she calls Critical Sankofa Planning to build healthy Black communities. She writes: "While students express interest in Black planning and placemaking in my classroom, planning educators compete with subtle imaginaries which lead students to believe that actualizing the equitable city is only a green infrastructure or complete streets project away. Alongside these concepts, find a home for Critical Sankofa Planning which privileges people over buildings, honors and critiques the past, and affirms Black communities' capacity to imagine and interpret their futures." Roberts, "Interpretations & Imaginaries: Toward an Instrumental Black Planning History," *Planning Theory and Practice* 19, no. 2 (2018): 283–288.

Urbanism journalist Brentin Mock asks critical questions regarding America's Chocolate Cities: "The critical questions for those in the school of Chocolate City preservation are: What does it mean to maintain a Chocolate City in an age of globalization? What is the leadership model for growing a Chocolate City? Can Chocolate Cities sufficiently provide sanctuary for their Black inhabitants?" Brentin Mock, "Wakanda: The Chocolatest City," CityLab, February 16, 2018, https://www.citylab.com/equity/2018/02 /wakanda-the-chocolatest-city/553259/.

43. BlackSpace NYC, "The BlackSpace Manifesto," *Multiple Cities*, February 14, 2019, https://www.multiplecities.org/home/2019/1/31/the-blackspace -manifesto. BlackSpace planning principles are as follows: (1) create circles, not lines; (2) choose critical connections over critical mass; (3) move at the speed of trust; (4) be humble learners who practice deep listening; (5) celebrate, catalyze, and amplify Black Joy; (6) plan with, design with; (7) center lived experience; (8) seek people at the margins; (9) reckon with the past to build the future; (10) protect and strengthen culture; (11) cultivate wealth; (12) foster personal and communal evolution; (13) promote excellence; and (14) manifest the future.

44. The solutions discussed here would work in concert with strategies and platforms proposed by advocates in the Movement for Black Lives across the nation. See Jesse A. Myerson and Michal Denzel Smith, "An Economic Program for #BlackLivesMatter," *The Nation*, 2016. See also the platform and demands of the Movement for Black Lives (M4BL): https://policy.m4bl.org /platform/. There are six overarching M4BL demands: (1) end the war on Black people, (2) reparations, (3) invest-divest, (4) economic justice, (5) community control, and (6) political power.

45. Sarah Malotane, *Invisible Violence, Invisible Wounding: Effects of Internalised Racism in South Africa*, Spring 2018. https://www.academia.edu/7323264 /Invisible_Violence_Invisible_Wounding_Effects_of_internalised_racism.

46. Sarah Malotane, *Disrupting Denial: Analysing Narratives of Invisible/Visible Violence and Trauma* (South Africa: New Adventure Publishing, 2018), 232–233.

Track 8. Outro: Organize!

1. Tactics of wealth extraction in redlined Black neighborhoods include reverse mortgages, predatory rents, tax lien confiscations, check cashing fees, payday loans, pawn shops, and regressive municipal taxation.

2. Alvin Chang, "White America Is Quietly Self-Segregating," Vox, January 18, 2017, https://www.vox.com/2017/1/18/14296126/white-segregated-suburb -neighborhood-cartoon. See also Brian Resnick, "White Fear of Demographic Change Is a Powerful Psychological Force," Vox, January 28, 2017, https:// www.vox.com/science-and-health/2017/1/26/14340542/white-fear-trump -psychology-minority-majority.

3. Lauren Camera, "The Quiet Wave of School District Secessions," *U.S. News & World Report*, May 5, 2017, https://www.usnews.com/news/education -news/articles/2017-05-05/the-quiet-wave-of-school-district-secessions.

4. Alexander Nazaryan, "Whites Only: School Segregation Is Back, from Birmingham to San Francisco," *Newsweek*, May 2, 2017, https://www .newsweek.com/race-schools-592637.

5. These groups include organizations such as Baltimore Bloc, CityBloc, the Baltimore Algebra Project, United Workers, Free Your Voice, Housing Our Neighbors, Unite Here!, Out for Justice, the Right to Housing Alliance, Communities United, the Baltimore Algebra Project, BMORE Caucus, Food and Water Watch, Jews United for Justice, the Energy Justice Network, and many, many others.

6. Ariel Guerrero, "How Baltimore Is Advancing Racial Equity: Policy, Practice & Procedure," citiesspeak, January 21, 2019, https://citiesspeak.org/2019/01 /21/how-baltimore-is-advancing-racial-equity-policy-practice-procedure/. The bill's lead sponsor was then City Councilmember Brandon Scott.

7. Baltimore City Council, "Equity Assessment Program (Council Bill 18-0223)," Baltimore Legistar, August 10, 2018, https://baltimore.legistar .com/Legislation.aspx.

8. Stokely Carmichael (Kwame Ture), *Stokely Speaks: From Black Power to Pan-Africanism* (Chicago: Chicago Review Press, 2007), 6. From his speech entitled "Who Is Qualified?"

9. Carmichael, *Stokely Speaks*, 50–51.

10. Ella Baker, "Developing Community Leadership," interviewed by Gerda Lerner, in *Black Women in White America* (New York: Pantheon, 1972), 347.

11. *Martin Luther King, Jr. Encyclopedia*, s.v. "Baker, Ella Josephine," 2018, https://kinginstitute.stanford.edu/encyclopedia/baker-ella-josephine. See also Criss Crass, "Organizing Lessons from Civil Rights Leader Ella Baker," Anarkismo, March 3, 2008, https://www.anarkismo.net/article/7645 ?userlanguage=de&save_prefs=true.

12. Ella Baker, "Ella Baker: Making the Struggle Every Day," speech addressing the Puerto Rico Solidarity Rally in 1974, YouTube video, 2:21, https://www .youtube.com/watch?v=t96fnyLMihA.

Index

Page numbers in *italics* refer to figures and tables.

Discussion Guide for Book Clubs and Educators

Introduction to Racial Equity

1. How have Black neighborhoods been treated by White Americans throughout American history? To probe further, ask about their treatment during the following time periods: during slavery, between 1865 and 1909, between 1910 and 1999, from 2000 to the present.
2. How does the stigmatizing language regarding Black neighborhoods or the "discursive redlining" affect how Black neighborhoods are treated?
3. Why is racial equity required in America?
4. Which one of the key terms (pages 8-14) stood out to you?

Track 1
The Trump Card

1. How does racial segregation impact American politics?
2. What is a "whitelash"?
3. What happens to a community, in terms of crime and violence, when it is starved of resources?
4. What is the relationship between hypersegregation and hyper-policing?
5. What are the factors that lead to urban uprisings in Black neighborhoods in America?

Track 2
This Is America

1. What were the First, Second, and Third American Whitelashes?
2. African Americans were subjected to the Seven Great Displacements throughout American history. What are the Seven Great Displacements?

3. What was the impact of white supremacist violence and White Redemption on Black neighborhoods during the First American Whitelash?

4. How did Black Freedom movements strike back?

5. At the same time that Black people were gaining civil rights from 1950 through the 1970s, what was happening to Black neighborhoods?

6. How is the Third American Whitelash connected with the events of January 6, 2021 (when a large mob of supporters of then US president Donald J. Trump stormed the Capitol Building attempting to stop Congress from affirming Joe Biden as the winner of the 2020 presidential election)?

Track 3
The "Negro Invasion"

1. What is the "Negro Invasion"?

2. What were the three justifications given by White Baltimoreans for racial zoning ordinances in the 1910s?

3. What role did Baltimore's mayors have in establishing and maintaining Baltimore Apartheid?

4. What was the role of the *Baltimore Sun* in supporting and maintaining urban apartheid in the city?

5. What role did officials with the Baltimore City Health Department play in supporting urban apartheid?

6. What was the role of White clergy and religious institutions in supporting Baltimore Apartheid?

7. What role did the United State government have in helping to solidify Baltimore Apartheid?

8. How did the Housing Authority of Baltimore City contribute to racial segregation in the city?

9. Describe the scope of Baltimore City's serial forced displacement with respect to Black neighborhoods.

10. How did Baltimore County contribute to a racially segregated metropolitan area?

Track 4
Ongoing Historical Trauma

1. How does Lakota scholar Maria Yellow Horse Brave Heart define historical trauma?
2. Why did desegregation fail?
3. How does Dr. Brown define *segrenomics*, a term coined by Noliwe Rooks?
4. How does hypersegregation affect redlined Black neighborhoods today?
5. How does hyperpolicing affect redlined Black neighborhoods today?
6. Describe how economic destruction and wealth extraction impact redlined Black neighborhoods in Baltimore City.
7. How does the removal of resources and repeated uprootings affect redlined Black neighborhoods in Baltimore City today?
8. What are the five stages of publicly subsidized gentrification?
9. What are the three tiers of organizational actors in Baltimore and how do they affect the economic agenda of the city?

Track 5
Black Neighborhood Destruction

1. While Black people were gaining civil rights in the 1960s and 1970s, what was happening to Black neighborhoods?
2. How do each of the following factors lead to Black neighborhood destruction?
   - Root shock
   - Internal colonization
   - Resource apartheid
   - Toxic lead exposure
   - Housing precarity
   - Racism-based traumatic stress
   - Homicides
   - Urban uprisings
3. How do you interpret the *Ecosocial Model of Black Neighborhood*

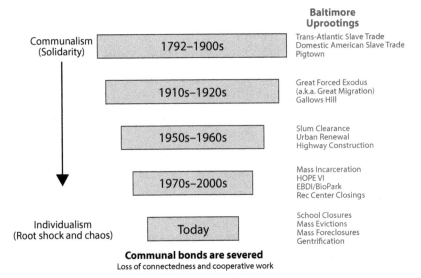

Figure 5.1. Ecosocial Model of Black Neighborhood Destruction

This model was drafted based on various insights and scholarship by the following scholars: Alexander Leighton, Mindy Thompson (Fullilove), Rodrick Wallace, Lawrence Brown,
Nyasha Grayman-Simpson, and Jacqueline Mattis<FIGS>

Destruction? (See page 173; see also the figure above.)

4. How does America's destruction of Black neighborhoods impact the
   health of communities?

5. What does the story of Lucille Gorham reveal about the effects of
   America's destruction of Black neighborhoods on the lives of Black
   people?

Track 6

Make Black Neighborhoods Matter

1. Black neighborhoods have received far fewer resources than White
   neighborhoods for decades. If a mayor makes the decision in a giv-
   en city to finally allocate resources equally among neighborhoods,
   would this constitute racial equity? Why or why not?

2. How does racial equity work to help redlined Black neighborhoods
   heal from ongoing historical trauma (see page 183)?

3. How can racial equity be fostered in:

- Public education?
- Community economic development?
- Housing and ending homelessness?
- Public health?
- Public transit?
- Public works?
- Tax policy?

4. What are the three wars that White America has waged on Black communities that racial equity seeks to heal?

5. The *Community Health Garden* model is shown on page 181. How does this model depict the factors that contribute to community health and well-being?

6. What do policymakers and public officials need to do in YOUR city to make Black neighborhoods matter?

Track 7
Healing the Black Butterfly

1. In the 1910s, the inception of racial segregation was described as "radical and far reaching" by the *New York Times Magazine*. Uprooting a Black community was described as a "radical measure" by the *Baltimore Municipal Journal*. Based on this, what kind of solutions are needed today to address urban apartheid?

2. Explain how each of the following can help heal the Black Butterfly:
   - A $3 Billion Racial Equity Social Impact Bond
   - Fund Freedom Budgets and Black Neighborhood Reparations
   - Create the Baltimore Peacebuilding Authority
   - Desegregate the city and the suburbs
   - Strengthen the Baltimore Office of Equity and Civil Rights
   - Bolster community wealth building and cooperative enterprises
   - Finance racial equity efforts with funds from the 1977 Community Reinvestment Act
   - Center Black Planning Principles in Redlined Black Neighborhoods

3. Dr. Brown arrives at a figure of $99 billion that's needed to make Black neighborhoods matter in Baltimore City. What is your reaction to this figure and his reasoning behind it?

Track 8

Outro: Organize!

1. Democrats are in charge of many large urban areas. How should organizers and activists address the Democratic Party given the urban history discussed throughout the book?
2. What obligation does the Democratic Party have in terms of dismantling urban apartheid in America?
3. Why is "Afrofuturistic ecological thinking" needed according to *The Black Butterfly*?
4. How does the Student Nonviolent Coordinating Committee (SNCC) serve as an example of the kind of organizing and activism needed today?
5. Describe the Ella Baker model of organizing. Which model of organizing do you think is more effective and sustainable for social movements, A or B?
   A. The group-centered leadership model (best practiced by Ella Baker)?
   B. Or the messianic/charismatic model of leadership (best practiced by Dr. Martin Luther King Jr.)?